T0230608

Also in the Variorum Collected Studies Series:

WILLIAM A. WALLACE
Galileo, the Jesuits and the Medieval Aristotle

GUY BEAUJOUAN
Par raison de nombres:
L'art du calcul et les savoirs scientifiques médiévaux

GERARD L'E. TURNER
Scientific Instruments and Experimental Philosophy, 1550–1850

FRANZ ROSENTHAL
Science and Medicine in Islam

ALLEN G. DEBUS
Chemistry, Alchemy, and the New Philosophy, 1550–1700:
Studies in the History of Science and Medicine

VIVIAN NUTTON
From Democedes to Harvey:
Studies in the History of Medicine

WALTER PAGEL
From Paracelsus to Van Helmont:
Studies in Renaissance Medicine and Science

WALTER PAGEL
Religion and Neoplatonism in Renaissance Medicine

CHARLES B. SCHMITT
Studies in Renaissance Philosophy and Science

CURTIS WILSON
Astronomy from Kepler to Newton:
Historical Studies

BRUCE S. EASTWOOD
Astronomy and Optics from Pliny to Descartes:
Texts, Diagrams and Conceptual Structures

DAVID A. KING
Islamic Astronomical Instruments

E. WILLIAM MONTER
Enforcing Morality in Early Modern Europe

PAUL GRENDLER
Culture and Censorship in Late Renaissance Italy and France

Quid pro quo: Studies in the history of drugs

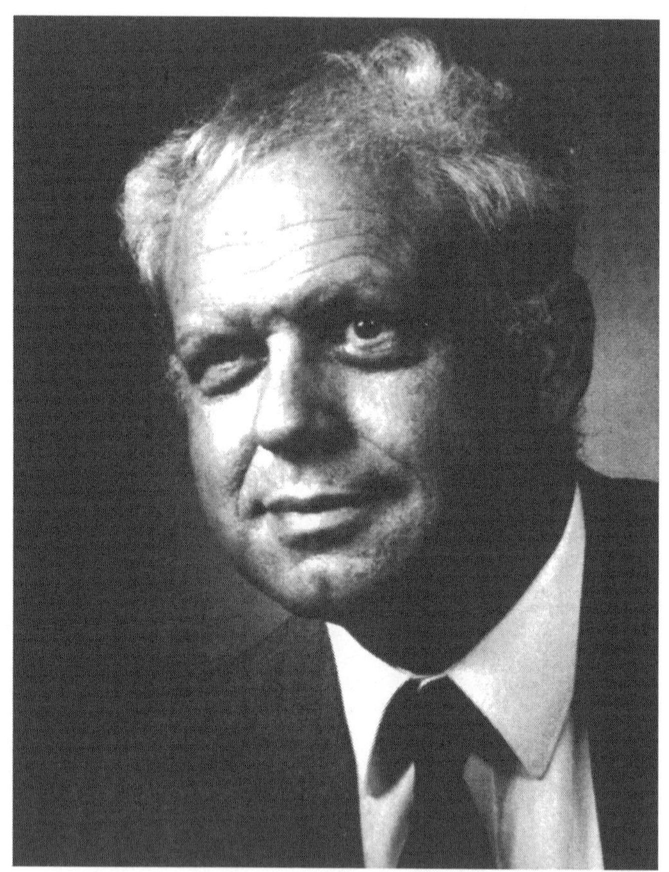

Professor John M. Riddle

John M. Riddle

Quid pro quo: Studies in the history of drugs

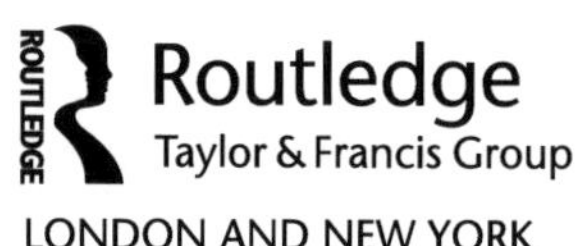

LONDON AND NEW YORK

First published 1992 by Variorum, Ashgate Publishing

Published 2017 by Routledge
2 Park Square, Milton Park, Abingdon, Oxon OX14 4RN
711 Third Avenue, New York, NY 10017, USA

Routledge is an imprint of the Taylor & Francis Group, an informa business

This edition copyright © 1992 by John M. Riddle

All rights reserved. No part of this book may be reprinted or reproduced or utilised in any form or by any electronic, mechanical, or other means, now known or hereafter invented, including photocopying and recording, or in any information storage or retrieval system, without permission in writing from the publishers.

Notice:
Product or corporate names may be trademarks or registered trademarks, and are used only for identification and explanation without intent to infringe.

A CIP catalogue record for this book is available from the British Library and the US Library of Congress.

ISBN 13: 978-0-86078-319-0 (hbk)

COLLECTED STUDIES SERIES CS367

CONTENTS

Preface vii–xi

Acknowledgements xii

I Pomum ambrae: Amber and Ambergris in Plague Remedies 111–122
Sudhoffs Archiv für Geschichte der Medizin und der Naturwissenschaften 48. (1964)

II The Introduction and Use of Eastern Drugs in the Early Middle Ages 185–198
Sudhoffs Archiv für Geschichte der Medizin und der Naturwissenschaften 49. (1965)

III Lithotherapy in the Middle Ages . . . Lapidaries Considered as Medical Texts 39–50
Pharmacy in History 12. (1970)

IV The Latin Alphabetical Dioscorides Manuscript Group 1–6
Proceedings of the XIIIth International Congress for the History of Science, Acts Section IV. (Moscow, 1971), pp. 204–209

V Amber in Ancient Pharmacy. The Transmission of Information about a Single Drug. A Case Study 3–17
Pharmacy in History 15. (1973)

VI Theory and Practice in Medieval Medicine 157–184
Viator 5. (1974)

VII Book Reviews, Lectures and Marginal Notes. Three Previously Unknown Sixteenth-Century Contributors to Pharmacy, Medicine and Botany – Ioannes Manardus, Franciscus Frigimelica and Melchior Guilandinus 143–155
Pharmacy in History 21. (1979)

VIII Albert on Stones and Minerals 203–234

(In collaboration with James A. Mulholland)

Albertus Magnus and the Sciences, Commemorative Essays 1980, ed. James A. Weisheipl. Toronto: Pontifical Institute of Mediaeval Studies, 1980

IX Pseudo-Dioscorides' *Ex herbis femininis* and Early Medieval Medical Botany 43–81
Journal of the History of Biology 14. (1981)

X Gargilius Martialis as a Medical Writer 408–429
Journal of the History of Medicine and Allied Sciences 39. (1984)

XI The Pseudo-Hippocratic *Dynamidia* 283–311
Sudhoffs Archiv für Geschichte der Medizin und der Naturwissenschaften 27. (1984)

XII Ancient and Medieval Chemotherapy for Cancer 319–330
Isis 76. (1985)

XIII Byzantine Commentaries on Dioscorides 95–102
Symposium on Byzantine Medicine, ed. John Scarborough = Dumbarton Oaks Papers 38. (1984)

XIV Folk Tradition and Folk Medicine Recognition of Drugs in Classical Antiquity 33–61
Folklore and Folk Medicines, ed. John Scarborough. Wisconsin: American Institute of the History of Pharmacy, 1987

XV Methodology of Historical Drug Research 1–19
First publication

Index 1–18

This volume contains xii + 316 pages

PREFACE

If one does not have acetaminophen, one takes acetylsalicylic acid. Or, in lay terms, if one does not have Tylenol, one takes Bayer aspirin. All of us have learned basic information about drug substitutes. In antiquity and, more abundantly, during the Middle Ages, there existed a genre, known as "Quid pro quo" or "This for that", that is, lists of drug substitutes. These treatises have not been studied in any detail by anyone and serve as an example of not what has been learned about the history of pharmacy but of how much there is yet to learn. What few times I have studied the "Quid pro quo" tracts, I have found that the substitutes are as rational as when we substitute one analgesic for another.

"Quid pro quo" is an appropriate title to my publishing career. I began graduate work in classical history under the late Professor Wallace Caldwell, a man of extraordinary learning and with whom I was staying as a student, when he died in October of 1961. Having taken away Prof. Caldwell, the "quid" in this case, the Fates led me to medieval medical history, specifically to Professor Loren C. MacKinney, for me a most fortunate "quo". Because medical history connected with an interest in science and because I had worked for three years in a biology laboratory, Prof. MacKinney secured for me a fellowship in the School of Medicine and instilled in me a deep love and an enthusiasm for the field of early medicine. Thereby, medical history was substituted for classical history.

From the beginning I was captivated by pharmacy as a branch of medicine. Although central to medicine, the history of drugs is a neglected area. From Roman history I had learned that an important reason for the Fall of the Western Empire had been the unfavourable balance of trade with the East. Romans imported items from the East, but there were few products that came from the West. Most of the items that the Romans imported were drugs. What made drugs so important to the Romans? Were drugs as important to earlier societies as they are to today's?

Medical tracts, especially those pertaining to pharmacy, are numerous in medieval manuscript collections. The treatises are by both classical and medieval authors. Only a small number have been studied. Those studies that have been conducted are an analysis of dating the treatise and a study of the text to determine the connection with previous works on the same subject. To be sure, this category of study, *Quellenkunde*, as the Germans call it, is valuable and necessary. Some of the studies in this volume reveal a desire to go beyond the descriptive phase of scholarship to an analysis of the pharmaceutical works in their relationship to medicine and, broader yet, intellectual history.

During the Black Death of the mid-fourteenth-century, people attributed the plague to corrupted air. The first study concerns an interesting preventive: a ball or, from the Latin, an "apple" of fragrant drugs and perfumes that were thought cleaned the air. There was a recognition that those who contracted the plague were often in close proximity to those who had it. They knew that, although one may not have touched the victim, one contracted the plague just the same. The cause was believed to be corrupted air and the solution was to clean the air.

In the first group of articles, the theme is descriptive detail from manuscripts about pharmaceutical literature. One article in this early period followed the information about one drug, amber, which was known from at least the Bronze Age and continued in the pharmacy of Mediterranean peoples down through the sixteenth century. The second article, however, is different from nuclear medical history in that the subject connects drug trade across continents. The dependence on eastern drugs that were present during the Roman Empire surprisingly continued after the collapse of political power in western Europe. The prescription literature during the early Middle Ages discloses a preference for eastern drugs. The trade in eastern drugs ultimately results in Christopher Columbus' expedition to the "Spice Islands". Even more surprising was the find that, when new drugs were discovered in the East, not only were they exported to Europe, but also the names for them were derived from eastern languages. At a time when Europe was supposedly isolated and in the dark throes of cultural regression, western culture was open to medical innovations from East Asia and southern Africa.

The period of research on drug trade was conducted at the History of Medicine Institute in Bonn, Germany, where I had the privilege of studying under Professor Johannes Steudel, a doctor of medicine and philosophy and a wonderful friend and mentor.

During the period of the 1970's and early '80's a number of extended manuscript searches were made in the various European collections, primarily in search of manuscripts attributed to Dioscorides, the leading writer on *materia medica* – an appropriate Latin name for drugs. The account of the manuscripts was published in the *Catalogus Translationum et Commentariorum* series (Washington: Catholic University

Press, 1981) and a monograph on Dioscorides by the University of Texas Press (1985). The article on the Latin alphabetical manuscript group of Dioscorides relates to this research and concerns a treatise of the eleventh century that, while based on Dioscorides, was a substantially new contribution to medicine. The work was disguised to belong to the classical author. Another pseudo-Dioscoridean work, very popular during the early Middle Ages, was called *Ex herbis femininis* or "Female Herbs". The rubric to some of the manuscript texts explains that these seventy-one herbs were those most often used in medicine.

Treatises falsely attributed to Dioscorides, however, are not the only way that manuscript studies reveal new knowledge passed through the authority of a classical author. In the article on Byzantine commentaries the marginal notes and textual alterations made to Dioscorides' text reveal still other ways in which information about drugs was first recognized and transmitted. Finally, the Latin Alphabetical Dioscorides manuscript group reveals that Latin texts reflect even greater alterations than did the Byzantine Greek texts.

While searching for Dioscorides manuscripts, often classified under the rubric "Herbals", I found another genre of manuscripts which had little attention. These were the lapidaries or treatises on stones, that I reported on in two articles reprinted here. The lapidaries were truly intended as medical guides for the use of minerals in medicine. The second article in this group explains about Albert the Great and his inquisitiveness about minerals. The study is coauthored with my colleague, James Mulholland, an historian of mineralogy and a trained metallurgist.

Following the Fulbright year of study under Professor Steudel, I met the person who became my fourth mentor, Professor Lynn White jr., scholar and gentleman. Prof. White's total involvement in the search for an understanding of science, technology, and society was an inspiration. Always in the background was his sometimes gentle, sometimes harsh insistence to me to relate the evidence found in early medicine with the broad themes of society. He pressed me to come to grips with what was a troubling anomaly. When medicine was reviving and returning to its classical roots during the period of scholastic medicine, why was it that the practical pharmaceutical texts indicate harmful prescriptions and a likely deterioration in medical practice? The resulting article, actively edited by Prof. White, has predictably caused comment and, in fairness, disagreement. The lasting value, I hope, from this study is to enter a caution to those historians who see medical theory as a positive indication of improvement in medicine but who fail to ask the practical questions about how the practitioner dealt with the theory. In the end, the empirical benefit to the patient is a necessary consideration in evaluating medicine, science and technology.

Especially during lectures to medical students about early drugs, the question is often raised: "Does it work?" For years I avoided answering this question on the basis that no one could possibly know for certain. Literally scores of factors must be known before a sure answer can be delivered and the nature of historical documentation always precludes finding the evidence. The last three published articles were written with the assertion that this question should no longer be ignored.

Credibility was lost with students who raised the question of effectiveness because they wanted to know whether, at the very least, answers were even attempted to evaluate ancient drugs. The first among these articles is a study of the writings of Gargilius Martialis that postulates his works were not high-level "professional" medicine of the late Roman Empire but instead useful medical knowledge for an estate leader. The fact that the writings were employed during the early Middle Ages as medical guides discloses information about both the time of the author and the Middle Ages. The death of a good friend led to an interest in cancer chemotherapy. I learned that the ancients employed the same drug against cancer that he took. The article that resulted stimulated a greater reaction in the medical and pharmaceutical communities than it did among historians. The message is that, when searching for new drugs, a scientist can profitably begin with the history of the drugs used against the affliction he wishes to probe. How folk practices may have discovered the medicinal uses of herbs, minerals and animal products is the subject of the last previously published article. The surprising disclosure was that there is a close correlation between the drugs we take today and those that the ancients had in their drug cabinets.

These studies provoked criticism, specifically about my methodology. Some critics claim that the use of the scientific knowledge of today is being applied to verify the ancient and medieval peoples' science, and that this is an application of historical positivism. The critics are absolutely incorrect about my intention and, I hope, wrong about the result. A forthcoming study in a monograph (*Contraception and Abortion from the Ancient World to the Renaissance*, Harvard University Press) claims that the ancients had effective chemical birth control measures and, moreover, the resulting historical demographic profile of the classical and medieval worlds reflects the importance of people exercising control over their reproduction. As a means of addressing concerns about how one today can make a judgement about the effectiveness of a drug, I have included an original essay, the last in this collection, to set forth my methodology of historical drug research.

This research was made possible through the assistance and good will of many people, too many to name, too cherished not to acknowledge. While my mentors, Caldwell, MacKinney, Steudel and White, cannot be held responsible for my errors in my work, they are the resources and the inspiration for my work. So too must I acknowledge my colleagues in the physical and biological sciences who over the years have answered my questions and given me so many tutorials in their specializations as I have sought to understand our ancestors and their use of drugs.

JOHN M. RIDDLE

North Carolina, 1991

PUBLISHER'S NOTE

The articles in this volume, as in all others in the Collected Studies Series, have not been given a new, continuous pagination. In order to avoid confusion, and to facilitate their use where these same studies have been referred to elsewhere, the original pagination has been maintained wherever possible.

Each article has been given a Roman number in order of appearance, as listed in the Contents. This number is repeated on each page and quoted in the index entries.

ACKNOWLEDGEMENTS

Grateful acknowledgement is made to the following publishers and journals for permission to reproduce in this volume the following articles originally published by them: Franz Steiner Verlag Wiesbaden GmbH (I, II, XI); the American Institute of the History of Pharmacy (III, V, VII, XIV); the Institute of the History of Sciences, Moscow (IV); the Regents of the University of California (VI); The Pontifical Institute of Medieval Studies (VIII); Everett Mendelsohn, editor of the *Journal of the History of Biology*, and Kluwer Academic Publishers (IX); Robert U. Massey, editor of the *Journal of the History of Medicine and Allied Sciences* (X); The History of Science Society (XII); and Dumbarton Oaks (XIII). Particular thanks are due to James Mulholland, co-author of study VIII.

I

Pomum ambrae

Amber and Ambergris in Plague Remedies*

Fashionable Roman ladies of the first and second centuries A.D. had a curious custom of carrying balls of amber in their hands. MARTIAL and JUVENAL reported that the practice of carrying amber (*sucinum*) was highly respected and that the sweet fragrance and warmth emitted was very pleasing, both to the bearer and her company[1].

After the lapse of more than a millenium amber balls appear once again in records of human behavior. At this time, however, it was more than a fashion. In the fourteenth century, amber was used for the very utilitarian purpose of warding off the dreaded pestilence then ravaging Europe. A great body of medical literature, *Pestschriften*, was produced during the century and a half following the catastrophic year 1348. KARL SUDHOFF collected and published the texts of numerous *Pestschriften* in his Archiv für Geschichte der Medizin. On the whole, the *Pestschriften* represent a highly intelligent and individualized effort by medical men to find protection against the plagues. SUDHOFF's collection provides most of our first hand material but several other important sources have also been used to supplement the *Pestschriften*.

In this study we propose to describe the following: (1) the use and manufacture of a unique "amber" product, *pomum ambrae* (ambergris balls or apples[2]), (2) ambergris (*ambra*) used as a fumigant, (3) the prevailing confusion concerning the two types of so-called amber, *i.e.* the animal substance, ambergris (*ambra*), and the vegetable amber, (4) a brief perusal of the pharmaceutical ingredients with which amber and ambergris were compounded, (5) the unusually high cost of ambergris, and (6) concluding statements.

* For his scholarly supervision of this paper, I am deeply indebted to LOREN C. MACKINNEY, Kenan Distinguished Professor, University of North Carolina. Mr. THOMAS HERNDON also has made helpful suggestions. I am also indebted to the School of Medicine of the University of North Carolina for a grant which enabled me to spend two years of research on amber and its medical uses.

[1] MARTIAL *Epi.* V. 37. 9—11; III. 65. 4—6; XI. 8. 6; and JUVENAL *Satires* VI. 573; IX. 50—53.

[2] Munich, Staatsbibliothek, MS Lat. 441, f. 244 (SUDHOFF, Archiv, 14, 87), partly in German, has the term *ein ambra apfel.*

I

1. The use and manufacture of Pomum ambrae

Pomum ambrae is a term which appears constantly in manuscript texts. In the interval between the fashionable Roman ladies and late medieval accounts, the usage, composition, and semantics of ambergris "apples" (*pomum ambrae*) became extremely complex. Actually, *pomum ambrae* was so-called because it was composed of ambergris (*ambra*) along with other ingredients which occasionally included amber (*karabe*). The semantic inconsistency is characteristic of the confusion which has surrounded amber through the ages and will be discussed more fully in Section 3 below.

Like his modern counterpart, the medieval physician was vitally concerned with protective medicine (*preseruatiua medicinalia*[1]). One source admonishes the reader to be cautious; "windows should be closed against the winds coming from the pestilent region and especially against the west wind since the pestilence now prevailing in our regions is from western neighborhoods[2]." *Pomum ambrae* was administered to protect against the corrupting influence of such foul and plague-ridden air. In leaving a house, one was urged to hold *pomum ambrae* before the nose, neck, and face[3]. Every day at dawn one should smell a pellet (*trociscus*) which included amber (*karabe*) and ambergris (*ambra*) along with numerous other ingredients[4]. In addition to rectifying the air, *pomum ambrae* also was supposed to uplift the spirit[5], aid the heart[6], help diges-

[1] Berlin, Staatsbibliothek, MS Lat. 60, f. 98 v (Archiv 16, 111); and *passim* throughout the *Pestschriften*.

[2] Nicolaus von Udine. Munich, Staatsbibliothek, MS Lat. 75, ca. 1390, f. 351 v (Archiv 6, 363): „Teneantur clausae fenestrae oppositae vento, venienti a regione pestilentica, ut non clauduntur fenestrae versus ventum occidentalem propter pestilenciam nunc regnantem in partibus nobis occidentalibus satis proprinquis."

[3] Leipzig, Universitätsbibliothek, MS 1179, 15th c., f. 29 (Archiv 6, 330): „In exitu ad populum de domo sit ante nares et collum et faciem et manus et pulsus cum eodem liniendo vel pomum ambrae vel huiusmodi."

[4] Joannis de Pinna. Breslau, Universitätsbibliothek, MS 111 F. 6, early 15th c., and Wiesbaden, Landesbibliothek, MS 61, ca. 1400 (Archiv 16, 164).

[5] Magister Berchtoldus. Heilbronn, Stadtbibliothek, MS M. 2002 Q, ca. 1440, f.93 v (Archiv 16, 91).

[6] Nicolaus von Udine. Munich, Staatsbibliothek, MS Lat. 75, ca. 1390, f. 352 v (Archiv 6, 367); unidentified MS in Vienna, Hofbibliothek, MS Palatinus latinus 2317, late 14th c., f. 35 (Archiv 5, 339); Hansen Wircker. Augsburg, Stadt- und Kreisbibliothek, MS 121, mid 15th c., ff. 63—64 v (Archiv 8, 198).

tion[1], comfort the principal membranes[2], strengthen the body to better resist disease[3], and fortify the brain[4]. Not all references mentioning *pomum* are concerned with *pomum ambrae* specifically. In fifty-two descriptions of a pomum that included ambergris (*ambra*), only thirty actually used the title *pomum ambrae* and only thirteen of these thirty were true *ambra* (ambergris) recipes. Furthermore the prescriptions that include *ambra* (ambergris) in a *pomum* show many variations. The thirteen recipes for *pomum ambrae* had a total of 124 ingredients including sixty-nine separate substances. This produces an average of 9.54 ingredients for each recipe. Thus, each recipe is unique—a surprising factor when one considers the medieval custom of borrowing freely.

Some of the compounds most used in *pomum* prescriptions are *lignum aloes* (in 7 out of 13 recipes), *camphor* (7), *storax* (7), *calamite* (6), *gariofilum* (6), *musca* (6), and *karabe* (2). A good example of a *pomum* recipe from a fifteenth century manuscript reads as follows:

> Pomum ambrae tempore pestis secundum fracinum doctorem R_x storacis, calamitae, florum buglossae, melissae ana ℈ ij, gariof. ʒ j, doronici, ben albi et rubei ana ℈ j, ligni aloes ℈ ij, calami aromatici, nucis muscatae, spicae, thuris vernicis, masticis ana ℈ j, ambrae, musti ana grana xij, carabe, croci ℈ semis, camphorae ℈ ij, sandalorum utriusque ana ʒ j, ro[sarum] ru[bearum] ʒ iij, succi portulacae, succi arancij ana ʒ iiij, nenufaris, corticum citri, coriandri correcti ana ʒ ij, corallorum rubeorum, spodij ana ʒ semis, syrupi de citro, boli armenici ana ʒ semis, terrae sigillatae ʒ i misce omnia pulverisanda, piretrum, ambra, muscus pulverisentur per se, demum misceantur cum praedictis, postea R_x laudani infusi in aqua ro[sarum] et aceto ℥ iiij, terbentinae lotae cum aqua rosarum, quantum sufficit ad faciendum pomum[5].

Though frequently employed as an aromatic substance, ambergris (*ambra*) was not indispensable in an odoriferous *pomum*. For in-

[1] NICOLAUS VON UDINE. Munich, Staatsbibliothek, MS Lat. 75, ca. 1390, f. 352 v (Archiv 6, 367).

[2] MAGISTER BERCHTOLDUS. Heilbronn, Stadtbibliothek, MS M. 2002 Q, ca. 1440, f. 93 v (Archiv 16, 91).

[3] Vienna, Hofbibliothek, MS Palatinus latinus 2317, late 14th c., f. 35 (Archiv 5, 339); see also NICOLAUS VON UDINE. Munich, Staatsbibliothek, MS Lat. 75, ca. 1390, f. 352 v (Archiv 6, 367).

[4] NICOLAUS VON UDINE. Munich, Staatsbibliothek, MS Lat 75, ca. 1390, f. 352 v (Archiv 6, 367).

[5] Leipzig, Universitätsbibliothek, MS 1179, 15th c., f. 28 v (Archiv 6, 328—329). The sign ℈ indicates scrupuli; ʒ indicates drachmae; and ℥ uncia.

I

stance, PRIMUS DE GORLICIO, a physician and professor of medicine at the University of Paris in the fifteenth century, in a recipe for a *pomum* included many of the usual ingredients in *pomum ambrae*, but left out the ambergris (*ambra*[1]). That substitutes were available is evident from the advice that "one should carry in his hand something odoriferous, such as *pomum generatum* or *pomum ambrae*[2]"; or, "before his mouth and nose one should hold *pomum ambrae* or a sponge soaked in wine, when going into the open air[3]."

A manuscript of the writings of JOHANNES JACOBI (fl. 1400—1420) affords unusual advice against the use of ambergris (*ambra*). JACOBI advises keeping rooms moist, especially in the summer, and the regular washing of the body with water and vinegar; careful selection should be made of the size of the living quarters, a medium size preferred, and (JACOBI continues) one should remain indoors during the plague. Smelling pleasant things is highly recommended, but JACOBI specifically warns against *pomum ambrae* lest it lead corrupt air to the heart[4].

Contradicting JACOBI is a note in the margin of the manuscript which was inserted by a survivor of the plague. This individual stated that on account of his poverty he had lived *outside* in everyday house-to-house begging. Even though he was daily exposed to the plague and filthy conditions, he had survived to the astonish-

[1] Hanover, Königliche Bibliothek, MS IV. 339, early 15th c., f. 175 (Archiv 17, 82—83).

[2] Munich, Staatsbibliothek, MS Lat. 19901 B., mid 15th c., f. 62 v (Archiv 14, 156): „Item portabitis in manu aliquid odoriferi sicud[t] pomum generatum uel pomum ambre."

[3] Breslau, Universitätsbibliothek, III. Q. 12, early 15th c., f. 281 (Archiv 9, 160): „Et in exitu ad aerem teneatis ante os et nares spongiam intictam in aceto vini aut pomum ambrae."

[4] Munich, Staatsbibliothek, MS Lat. 6018; Erfurt, Stadtbibliothek, MSS Q 194, Q 217; Wolfenbüttel, Herzogliche Bibliothek, MS Helmstädt 429 (Archiv 17, 26): „Istis visis videamus qualiter quis debeat preseruari. primo precauet ab aere corrupto fetido uel infecto et eligatur domus munda. Camera sit media, non inferior reumatica, quia aliter si non esset reumatici, esset melior, sed superior non habitetur; melius enim attingitur ab influencia dicta tempore turbido et nebuloso, melius est stare infra domum quam extra. ymmo non est bonum ire per villam sed in aliquo occupari infra domum in qua sint pauci. Domus irroretur, specialiter in estate cum aceto et rosis uel folijs vitis; ymmo est bonum ualde frequenter in die lauare manus cum aqua et aceto et post tergere faciem et odorare acetosa, si est mortalitas, quia timemus cordis calefactionem et ideo non laudo pomum ambre, ymmo [quia] forte ducit ad cor aerem corruptum."

ment of his friends. On AVICENNA's recommendation and his own experience this survivor praised the use of *pomum ambrae*[1].

"Water of roses" (*aqua rosata*) and sometimes *buglossae* were used to give the *pomum* or "apple" its form[2]. Apparently the pulverized ambergris (*ambra*) and, sometimes, amber (*karabe*) and musk (*muscus*) were dissolved in "water of roses," the other ingredients added, and then the mixture was allowed to harden into a *pomum* or "apple[3]." Very similar to the amber (*sucinum*) necklaces and amulets mentioned by PLINY[4], *pomum ambrae* may have had a hole bored through so that it could be worn and perforated for maximum exposure to the air[5].

2. Ambergris as a fumigant

When medieval physicians adopted the method of purging the air of plague infestation by burning aromatics, ambergris (*ambra*) was widely used. Mixed with other substances, it was burned to fumigate rooms before and after pest visitation[6]. One unusually

[1] Ibid., Archiv 17, 31: „Ergo dicit magister Jacobus, quod quondam fuit pestilencia in Montepessulano et ego non potui vitare communitatem, quia transivi de domo in domum ad curandum infirmos causa paupertatis, attamen portaui panem uel spongiam uel pannum intinctum in aceto in manu mea et tenui prope os et nasum et sic euasi talem pestilenciam. Socii autem mei, non credentes me vitam retinere, quia acetosa opilant meatum humorum nec faciunt venenosa intrare. Et si eciam haberes pomum ambre, qui habetur in apotecis iuxta dictum Avicenne qui dicit, quod pomum ambre attrahit malos humores. Et omnia hec remedia per me ipsum probaui." Standard AVICENNA MSS fail to mention *pomum ambrae*.

[2] Munich, Staatsbibliothek, MS Lat. 75, ca. 1390, f. 352 v (Archiv 6, 367), which says to use *buglosa* water in the winter and rose water in the summer.

[3] *e.g.*, see above R_x on p. 113. [4] *Natural History* 37. 11. 3.

[5] Berleburg, Schloßbibliothek MS F. 4, late 15th c., ff. 211 v—212 (Archiv 16, 17): „Ir sullent alle zijt bij uch tragen camphoram vnd pomum [f. 212] ambre, der dorch hol ist"; see also Archiv 17, 15, for text of an unidentified MS which has „... fiat pomum in medio perforatum...."

[6] *e.g.*, JOANNES DE PENNA. Wiesbaden, Nass. Landesbibliothek, Codex 61, early 15th. c., f. 50 v (Archiv 16, 164): „Fumigium bonum R_x rosarum rubearum prolzandi [?] citri ʒ 20 [?], ligni aloes, ambre, camphore ana ʒ semis. Ambra soluatur in aqua rosarum et alie medicine conficiantur cum ea et fiant pilule, quarum vna post vnam fumigatur in pestilencijs et ante et post." See also Munich, Staatsbibliothek, MS Lat. 323, late 14th c., f. 119 (Archiv 6, 318 to 319); Florence, Biblioteca Riccardiana, MS 1219, late 14th c., f. 18 v (Archiv 5, 373); JOHANNIS DE NOCTHO of Sicily. Florence, Biblioteca Riccardiana, MS 2114, late 14th c., f. 4 r & v (Archiv 5, 386); Bern, Stadtbibliothek, MS 556, late 15th c., f. 161 v (Archiv 16, 62); MAGISTER BERCHTOLDUS. Heilbronn,

elaborate concoction for fumigation contained thirty-four separate ingredients including ambergris (*ambra*[1]). Some sources warn against the intensive use of burning aromatics[2]. It was thought that the strong odors emitted by ignition might be damaging in a small room[3], and it was urged that the quantity of ambergris (*ambra*) should be closely restricted[4]. Twenty-four per cent of the ambergris (*ambra*) recipes are fumigants.

Revealing the individuality of late medieval, medical writings, one manuscript contains a lengthy explanation of the method of burning ambergris in the sick room and then specifically admonishes the user not to smell the *pomum ambrae*[5]. In contrast, JOHANNES DE NOCTHO (ca. 1398) asserts that a room needs the good odors produced by burning ambergris but includes a recipe for an aromatic ball that does not contain ambergris (*ambra*[6]).

3. The confusion between amber and ambergris

Words in pharmaceutical texts are like the labels of modern drugs and, like labels, can convey wrong meanings. Amber and ambergris, though chemically unlike, have approximately the same pharmaceutical value when used as aromatic stimulants. Consequently the confusion between them is not entirely illogical.

Ambra, an Arabic word meaning ambergris, was introduced into medieval Latin by the translators of the Arabic medical works.

Stadtbibliothek, MS M. 2002 Q, mid 15th c., f. 91 (Archiv 16, 83); BLASIUS OF BARCELONA. Florence, Biblioteca Nazionale Centrale, MS XV. 150, ca. 1400 ?, f. 3 v (Archiv 17, 107); COSTOFFORUS OF OXFORD. Florence, Biblioteca Riccardiana MS 2114, 14th c., f. 11 v (Archiv 17, 122); Wolfenbüttel, Herzogliche Bibliothek. MS Helmstädt 784 (Archiv 17, 73); MAGISTER HENRICUS DE BREMIS (or de Ribbenicz). Prague, Universitätsbibliothek, MS I. F. II, late 14th c., f. 141 v (Archiv 7, 86).

[1] BLASIUS OF BARCELONA. Florence, Biblioteca Nazionale Centrale, MS XV. 150, ca. 1400 ?, f. 3 v (Archiv 17, 107). This MS was allegedly written for KING MARTIN OF ARAGON (1396—1410).

[2] MAGISTER BERCHTOLDUS. Heilbronn, Stadtbibliothek, MS M. 2002 Q, ca. 1440, f. 91 (Archiv 16, 83) and f. 93 r & v (Archiv 16, 90—91).

[3] Bern, Stadtbibliothek, MS 556, late 15th c., f. 161 r & v (Archiv 16, 62).

[4] Florence, Biblioteca Riccardiana, MS 1219, late 14th c., f. 18 v (Archiv 5, 372); MAGISTER BERCHTOLDUS, Heilbronn, Stadtbibliothek, MS 2002 Q, ca. 1440, f. 91 (Archiv 16, 83).

[5] Bern, Stadtbibliothek, MS 556, late 15th c., f. 161 v (Archiv 16, 63).

[6] JOHANNES DE NOCTHO. Florence, Biblioteca Riccardiana, MS 2114, late 14th c., f. 4 (Archiv 5, 386).

Karabe (amber) is the basic Persian word adapted into Arabic and subsequently into Latin by the same route. In the centuries that followed the arrival of Arabic medicine in western Europe, there was confusion between amber and ambergris. Western Europe had many words meaning amber, *e.g. sucinum, electrum, lyngurion,* and *bernstein*; and presumably there was only one word for ambergris, *ambra*, the derivation of which in many Western tongues now means the resinous substance and not the secretion of the sperm whale.

The *Pestschriften* maintain a relatively clear distinction between amber and ambergris by employing only the words *ambra* and *karabe*; other types of literature, both medical and non-medical, show more confusion. In some *Pestschriften* the Latinized Arabic word *ambra* is expanded into *ambra-grisse*—the suffix "grisse" meaning "grey". Of significance is the fact that seventy-six per cent of the examples of *ambra-grisse* occurred in the same recipe with *karabe*. This would imply that the authors of the *Pestschriften* felt some sort of color distinction was necessary when both amber and ambergris were used together.

In the *Pestschriften* in German there is a greater tendency to use the full title *ambra-grisse* than in Latin writings; however, the number of examples is too small for an absolute evaluation. Great importance can be attached to the fact that in no *Pestschriften* in German is the German word *Bernstein* used for amber; always it is the non-German term *karabe*. Being native to the Baltic shores, amber was well-known to Germans. In other writings at the same time as the *Pestschriften*, they often referred to it in their native tongue as *Bernstein*[1].

References to ambergris show much variation in spelling. It is spelled "lambra[2]," "dyambra[3]," "mambrae[4]," and, in English

[1] *e.g.* ALBRECHT VAN BORGUNNIEN (13th c. or possibly 14th c.). *Treatise on Medicine.* Edited by W. L. WARDALE (London 1936 [London, B. M. Sloane MS 3002]), II, 1: "Bernstein is gut tegen(n) allerha(n)de sten." PLINY (*N.H.* 37. 11. 3) mentions that the Germans used amber as a fuel, hence probably the word *bernstein* stems from "burning stone."

[2] MARIANO DE SER JACOBI DE SIENA. Modena, Biblioteca Estense, MS Lat. 606, f. 51 (Archiv 16, 145).

[3] *e.g.* MAGISTER BERCHTOLDUS. Heilbronn, Stadtbibliothek, MS M. 2002 Q, ca. 1440, f. 94 v (Archiv 16, 95).

[4] MAGISTER GALLUS. Prague, Universitätsbibliothek, MS IX. A. 4, early 15th c., ff. 168 v—169 (Archiv 7, 60).

I

manuscripts, "pomamber[1]." Further distinctions appear in various adjectives introduced to modify the noun, e.g. *electa ambra*[2], *bona ambra*[3], *pura ambra*[4], and *pura et optima ambra*[5].

The usage of *karabe* (amber[6]) is somewhat different. Sixty-two per cent of the recipes containing amber (*karabe*) occur in prescriptions in which ambergris (*ambra*) is not mentioned. Amber (*karabe*) is apt to be used internally, ambergris (*ambra*) externally[7]. Amber (*karabe*) is often prescribed for the stomach[8]—a significant fact since AVICENNA prescribed the animal substance, ambergris (*ambra*), not amber (*karabe*[9]).

For internal medicine (*ex medicinis vero administrandis interius*) MAGISTER ALBERTUS writes a recipe for a syrup which contained both amber (*karabe*) and ambergris (*ambra*); but in another preparation (*confectio*) for the same purpose he includes only amber (*karabe*[10]). Both amber (*karabe*) and ambergris (*ambra*) were used in pills[11]. An unusual prescription for preserving the air against plague corruption recommends a syrup containing thirty-eight separate ingredients including *karabe* (amber) but not the scarce *ambra* (ambergris[12]).

[1] WILLIAM BULLEIN, *A Dialogue against the feuer Pestilence* . . . Edited by MARK W. BULLEN and A. H. BULLEN (London 1888), pp. 49—50.

[2] Vienna, Hofbibliothek, MS 5312, f. 244 (Archiv 6, 360).

[3] Leipzig, Universitätsbibliothek, MS 1179, 15th c. (Francinus doctor), f. 28 v (Archiv 6, 329).

[4] *e.g.* Wolfenbüttel, Herzogliche Bibliothek, MS Helmstädt 783, early 15th c., f. 23 (Archiv 11, 90).

[5] *e.g.* MAGISTER BERCHTOLDUS. Heilbronn, Stadtbibliothek, MS M. 2002 Q, ca. 1440, f. 93 (Archiv 16, 91).

[6] *karabe* is often spelled *carabia* or *carabe*, e.g. Breslau, Universitätsbibliothek, MS III. Q. 4, early 15th c., f. 173 (Archiv 9, 151); and RUFINUS, *Herbal*, f. 37 r a (*Thorndike edition*, p. 75).

[7] *e.g.*, Munich, Staatsbibliothek, MS 372, mid 15th c., f. 2 v (Archiv, 14, 160); NICHOLUS DE BURGO. Bologna, Universitätsbibliothek, MS 1887, ca. 1400, f. 90 (Archiv 5, 360); MAGISTER ALBERTUS, Vienna, Hofbibliothek, MS Lat. 2317, f. 34 v (Archiv 6, 316).

[8] NICHOLUS DE BURGO. Bologna, Universitätsbibliothek, MS 1887, ca. 1400, f. 90 (Archiv 5, 360).

[9] AVICENNA, *Canon* II. 337 a. 26 (1564 ed.).

[10] MAGISTER ALBERTUS. Vienna, Hofbibliothek, MS Lat. 2317, f. 34 v (Archiv 6, 316—317); see also BERTOLD OF BASEL. Wolfenbüttel, Herzogliche Bibliothek, MS Helmstädt 429, f. 71 v (Archiv 17, 259).

[11] *e.g.*, Munich, Staatsbibl., MS Lat. 372, mid 15th. c., f. 2 v (Arch. 14, 160); Bologna, Universitätsbibl., MS 1887, f. 90 v (Archiv 5, 360), by implication.

[12] Erfurt, Stadtbibliothek, MS Amploniana 222, mid 14th c., f. 213 (Archiv 11, 64—65). cf. Breslau, Universitätsbibliothek, MS III. Q. 4, early 15th c. f. 173 (Archiv 9, 151).

4. Other pharmaceutical ingredients

Variation of ingredients in amber and ambergris recipes is noteworthy. Thirty-one prescriptions, containing either amber or ambergris, were examined; therein was a total of 446 items, involving 126 separate ingredients. Of these, eighty-three were used only once or twice. Those most widely used were *lignum aloes* (79 %[1]), *gariofilum* (79 %), *storax* (54 %), *laudanum* (31 %), *rubeus sandalus* (34 %), *thus* or frankincense (38 %), *camphora* (54 %), *muscus* (69 %), and *karabe* (28 %).

Of significance is the fact that *lignum aloes, laudanum, camphora, gariofilum, rubeus sandalus*, and *thus* are all eastern products. These are mostly aromatic substances, an illustration of the large scale employment of odoriferous stimulants in late medieval medicine.

5. Cost of ambergris

A relatively large number of sources note the expense of ambergris[2]. Frequently recipes containing ambergris (*ambra*) are specifically recommended for rich patients; for the poor, recipes substituting myrrh and mastic or an entirely different recipe may be offered[3]. In three instances ambergris (*ambra*) is specifically pre-

[1] The percentages were computed by the number of times the substance appears in recipes with ambergris.

[2] *e.g.* Wolfenbüttel, Herzogliche Bibliothek, MSS 784 and 217 (Archiv 17, 73, correlated text of both MSS): "... subfumigaciones aerem rectificantes cum ligno aloes, ambra, musco quo ad divites et potentes ...."; Berlin, Staatsbibliothek, MS Lat. 60, f. 99 v (Archiv 16, 111—112): "Et si apposueris de ambra ʒ iij vel iiij erit preciosissime et conueniens multum"; Giovanni Santa Sofia. Munich, Staatsbibliothek, MS Lat. 250, ca. 1400, f. 214 (Archiv 6, 348): "... si ambra inveniri non potest vel sine ambra vel musco pro pauperibus laudani optimi quantum sufficit...."; Berlin, Staatsbibliothek, MS Lat. 60, f. 98 v (Archiv 16. 111): "Primum debent homines et mane bibere acetum in quo posita sunt pulveres de mirra et thure ... Diuites ... omni mane acetum tepidum in quo resoluta sit ambra ... camphora ... bdellium ... tyriaca ... pill. pestilenciales quinque...."

[3] *e.g.* Paris, Mazarine, MS 3599, late 13th c., f. 65 v: "Pomum ambre est duplicatum .... Item per pauperibus .... " The following MSS are collated in Archiv 5, 63f.: London: B. M. Sloane, MS 2320, ca. 1400, ff. 13 v—16; Cambridge, Gonville and Caius College, MSS 336 and 725, ff. 144 v—148; Cambridge, Trinity College, MS O. I. 77, 15th c., ff. 53—72 v, *et al.* It reads (p. 63): "... si dives est, utatur dyambra, dyamusco, dyanthos, et consimilibus. Si vero pauper est...."; see also, Wolfenbüttel, Herzogliche Bibliothek, MS Helmstädt 783, early 15th. c., f. 13 v (Archiv 11, 76).

scribed for royalty[1]; in two others papal physicians recommended it for the pope[2]. That ambergris was scarce in the middle ages is understandable; similar conditions prevail in modern times.

A French manuscript, bearing the date 1348 and written to protect against the dreaded pestilence (Compendium de epidemia per collegium Facultatis Medicorum Parisius ordinatum), affords an interesting example of the importance and costliness of amber:

> A description of amber apples: for the king or queen let them be solely of the purest and best ambergris, because by itself it has the powerful qualities of soothing and comforting. In this form it is stronger and, because of its fortitude as an aromatic, it consequently gives substantial comfort to the spirit and the principal membranes and increases them. Because pure amber is very expensive it can be compounded into an apple with other substances less expensive and sufficiently convenient. Another description of amber apples: R_x...[3]

The high price of ambergris doubtless accounts for its scarcity in prescriptions; for an example, an electuary to prevent the plague contains forty-three ingredients but neither amber nor ambergris[4]. Throughout the late medieval writings there are many recipes for which amber and ambergris would have been suitable but from which they are totally absent[5].

[1] Magister Berchtoldus. Heilbronn, Stadtbibl., MS M. 2002 Q, ca. 1440, f.93 (Archiv 16, 91): "Descriptio pomi ambre pro rege et regina...."; Paris, Bibliothèque Nationale, MS 12233, 15th c., f. 119 (Archiv 17, 71): "Descripcio pomi ambre: pro rege aut regina fiat de ambra sola pura et optima...."; Blasius of Barcelona. Florence, Biblioteca Nazionale Centrale, MS XV 150, f. 3 v (Archiv 17, 107): MS written for King Martin of Aragon (1396—1410).

[2] John of Saxony, Gotha, Landesbibliothek, MS A 501, early 15th c., f. 10 r & v (Archiv 16, 27): "... cum electuario nobilissimo magistri Guidonis phisici Urbani papae quinti... [f. 10 v] 10° valet pomum ambre..."; also Berlin, Königliche Bibliothek, MS Lat. 88, early 15th c., f. 151 v for pope Clemens V. (Archiv 11, 59).

[3] Paris, Bibliothèque Nationale, MS 12233, 15th c., f. 119 (Archiv 17, 71): "Descripcio pomi ambre: pro rege aut regina fiat de ambra sola pura et optima, ipsa enim habet vehementem proprietatem letificandi et confortandi simul et est ad hoc pocior siue potentior propter fortitudinem sue aromacitatis et ideo confortatiuum est substancia cuiuslibet spiritus et membrorum principalium et multiplicatam ipsius. Quia cum ambra pura esset nimis cara ideo potest componi ad pomum minus carum et satis conveniens. Alia descripcio pomi ambre: R_x...."

[4] Munich, Staatsbibliothek, MS Lat. 963, late 15th c., f. 186 (Arch. 16, 179).

[5] Munich, Staatsbibliothek, MS Lat. 372, f. 1 (Archiv 17, 51—52); Primus de Gorlicio. Hanover, Königliche Bibliothek, MS IV 339, early 15th c., ff. 171—182 v (Archiv 17, 82—83).

6. Conclusions

Since Roman times at least, amber has been employed in materia medica[1]. After the appearance of Latin translations of Muslim medical works, especially in the *Pestschriften*, ambergris was given a more important place. It was believed that aromatic stimulants, such as amber and ambergris, rid the air of plague infestation. Being by far the more powerful of the two stimulants, ambergris eclipsed amber in materia medica. This is evident in *pre-Pestschriften* manuscripts which we have merely cited in passing in this survey. From the thirteenth century there are two important examples in which *pomum ambrae* appears as the title of a brief treatise. In one of them[2] a historiated capital letter and an "*Incipit tractatus de pomo ambre*" introduces a sixteen line description, below which is a marginal miniature picturing three stages in the compounding of the *pomum* (Fig. 1). A similarly brief treatment is found in another manuscript (cf. p. 119, n. 3), which has a marginal miniature of a man manufacturing a *pomum ambrae* while a younger man watches[3]. However, previous to these thirteenth century manuscripts, Avicenna and Mesue (the Third) had mentioned *pomi* ("apples") of this sort without the name *ambra*[4].

Even modern purchasers have difficulty in recognizing ambergris at first glance. In pre-modern times the two substances were confused to such an extent that the Arabic word for ambergris (عنبر) was first translated into Spanish, Italian, French, and English as a designation for both amber and ambergris, later to be used for

[1] Pliny, *N.H.* 37. 12. 1; Dioscorides, *Herbal* II. 100 [II. 81, Wellmann ed.]; Galen, *Opera* XII, 549 (p. 86 Kühn).

[2] Kraków, Bibliotheca Jagellonica, MS 816, ff. 101 v—113. We have studied this MS in a microfilm of Professor Loren C. MacKinney's collection of medical miniatures. This MS, with photoreproduction of the folio in question, is described in Zofia Ameisenowa, *Rekopisy I Pierwodruki Iluminowano Biblioteki Jagiellonskie* (Wroclaw 1958), fig. 107.

[3] Paris, Mazarine, MS 3599, late 13th c., f. 65 v.

[4] Avicenna, *Canon* II. 1 (1564 ed.); Mesue, *De medicinis aegritudinum capillorum*, ff. 225 r & v, 235 v, 253 (1581 ed.); the text of John of Gaddesden (*Rosa Anglica*, p. 141, Lat. ed. 1595) has a mention of *pomum ambrae* but this appears to be a later insertion. The Salernitan writer, John of Procida (d. ca. 1266), compiled a list of maxims which includes a quotation allegedly from Alexander the Great but what is obviously a version of the Alexandrian Romance. John of Procida cites Alexander as having said he took one hundred *pomi ambrae* from the king of Tyre. — *Placita Philosophorum* ..., as published in *Collectio Salernitana* 5, III, 125.

amber alone. Surprisingly, however, the authors of the *Pestschriften*, using the distinctive terms *ambra* and *karabe*, did not succumb to this common confusion. In spite of the *Pestschriften*'s semantic consistency, one finds a medical glossary of the Salernitan school (*Alphita*, late 14th c. or early 15th c.) which reports that "*karabe* is called ambergris by the common people (*karabe a vulgo dicitur lambra est* ...[1])." It appears that, whereas the differences between amber and ambergris were recognised by the relatively well-informed authors of the *Pestschriften*, other supposedly well-informed medical men along with contemporary readers of the *Pestschriften* often confused the two substances. Perhaps there were those who deliberately confused the two because of the high price of ambergris ("grey" *ambra*) and the abundance of amber ("yellow" *ambra*). It is obvious that the cost of ambergris was a serious problem for the rank and file of medieval people.

The *pomum* form of aromatic stimulants was prominent in medieval materia medica. This "apple" provided a portable remedy that could be used as both a preventative and a curative and by both ambulatory and bed-ridden patients. The term *ambrae*, often only one of the many ingredients, may have been used because its relatively high cost gave a certain prestige[2].

[1] as published in *Collectio Salernitana* III, 281.

[2] In the near future we hope to publish in detail the results of our intensive research on all aspects of the use of amber and ambergris in materia medica during antiquity and the middle ages.

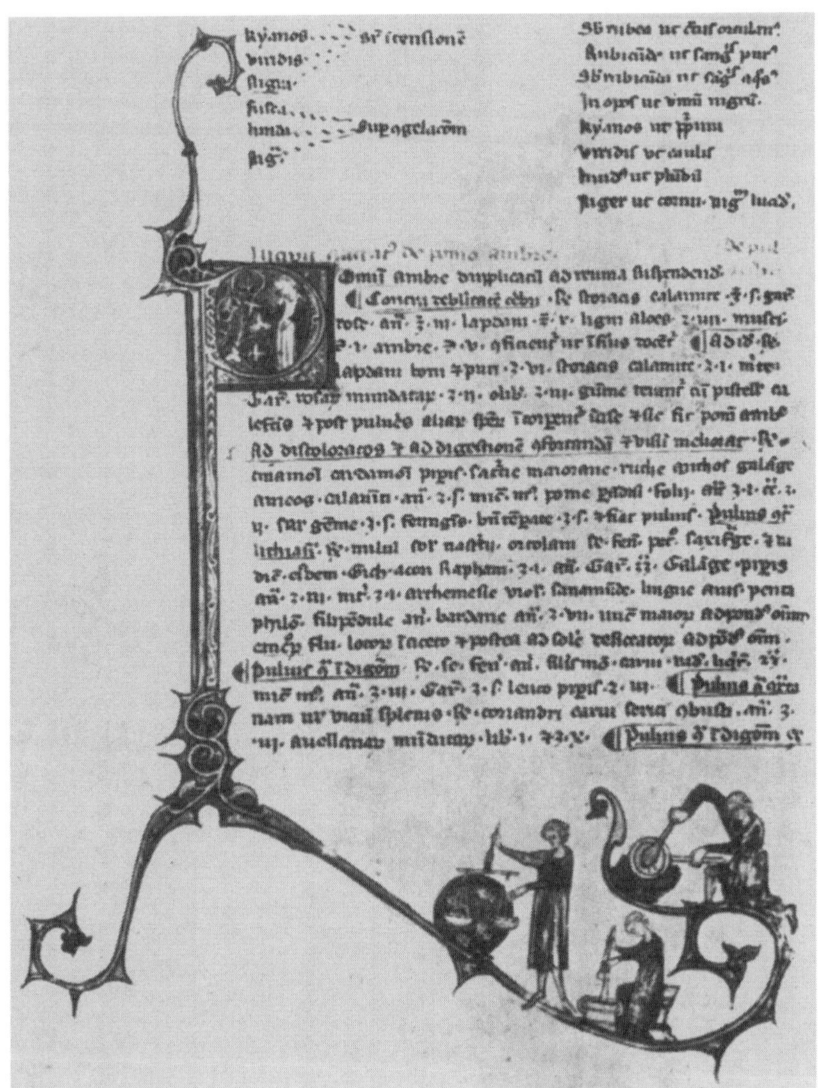

Fig. 1. Tractatus de pomo ambrae. Bibliotheca Jagellonica Ms. 816, fol. 101 v.

II

The Introduction and Use of Eastern Drugs in the Early Middle Ages*

Medical recipes are scattered in numerous manuscripts both in Latin and the vernacular. Many date from the so-called „dark ages", that is, pre-Salernitan Europe before the first translations of the Islamic medical writings[1]. Examination of the nature and sources of this early medieval recipe literature has disclosed an interesting connection with eastern drugs. The importance of this connection is grasped when we note that the large amounts of oriental products mentioned in western texts indicates both extensive trade contact and a type of communication about new drugs. This development comes prior to any known translations of medical texts and when, according to the old PIRENNE thesis, Europe was introverted and isolated from contact with the Islamic east.

Before launching this study it might be wise to make some introductory comments about the nature and content of the medieval recipe literature. Few existing manuscripts are completely devoted to the antidotaries and receptaries, words used to describe the Latin recipe literature, although numerous medical and non-medical manuscripts contain folios of prescriptions for all sorts of afflictions[2]. The authorship is always anonymous. SIGERIST and JÖRIMANN agreed that the antidotaries were compiled by monks having some medical knowledge[3]. Most recipes are derived directly out of the

* For his scholarly supervision and many aids, I am deeply indebted to Prof. JOHANNES STEUDEL. Also I wish to express my appreciation to the Fulbright Kommission for making my studies under Prof. STEUDEL possible.

[1] In the last century the Rev. THOMAS OSWALD COCKAYNE published an extensive collection of the Anglo-Saxon recipe literature (*Leechdoms, wortcunning, and starcraft of early England*, re-issue 3 vols. [London 1961].) which has been subsequently re-examined in book form by J. H. GRATTAN and CHARLES SINGER (*Anglo-Saxon magic and medicine* [London 1952]) and, still more recently, by WILFRID BONSER (*The medical background of Anglo-Saxon England. A study in history, psychology, and folklore* [London 1963]). Early in this century HENRY SIGERIST (*Studien und Texte zur frühmittelalterlichen Rezeptliteratur* [Leipzig 1923]) and his pupil JULIUS JÖRIMANN (*Frühmittelalterliche Rezeptarien* [Zürich 1925]) published the texts of some of the early Latin recipe literature.

[2] LOREN C. MACKINNEY, *Early medieval medicine: with special reference to France and Chartres* (Baltimore 1937), p. 136.

[3] SIGERIST, *Rezeptliteratur*, p. 168; JÖRIMANN, *Rezeptarien*, p. 1.

works ancient authors, especially ALEXANDER OF TRALLES, AETIUS OF AMIDA, and PAUL OF AEGINA, but not two antidotary or receptary are alike. Individuality and originality are present in so far as the compiler had to make the selection himself from the plentiful supply of prescriptions in ancient texts and, therewith, came personal judgment[1]. GALEN was the most named author, HIPPOCRATES being in the background, but many classical names were attached to the prescriptions. Some have emperors' names, *e. g.*, VESPASIAN and ALEXANDER OF MACEDONIA, and other writers of the early middle ages, *e. g.*, AFRODISIUS, THOMAS, GENTILIS, NEUCLERIUS, and EUGENIUS[2]. There is evidence that new material was translated from the Greek[3]. Still some recipes cannot be attributed to extant classical works, and it is certain there were new additions. What we have in most cases are original compilations, SIGERIST said, which the writer has gathered for the necessity of his monastic needs[4].

For the most part the recipes pertain to things of everyday life, *e. g.*, remedies for coughing and removing lice, and for headaches, pain in the stomach, and wounds. Most recipes are not for specific diseases. Early medieval medicine was unprepared for advanced diagnostic techniques required for such prescriptions. The recipes were mostly for what today would be called patent medicines purchased across counters[5].

Recipe literature is found in Anglo-Saxon England and written in the old English vernacular. These numerous manuscripts, mostly pre-Salernitan, are not translations but compilations by herbalists (leeches) mainly from Latin sources but with unusual amounts of folklore sprinkled throughout. The folklore is derived from Roman, Celtic, and Teutonic cultural strands. Additionally these leechbooks show evidence of southern Italian and Byzantine influence, chiefly via Benedictine transmission[6].

In attempting to obtain an insight into the extensiveness of drugs in early medieval, western pharmacopoeia, I took a statistical analysis of the 9th century antidotary, St. Gall MS 44, ff. 228–255[7]. The manuscript is divided into sections according to the form of the

[1] SIGERIST, *Rezeptliteratur*, pp. 185–6; JÖRIMANN, *Rezeptarien*, pp. 1–2.

[2] SIGERIST, *Rezeptliteratur*, pp. 182–4.

[3] *Ibid.*, p. 186. [4] *Ibid.*, pp. 185–6. [5] *Ibid.*, p. 170.

[6] CHARLES SINGER, „Introduction", to COCKAYNE, *Leechdoms* . . ., I, xxvi–xl; BONSER, *The medical background of A. S. Engl.*, pp. 34–47.

[7] The text is published in SIGERIST, *Rezeptliteratur*, pp. 78–99.

recipe, *e. g.*, salves, poultices, and the like. This antidotary has a total of 123 recipes involving some 361 different ingredients used a total of 944 times, thereby, illustrating at once the large number of drugs. Since the drugs were not often repeated, just a few accounting for the majority, we can see the specialized nature attributed to each simple. In our analysis we eliminated honey, wine, wax, and rose water, substances used as emollients, flavoring agents, and solvents. From a list made of the substances, the following are those appearing in eight or more recipes (The number of times per recipe is in parenthesis): *aloes* (15), *ammonicum* (11), *amomum* (9), *apium semen* (10), *cassia* (12), *ciminum* (8), *colofonia* (14), *fenuogrecum* (10), *libanus* (12), *linum* (11), *mastice* (16), *murra* (17), *piper* [white, long, and black] (33), *petroselinum* (17), *picea* (10), *scamonia* (14), *storace* (13), *terebentina* (17), *and zinzibar* (8).

An examination of the identities of these drugs reveals a startling fact: *most can only be found in the orient.* Eastern drugs seemed to have been the „miracle drugs" of the Age[1]. Though it is impossible always to identify each according to the exact plant species, one can be fairly certain of the family or, at least, genus[2].

Amomum is an aromatic scrub said by PLINY to come from India, Persia, and the Aral Sea region and presently attributed to Persia and the Aral Sea region[3]. *Ammonicum*, a salt, is ammonium chloride and apparently associated in antiquity with the oracle Hammon in the desert regions of Africa where *ammonicum* is found. Both PLINY and GALEN note its use in early medicine[4], but it is known to have been manufactured in the late middle ages from the

[1] I roughly define *eastern* as those regions either controlled by Islam or east of it and excluding Spain. This includes northeastern Africa.

[2] The confusion over nomenclature, plant identities, and taxonomic categories in ancient-medieval medicine is illustrated in an excellent study by JERRY STANNARD, „The plant called moly", *Osiris*, 14 (1962), 254–307.

[3] PLINY, *Natural History* 12. 28. 49–9; HEINRICH ZÖRNIG, *Arzneidrogen. Als Nachschlagebuch für den Gebrauch der Apotheker, Ärzte, Veterinärärzte, Drogisten und Studierenden der Pharmazie*, 2 vols. (Leipzig 1909), I, 7. Of course, seeds scatter and species are unable to survive in some regions. This causes differences in the distribution of plants between ancient and modern times, but I shall assume in this study that plants, presently found only in the warm, moist climate of southern Asia were there also in antiquity. In most cases, I have been able to cite ancient sources collaborating modern botanists.

[4] PLINY, *N. H.* 31. 39. 78–9; GALEN, *Opera*, K. XIX, 724, 734.

distillation of the horns and hoofs of oxen[1]. *Aloes*, employed extensively in ancient medicine, is found in south Africa but mostly in India where there exists a variety of species[2]. Medicinal aloes is a resin described in the *Materia Medica* of DIOSCORIDES[3]. *Cassia*, probably a product of *cinnamomum pauciflorum nees*[4], is said by PLINY to be the „skin" of a scrub[5], and it is known to be found only in the far east[6]. *Crocus* is simply the Latin and Greek form for saffron, an oriental product[7]. *Libanus*, or frankincense, is a product of the orient, though one variety of the tree bearing this gum is indigenous to the Somilia region[8]. *Murra*, or myrrh, remembered along with frankincense as two of the Magi's gifts, is the gum resin product of *commiphera myrrha*, found only in Arabia and Abyssinia[9]. On the other hand, *mastice* or mastic, a resinous exudation obtained from the lentisk plant, is presently grown in the entire Mediterranean area though evidence shows that in antiquity and the middle ages it was imported from the eastern Mediterranean[10]. *Pepper*, of course, is a product of the far east, a fact widely recognized in antiquity[11]. Derived from the plant *convolvulus scam-*

[1] LUDWIG FREDERICK AUDRIETH, „Ammonia", *Encyclopaedia Britannica* (1962 ed.), I, 815.

[2] ZÖRNIG, *Arzneidrogen*, I, 1–7; ALEXANDER TSCHIRCH, ed., *Handbuch der Pharmakognosie*, 3 vols. (Leipzig 1910), I, pt. 2, 1420ff.; 2nd ed.

[3] *M. M.* 3. 22 (WELLMANN, ed.); see also ISIDORE. *Ety.* 17. 8, 9, 28; and GRATTAN AND SINGER, *A.-S. magic and med.*, pp. 97–8. TSCHIRCH (*Pharmakognosie*, II, pt. 2, 1441) reports that aloes was mentioned in a letter between the PATRIARCH HELIAS of Jerusalem and ALFRED THE GREAT of England.

[4] GEORG DRAGENDORFF, *Die Heilpflanzen der verschiedenen Völker und Zeiten* (Stuttgart 1898), p. 239; TSCHIRCH, *Pharmakognosie*, II, pt. 2, 1261ff.

[5] PLINY, *N. H.* 12. 43. 95–8.

[6] DRAGENDORFF, *Die Heilpflanzen*, p. 239.

[7] ZÖRNIG, *Arzneidrogen*, I, 97; DRAGENDORFF, *Die Heilpflanzen*, p. 139.

[8] DRAGENDORFF, *Die Heilpflanzen*, p. 366; *Enc. Brit.*, (1962 ed.), IX, 689. The word *libanus* is derived from the Greek form, but also the Latin word for frankincense, *thus*, is found twice in this same manuscript. For ancient authorities, see PLINY, *H. N.* 12. 30. 51–65; 20. 64. 172; and THEOPHRASTUS, *On Plants* 9. 4. 4–9.

[9] DRAGENDORFF, *Die Heilpflanzen*, pp. 367–8; see also PLINY, *N. H.* 12. 30. 71, and THEOPHRASTUS, *On plants* 9. 4. 1–10.

[10] DRAGENDORFF, *Die Heilpflanzen*, p. 396; *Enc. Brit.* (1962 ed.), XV, 44; W. HEYD, *Histoire du Commerce du Levant au Moyen-Age*, 2 vols. (Amsterdam 1959), II, 633–5.

[11] See below, p. 192; also HEYD, *Histoire du Commerce . . .*, II, 658–64; and PLINY, *N. H.* 12. 14. 26–29.

monia, scammony is found only in the eastern Mediterranean area especially Asia Minor[1]. *Storace* or storax, widely employed in ancient medicine, comes from Asia Minor, Syria, and the far east[2]. Described by many ancient writers, *zinziber* or ginger is a native to the warm parts of Asia[3]. The remaining substances, *apium semen* (parsley seeds), *colofonia* (a resin product), *ciminum*[4], *fenogrecum* (or *fenum Grecum*, a plant), *linum* (flax), *petroselinum* (rock-parsley), *picea* (various forms of pitch), and *terebentina* (terebinth) are all found in western Europe. Thus, the evidence from this typical antidotary of 9th century Europe discloses a large use of eastern products which had to have been imported. That is to say, the drugs WERE imported if the manuscripts of recipe literature were in actual use.

Convincing evidence can be shown to those who with laudable stubbornness refuse to believe that the recipe literature was anything but handwriting exercises for monks with no medical knowledge. FULBERT wrote a letter to a bishop urging him to consult the antidotaries for proper medicines[5]. ALCUIN states that physicians (*medici*) collected and compounded drugs[6]. Prescribed ceremonies were probably performed while collecting herbs[7]. Intermittently medieval writers have appended their own observations onto

[1] DRAGENDORFF, *Die Heilpflanzen*, p. 553; TSCHIRCH, *Pharmakognosie*, II, pt. 2, 1333–5.

[2] DRAGENDORFF, *Die Heilpflanzen*, pp. 270–1; PLINY, *N. H.* 12. 55. 124–5.

[3] DRAGENDORFF, *Die Heilpflanzen*, p. 141ff.; *Enc. Brit.* (1962 ed.), X, 365; TSCHIRCH, *Pharmakognosie*, II, pt. 2, 1044–58. See also PLINY, *N. H.* 12. 14. 28; CELSUS, *De re medica* 5. 23; GALEN, *Opera*, XI, 880ff.; DIOSCORIDES, *M. M.* 2. 160 (WELLMANN, ed.). For trade in ginger, see HEYD, *Histoire du Commerce* . . ., II, 619–23.

[4] Though the plant is said to be found in modern, southern Europe as well as Egypt and Asia, PLINY spoke only of a species from Ethiopia. (Pliny, *N. H.* 20. 55. 161; DRAGENDORFF, *Die Heilpflanzen*, pp. 499–500) We know, however, that in the year 820 A. D. *ciminum* was growing in the herbal garden at St. Gall. — P. JUNG, „Das Infirmarium im Bauriß des Klosters von St. Gallen vom Jahre 820", *Gesnerus* 6 (1949), 5. There is some evidence that it may have been imported also. — see the list on p. 194.

[5] *Ep.* 4 (*P. L., lat.*, CXLI, 195–6).

[6] *Ep.* 213 (*M. G. H., Ep.* IV, 356–7): „Solent namque medici ex multorum speciebus pigmentorum in salutem poscentis quoddam medicamenti conponere genus, nec se ipsos frateri praesumunt creatores herbarum vel aliarum specierum, ex quarum conpositione salus efficitur egrotantium . . . ".

[7] BONSER, *The medical background of A.-S. Engl.*, p. 314–6.

ancient texts to clarify plant identities and to add where they are to be found[1]. As a final proof of the use of the recipe literature and of eastern products in them, the manuscripts contain new drugs recently discovered in the east. These new drugs were unknown in antiquity and were actually introduced into western Europe during the early middle ages. For example, the St. Gall MS 44 on folio 247 contains the word *ambar*, from the Arabic meaning ambergris, the biliary concretion of the sperm whale.

Unknown in antiquity, the pharmaceutical values of ambergris were discovered by the Arabs, though possibly they borrowed it from other eastern sources[2]. ABU ZAKARIYA IBN MASAWAIH (777–857 A.D.), the last great physician of the school at Jundišapur, named ambergris as one of the five principal aromatics[3]. A manual for traders, composed possibly in the 11th century or even earlier, lists ambergris along with camphor, musk, aloes, pepper, cinnamon, and ginger[4]. By the 12th century ambergris was confused with amber in western Europe. Thus, the knowledge of ambergris and its Arabic name were introduced into western Europe by the 9th century or two centuries before the first Latin translations of Islamic medical writers.

The word *cafora*, coming from the Arabic *kâfoûr*[5], is found in the same manuscript as ambergris and also in an antidotary written in Lombardic script in the 9th or 10th centuries[6]. As a product of the plant *cinnamomum camphora nees*, *cafora* or camphor is found

[1] JÖRIMANN, *Rezeptarien*, p. 81; MACKINNEY, *Early medieval med.*, pp. 35–6.

[2] JOHN M. RIDDLE, „Pomum ambrae: Amber and ambergris in plague remedies", *Sudhoffs Archiv*, 48 (1964), 121–2; and „Amber in antiquity: Philological variants", *Laudatores temporis acti. Studies in memory of Wallace Everett Caldwell* (Chapel Hill 1964), pp. 110–20.

[3] MARTIN LEVEY, „Ibn Masawaih and his treatise on simple aromatic substances", *Journ. hist. med.* 16 (*1961*), 394.

[4] *Kitāb al-ishārati ilà mahāsini 't-tjāra* (Cairo A. H. 1318), as cited by T. W. ARNOLD, „Arab travellers and merchants, A. D. 1000–1500", Chapt. 5 of: ARTHUR PERCIVAL NEWTON, *Travel and travellers of the middle ages* (New York 1926), 93–4 [The word *amber* is mistranslated].

[5] TSCHIRCH, *Pharmakognosie*, I, pt. 2, 611ff. Camphor is included in a list of drugs introduced by the Arabs and Persians by both TSCHIRCH (*Ibid.*, I, pt. 2, 614) and ERIC JOHN HOLMYARD („Medieval Arabic pharmacology", *Proceedings Royal Soc. Med.* 29 (1936), 107.

[6] Glasgow, Hunterian MS T. 4. 13, f. 168, as published in SIGERIST, *Rezeptliteratur*, p. 147.

only in the orient[1]. The Arabs discovered camphor in the booty taken in the Persian Sassanides capital[2]. IBN MASAWAIH classified it as a principal aromatic[3]. Unknown in antiquity[4], camphor is mentioned in the early 7th century and subsequently its use became widespread in the middle ages[5]. According to ALEXANDER TSCHIRCH, SIMON SETH (11th c.) was the first to mention camphor in Greek[6]. Like ambergris, camphor was first known in pre-Salernitan Europe.

An Anglo-Saxon monk, living in the 9th century, compiled a series of recipes which we now call the *Lacnunga*. It contains three prescriptions with the word *zedoary*[7]. The word recurs in the Glasgow MS T. 4. 13 of the 9th or 10th centuries[8]. Zedaory, from the Arabic *zedwar*, is an aromatic root of a species of tumeris (*curmuma zedoaria*) found in the orient[9] and completely unknown to the ancients[10]. HILDEGARD (fl. 1099) mentions it[11]. According to

[1] DRAGENDORFF, *Die Heilpflanzen*, pp. 240–1; ZÖRNIG, *Arzneidrogen*, I, 35; TSCHIRCH, *Pharmokognosie*, II, pt. 2, 1110ff.; *Enc. Brit.* (1962 ed.), IV, 679–80.

[2] HEYD, *Histoire du commerce . . .*, II, 590.

[3] LEVEY, „Ibn Masawaih", *Journ. hist. med.* 16 (1961), 394.

[4] The word ἡ καψουρά is found in GALEN, *Opera*, XIV, 761 and AETIUS OF AMIDA, *Libri medicinales* 12. 63, 16. 130. Even though accepted as legitimate by ZÖRNIG (*Arzneidrogen*, I, 35), the Arabic term *kâfoûr* is considered by modern scholarship to be interpolations whenever found in classical MSS texts. See LIDDELL and SCOTT, *Greek-English Lexicon* (9th ed.).

[5] ALBERICO BENEDICENTI, *Malati-Medici e Farmacisti*. 2nd. Ed. (Milan 1947), I, 285, 295ff.

[6] *Pharmakognosie*, I, pt. 2, 593–4.

[7] *Lacnunga*, London, MS Harley 585, ff. 137b, 138b, 142a, as published in GRATTAN and SINGER, *A.-S. magic and med.*, pp. 108, 110, 114.

[8] SIGERIST, *Rezeptliteratur*, p. 164.

[9] DRAGENDORFF, *Die Heilpflanzen*, p. 143; HEYD, *Histoire du commerce*... II, 676; ZÖRNIG, *Arzneidrogen*, I, 558; TSCHIRCH, *Pharmakognosie*, II, pt. 2, 1058–63.

[10] ZÖRNIG (*Arzneidrogen*, I, 558) says the word is found in the works of AETIUS OF AMIDA and PAUL OF AEGINA. I have been unable to find the substance in any works currently attributed to these authors. DRAGENDORFF (*Die Heilpflanzen*, p. 143) states: „Wird von neuern griechischen Autoren als Zerumbed benannt, ist aber nicht der Zedoar des Aetius oder Macer Floridus". The Latin translation of Aetius made by JANUS CORNARIUS (Bale 1533–5) has: „Zedor id est zeduarie . . .". In a letter published as a preface to the 1535 edition („Epistolae ad Carolum V"), Cornarius clearly asserts that a good medical man will use his knowledge of Arabic pharmaceuticals when the Greek interpretation is unclear. Although I am not certain, I suspect that ZÖRNIG was using the old FRANCIS ADAM'S edition

Grattan and Singer, zedoary along with *gallenger* are probably the earliest Arabic words traceable in old English[1]. *Gallenger*, or galingale, is another oriental, aromatic plant, again unknown in antiquity, but found in the recipe literature in both Latin and old English, dating from a least the 9th century[2].

Generally throughout the early medieval recipe literature other products of eastern origin are scattered in countless prescriptions. Pepper was the most widely used substance[3]. Musk, a product of Tibet and China, is found repeatedly as are *galbanum, costus, balsam, cardamomum*, all eastern products[4]. Such items as myrrh, gariofilum, ginger, storax, aloes, opium, cinnamon, frankincense, mastic, and saffron are often found in the recipes[5].

(London 1844) of Paul of Aegina, an edition known to accept many interpolations as Paul's own writing. I have been unable to find zedoary in such standard authors as Pliny, Isidore, Theodore Priscian, Marcellus, and Galen. See also, J. H. Baxter and Charles Johnson, *Medieval Latin word-list* (Oxford 1934), p. 61, and DuCange, *Glossarium*, VIII, 428, for their entries on *zedoary*. Tschirch (*Pharmakognosie*, I, pt. 2, 614, 1063) includes zedoary in his list of substances introduced by the Arabs and Persians.

[11] *Physica* 1. 14 (*P. L.*, CXCVII, 1127).

[1] *A.-S. magic and med.*, p. 108.

[2] *Galanga* is found in Karlsruhe, Bibliothek, MS Augiensis CXX, 9th or 10th c., f. 10v (Sigerist, *Rezeptliteratur*, p. 54); Glasgow, Hunterian T. 4. 13, 9th or 10th c., f. 169 (*Ibid.*, p. 150); Cambridge, MS G. g. V. 35, 11th c., f. 429 (*Ibid.*, p. 163); London, B. M. MS Harley, 9th c., f. 138b (Grattan and Singer, *A.-S. magic and med.*, p. 110). See also Zörnig, *Arzneidrogen*, I, 517; Heyd, *Histoire du commerce . . .*, II, 616–8; Dragendorff, *Die Heilpflanzen*, p. 144; Tschirch, *Pharmakognosie*, II, pt. 2, 1063–71.

[3] In the leechbooks published by Cockayne (*Leechdomms . . .*, 3 vols.), I have found the use of pepper seventy-two times. Sigerist's *Rezeptliteratur* and Jörimanns *Rezeptarien* contain an equal abundance of usage. See a discussion on pepper in Aldhelm, *Aenigmatum* 3. 5. (*P. L.*, LXXXIX, 188).

[4] I shall cite only the references in the old English leechbooks (Cockayne, *Leechdomms . . .*) because they are not indexed as are the texts published by Sigerist and Jörimann; *galbanum*, II, 44, 174; III, 88, 112, 124, 134; *balsam*, II, 28, 174, 288; III, 90; *costus*, II, 238, 276; III, 6, 70, 72. As items of trade, see Heyd, *Histoire du commerce . . .*, II, 610–8, 636–40, 601–2, For the habitats and origins of these products, see Dragendorff, *Die Heilpflanzen*, 140–1, 144–6, 368–9, 495–6; Tschirch, *Pharmakognosie*, II, pt. 2, 1010–1, 1071–84, 1156–62. It is most difficult to identify the exact substance meant by the Latin word *balsam*. See the various discussions in Pliny, *N. H.* 12. 25. 41, 29. 50, 54. 111, 56. 126–7.

[5] See the texts of Cockayne, *Leechdomms . . .*, 3 vols.; Sigerist, *Rezeptliteratur*; and Jörimann, *Rezeptarien*, Benedictus Crispus (d. ca.

Generalizations about the pharmaceutical usage of these eastern drugs are next to impossible without treating each separately. A large number, however, are aromatic substances, which seemed to have received emphasis in Arabic medicine, a fact perhaps dating back to the time when the Nabatean Arabs, living along the famous „incense road", controlled much of the trade route between the Hellenistic-Roman world and India. Often these aromatics were used as stimulants for such things as syncope and chronic catarrh, as an antispasmodic and a „comforter" of stomachic and intestinal disorders, and as a remedy for various nervous afflictions. Aloes, for example, was often used as a cathartic[1]. Camphor is known to have mild antiseptic and anesthetic properties, but probably these qualities as such were not recognized by medieval medical men. Most of the substances so far mentioned are to be found in early 20th century pharmaceutical guides. Even though synthetic drugs have mostly replaced these natural products, pharmacy nonetheless attributes some beneficial physiological action to them. Surpri-

725), *Poematium medicum* (*P. L.*, LXXXIX, 369–74), mentions myrrh and cinnamon. The *Lacnunga* (Grattan and Singer, *A.-S. magic and med.*) has prescriptions for aloes, pepper, myrrh, zedoary, galingale, ginger, storax, and incense.

The Arabic word *saffron*, which gradually replaced the Greco-Roman word *crocus*, meaning the same substance, is found in a late leechbook (Cockayne, *Leechdomms* . . ., 96), but this particular manuscript seems to be a translation or, at least, heavily influenced by an earlier Salernitan work (See Singer, „Introduction", to Cockayne, *Leechdomms* . . ., xxiv.). Holmyard („Medieval Arabic Pharmacology", *Proc. Roy. Soc. Med.*, 29 [1936], 107) erred when he stated that *crocus* and *saffron* were introduced by the Arabs and Persians. According to Zörnig (*Arzneidrogen*, I, 97), saffron is mentioned in the Papyrus Ebers. A. C. Crombie (*Augustine to Galileo, the history of science A. D. 400–1650* [London 1952], p. 21) was mistaken also when he stated that saffron was introduced from the Arabs. There can be no doubt that the Latin *crocus* and the Greek *κρόκος* is saffron. For example, see the entries in Lewis and Short, *A Latin dictionary* (Oxford), and Liddel and Scott, *A Greek-English lexicon* (9th ed., Oxford). I have systematically excluded *nard* from the accounts because, although the best probably comes from the orient, a Gallic *nard* exists.

[1] Other uses are to be found. For example, aloes was employed for diseases of the head in the *Secreta secretorum*, 1681 (*Early English Texts Society* [London 1894], extra series LXVI, 55), which was probably originally a Syriac work of the 7th, 8th, or 9th centuries and, subsequently, widely translated in the west. — George Sarton, *An introduction to the history of science*, I, 556–7.

singly often, however, the substances in the recipe literature are used in ways which modern pharmacy can see no value. For example, zedoary, a carminative, is employed in a prescription against elf-enchantment[1], and aloes, zedoary, and pepper, all aromatic condiments, were used for inflammation of the eyes[2]! It would be a mistake to attribute a high prestige to the recipe literature in light of modern pharmacology; but despite superstition, faulty theories, and semantic problems, the early middle ages had a working pharmacopoeia.

Since western pharmacopoeia included large numbers of eastern products, what then is the relation between pharmacy and trade during the early middle ages? Noting oriental products in the old English recipes, WILFRID BONSER posited that this did not necessarily mean that the products were imported to England because the recipes with these particular articles may have been copied from manuscripts in the south.[3] We know that the monks of Corbie in the 9th century planned to buy the following herbs and spices *at the market:* „piper, ciminum, gingember [ginger?], gariofile, cinamomum, galingan, reopontico, costus, spicum, mira, sanguinem draconis, indium, percrum, pomicar, zedoarium, styrax, calaminta, apparment, thyme, gotyumber, clove, sage, and mastick."[4] A similar but shorter list comes from Mainz in the 10th century.[5] These lists can be compared with the lists of herbs grown on the villas of CHARLES THE GREAT, in the monastic garden of St. Gall (820 A. D.), and in the private herbal garden of WALAFRID STRABO.[6] The existence of such lists points to the definite use of

[1] *Lacnunga,* London, B. M. MS Harley 585, f. 137b, as published in GRATTAN and SINGER, *A.-S. magic and med.*, p. 109ff.

[2] *Ibid.*, f. 142a, p. 115. This caused GRATTAN and SINGER (p. 115) to comment that they could not see how this prescription could fail to make the affliction worse. The use of aloes, saffron, pepper, myrrh, and camphor are found in prescriptions, mostly salves, for the eyes as recorded by IBN MASAWAIH. — C. PRÜFER and M. MEYERHOF, „Die Augenheilkunde des Johannia b. Masawaih", *Der Islam*, 6 (1916), 248ff.

[3] BONSER, *The medical background of A.-S. Engl.*, p. 45.

[4] This list is found in the appendix of B. GUÉRARD, *Polyptigue de l'abbé Irminon . . .* (Paris 1886), II, 336. For drawing attention to this list I am grateful to the late Professor LOREN C. MACKINNEY.

[5] A. SCHULTE, *Geschichte des mittelalterlichen Handels und Verkehrs zwischen Westdeutschland und Italien* (Leipzig 1907), I, 73.

[6] Capitulary *de villis*, lxx (*M. G. H., cap. regum Franc.*, I, 90): P. JUNG,

the recipe literature and the importation of eastern drugs. Before the 12th century at Westminister Abbey, the Chamberlain was charged with the duty of supplying medicine to the poor.[1] One recipe in a 9th century manuscript mentions that the drug cannot be found locally but had to be imported from the orient.[2] ALCUIN mentions a doctor *(medicus)* who delivered medicaments en route to Rome.[3] If the drugs were not imported into western Europe, what possible explanation can there be for the appearance of new drugs, such as ambergris, galingale, zedoary, and camphor, in the western recipe literature? Contrary to BONSER's doubts, the evidence is convincing that western Europe maintained continuous contact with the east in respect to pharmaceutical items. The business of the preservation of health was not likely to have declined so drastically as to have been bankrupted completely.

According to ROBERT LOPEZ, the spice trade between east and west never ended, as HENRI PIRENNE has postulated.[4] W. HEYD's study of east-west trade proves that the Arabs continued trading in far eastern products after the sweep of Islam. They found a good market for spices with the Germans.[5] Many of the products, *e.g.*, aloes, storax, and frankincense, were the same as are found in a 1st century B.C. (?) sailor's guide to trade in the Red Sea.[6] LOPEZ reports a Muslim traveler from Spain in 973 A.D. „was surprised at the quantity of ‚Indian' spices" he found in Mainz.[7]

„Das Infirmarium im Baurіß des Klosters von St. Gallen vom Jahre 820", *Gesnerus*, 6 (1949), 5; WALAFRID STRABO, *Hortulus* (*P. L.*, CXIV, 1119–50).

[1] NANCY JENKINS, „Medieval monastic accounts, medicines and spices", *The Pharmaceutical Journal*, 118 (1954, 4th ser.), 515.

[2] St. Gall MS 44, f. 242: „Emplastrum diauotanus utilis. Diatanos recipit haec: sinuitu albu orientale quia hic non inuenitur . . ." (SIGERIST, *Rezeptliteratur*, p. 84.) To be sure these words may have been copied from some ancient text but a reader in the middle ages would learn from them where the drug was to be found.

[3] *Ep.* 45 (*M. G. H.*, *ep.*, IV, 91): „Nam Basilius medicus, qui vobis in montanis, Romam pergenti, medicamenta tradidit, jam mortuus est." See also *Ep.* 77 (*M. G. H.*, *ep.* IV, 119) which mentions a „negociatorem, Italiae mercimonia ferentem . . .".

[4] ROBERT S. LOPEZ, „The trade of medieval Europe: the south", *The Cambridge economic history of Europe* (Cambridge 1952), II, 261.

[5] W. HEYD, *Histoire du commerce* . . ., I, 6ff., 17–8, 22, 89ff.

[6] *The periplus of the Erythraean Sea.* WILFRID H. SCHOFF, ed. (New York 1912) *passim.*

[7] LOPEZ, „The trade of med. Eur.", *Cam. econ. hist.*, II, 273.

The best illustration of trade in drugs is exemplified in the derivation of the word *apotheca* or apothecary. The Byzantines had local depots, called ἀποϑῆκαι, in the main harbors and road termini of the Mediterranean area.[1] Just how or when the word changed from a general depot to a dispensory of drugs is unknown,[2] but some clues can be found. An edict of FREDERICK II, regulating medical activity, referred to *apotheca* apparently in the sense of a store house for drugs.[3] During the 13th century, at least, the word *apotheca* comes to have the specialized meaning of the modern word.[4] The very fact that the word for an import-export house came to be associated entirely with the meaning „drug-store" demonstrates vividly the relation between trade and drugs.

Placing its trust in faith, the early medieval church refused to turn its talents towards the field of medicine. Apparently the church looked mostly after its own clerics for physical cures. The well regulated profession of Roman medicine returned to the hands of the general people, the rustics.[5] Just as in all societies which lack sophisticated medical institutions, a semi-professional class rose to attend the needs of people in pain and sickness. These medical men are often practioners of a lower sort, such as, *harioli*, *leeches*, *midwives*, and the such. They were even consulted by ecclesiastics.[6]

[1] *Ibid.*, II, 275.

[2] HENRY ALAN SKINNER, *The origin of medical terms* (Baltimore 1949), p. 32; LUDWIG AUGUST KRAUS, *Kritisch-etymologisches medicinisches Lexikon* (Göttingen 1844), 115.

[3] WOLFGANG-HAGEN HEIN and KURT SAPPERT, *Die Medizinalordnung Friedrichs II.* (Veröffentl. d. Intern. Ges. f. Gesch. d. Pharmaz. N. F. 12, Eutin 1957), p. 51 (also see pp. 18–20): „Lucrabitur autem stationarius confectionibus suis secundum istum modum: de confectionibus vero et simplicibus medicinis, que ante non consueverunt teneri in apothecis ultra annum a tempore emptionis, pro qualibet uncia poterit et licebit tres tarenos lucrari. De aliis vero, que ex natura medicaminum vel ex alia causa ultra annum in apotheca tenentur, pro qualibet uncia sex tarenos lucrari licebit". (*Novae constitutiones, titulus* 46.)

[4] RUDOLF SCHMITZ, „Über deutsche Apotheken des 13. Jahrhunderts. Ein Beitrag zur Etymologie des apoteca-apotecarius-Begriffs", *Sudhoffs Archiv* 45 (1961), 290ff.

[5] MACKINNEY, *Early medieval med.*, pp. 68–9, 71, 79; BONSER, *The medical background of A.-S. Engl.*, p. 171ff.

[6] GRATTAN and SINGER (*A.-S. magic and med.*, p. 17, citing BEDE, *Life of St. Cuthbert*, 32–45; *Ecclesiastical history* 4. 32, 5. 2.) note that certain monasteries had resident leeches. GREGORY OF TOURS (De *miraculis Sancti Martini* 1. 26, cited by MACKINNEY, *Early medieval med.*, p. 71) refers to

In a certain sense it is not fair to say folkmedicine because a degree of training must have been required to enable the practitioner to use the recipe literature. Not every reader of the recipe literature would know every drug; in fact, maybe no one was familiar with every item. Still the practitioner had to have had a large knowledge of plant identities; and, because the amounts of the various ingredients are infrequently and poorly given, he had to have experience in the prescription manufacture.

By what process were new eastern drugs introduced to the west when „communication“ was at a low ebb? The best explanation suggests that mysterious process, almost silent in our records, called folk-communication. Just as trade in amber and tin occurred from northern Europe to the Mediterranean area in pre-history, so also continued a trade in pharmaceuticals between the Islamic and Christian sides of the Mediterranean.[1]

The method of folk-communication is illustrated by a statement of MARCELLUS, a late Roman writer, who said he included in his works „even remedies chanced upon by rustics and the populace and simples which they have tested by experience.“[2] ALEXANDER OF TRALLES confesses that he too borrowed prescriptions from rustics.[3] The spread of drugs from east to west is similar to the

harioli whom the general populace consulted about sorcery, potions, and *ligamenta*. GREGORY OF TOURS (MACKINNEY, *Early medieval med.*, p. 71, citing *Historia Francorum* 10. 25) „... vented his spite most bitterly on a miracle-working hermit who claimed to be Christ and who wandered about like a primitive medicine man with a mob of hysterical folk in his train.“

[1] ALBERICO BENEDICENTI (*Malati-medici e farmacisti*, I, 308.) credits the period of 'ABD-AR RAHMAN II (d. 961) as the time when many oriental products, *e. g.* ginger, saffron, and myrrh, were introduced into Spain and, hence, into Europe. The evidence in the recipe literature pre-dates this more formal, cultural communication at court level. GRATTAN and SINGER (*A.-S. magic and med.*, p. 5) noted the appearance of the Arabic words *zedoary, gallenger*, and *ginger* (!) in the Anglo-Saxon prescriptions. They state that „... the advent of these in England was unrelated to the ,Arabian' scholastic learning. They came with quite other cultural streams.“ They seem to suggest „hisperic elements“, but it is not clearly seen, by me, at least, how this is related to medical practices. GRATTAN and SINGER were wrong, however, in thinking ginger is from the Arabic. Actually the word is probably derived from the Greek ζιγγίβερι (see GALEN, *Opera*, XI, 880ff.).

[2] *De medicamentis* 2 (p. 1, NIEDERMANN ed.): „... sed etiam ab agrestibus et plebeis remedia fortuita atque simplicia, quae experimentis probauerant, ...“

[3] *Opera*, II, 563 (PUSCHMANN ed.), as cited by LYNN THORNDIKE, *A history of magic and experimental science* (New York 1923), I, 578.

discovery of the stirrup in 5th century A.D. China and its introduction to the Franks in the 8th century.[1] Perhaps too much emphasis has been placed on medieval „reading" and „writing" and not enough on medieval „doing".

The medieval disbelief in sense perception, however, caused a failure to recognize that which was new. We find what today we would regard as medical practice mostly by semi-literate, medical men. Despite the authoritarianism in relation to ancient writings and the paucity of manuscriptions, we can catch glimpses of movement in the so-called „dark-ages" when it was previously believed all stood still. Significantly new eastern drugs were certainly introduced into western medicine before and separate from the intellectual recognition of the Islamic contributions to medicine. This necessarily implies not only a continued trade contact, contrary to the PIRENNE thesis, but a type of communication between Islam and Christianty over new discoveries.

[1] LYNN WHITE, Jr., *Medieval technology and social change* (Oxford 1962), pp. 15, 27.

III

LITHOTHERAPY IN THE MIDDLE AGES

Lapidaries Considered as Medical Texts

THE USE of stones and minerals in medieval therapeutics has been overshadowed in the literature by a fascination with the lore of herbs. This circumstance is reinforced by the fact that in medieval manuscripts the treatises on stones are ordinarily separate from those on plants; moreover, the presumed medicinal virtues often are buried among other kinds of lore about stones.

Perhaps the limited attention given by historians to these treatises, called lapidaries, is partly because it is harder to see them as an antecedent to a line of development in modern "scientific" materia medica. In any event, the only attempt to understand the specifically medical aspect of medieval stone lore, of which I am aware, is a doctoral dissertation by Herman Führer, published in Berlin in 1902.[1] Führer's reliance solely on published sources limited his pioneering effort severely. That manuscript lapidaries abound in the major European collections became apparent during a study tour I completed in 1968.

There we find convincing evidence that stones were used by medical men as an important part of therapeutics. Indeed, statements are made that stones were more important and useful than herbs.[2]

In general, there are three types of lapidary literature.[3] The "scientific" lapidary was derived from such writers as Theophrastos, Dioscorides, Damigeron, and Galen. Secondly, the magical or astrological lapidary, which some authors

*This study was sponsored by grants from the National Arts and Humanities Foundation and The Professional Research Fund of North Carolina State University.

This paper was delivered to the American Institute of the History of Pharmacy meeting in Montreal, May, 1969.

Where I have actually seen a manuscript the reference is marked by an asterisk (*) and where I have seen only a microfilm it is noted by a (‴). Abbreviations to libraries are those employed by L. Thorndike and P. Kibre, *A Catalogue of Incipits of Mediaeval Scientific Writings in Latin*. Revised, (Cambridge, Mass., 1963). I hope soon to produce a catalogue of lapidary manuscripts. Unless otherwise noted the references are to the Latin manuscript collections, e.g., *BN* means Bibliothèque Nationale, Latin.

Key to Abbreviations on Page 48

[1] *Lithotherapie, Historische Studien über die medizinische Verwendung der Edelsteine* (Berlin, 1902, 150pp.).

[2] For instance in the Preface of Marbode's *De lapidibus* (Migne, *P.L.*, vol. 171, 1739): "Nec dubium cuiquam debet falsumve videri, / Quin sua gemmis divinitus insita virtus. / Ingens est herbis virtus data, maxima gemmis." The Rubric to a lapidary states this also in Turin Nazional Bibl. MS D. IV.5, 14th c., f. 179. BL Douce 291, 14th c., f. 121 (and published by Joan Evans and Mary S.

trace to Alexandrian writings, did not enjoy the general popularity of the scientific type. Finally, the Christian lapidary or Christian symbolic lapidary was a persistently popular form, especially in the early Middle Ages. These lapidaries describe the twelve stones mentioned for Aaron's breastplate in Exodus or in the Apocalyptic literature.[4] Although formulated by such scholars as Joan Evans and George Sarton,[5] these three categories are handy for casual classification; but they are not mutually exclusive, and in fact often overlap. Some late medieval lapidarists prefer to view knowledge of stones as a composite in attempting to integrate knowledge.

In this study a total of 616 lapidary manuscripts have been collected. Most of them are in Latin, although vernacular manuscripts were recorded whenever found. Of the total, a majority have been seen (a few only on microfilm), while the others are described from information from manuscript catalogues and secondary works. Three hundred and ten are classified as to author, generally associated with such well known names as Marbode, Albertus Magnus and Thomas of Cantimpré. Ninety-four are of the Christian symbolic category, which has little medical interest. But there are 164 anonymous Latin lapidaries, of which many are primarily medical. In the latter there are wide variations in the numerous texts. These differences reveal that lapidaries were an ever-changing, popular mode of medieval medical and scientific expression.

Magic, superstition, and pharmacology are intertwined — but such distinctions are modern. For an instance of "enlightened usage," red ferrous oxide is prescribed for eye salves, while matallic sulphates are used for eyes, gout, dimness of the eyes, and kidney trouble.[6] Elsewhere a lapidary says if a doctor (*medicus*) carries a sculptured *iaspis* he can know the causes of disease and have a knowledge of medicine and herbs.[7] A Spanish

---

Serjeantson, *English Medieval Lapidaries*, p. 17) states: "The vertues of stones . . . in many places shulde have myghte where misse ne herbe ne rotis may not auaile ne helpe."

[3]Previous studies of lapidaries, published texts, and stone lore in general include: Paul Studer and Joan Evans, *Anglo-Norman Lapidaries* (Paris: Edouard Champion, 1924); Leopold Pannier, *Les Lapidairies Françai*s . . . (Paris, 1882); Paul Meyer, "Les plus anciens lapidaires français," *Romania*, vol. 38 (1909), 44-70; 254-552; Robert Max Garrett, *Precious Stones in Old English Literature* (*Münchener Beitrage zur romanischer und englischen Philologie* (Leipzig, 1909); Joan Evans and Mary S. Serjeantson, *English Medical Lapidaires* ("Early English Text Society, No. 190, Oxford, 1960 rpr.); C. W. King, *Antique Gems: Their Origin, Uses, and Value* (London, 1860); Urban T. Holmes, "Mediæval Gem Stones," *Speculum*, vol. 9 (1934), 195-204; and George F. Kunz, *The Curious Lore of Precious Stones* (Philadelphia & London, c. 1913).

[4]The most recent attempt to identify the actual stones is by E. L. Gilmore, "Gemstones of the First Biblical Breastplate?", *Lapidary Journal*, vol. 22 (1968), 1130-4.

[5]Evans, *Magical Jewels*, p. 38 and *passim;* Sarton, *Introduction to the History of Science*, vol. 1, p. 764.

[6]For instance, see Marbode *Emathite*, No. 32,(*P.L.* vol. 171, 1759) and *Medus*, No. 36 (1760-1); Damigeron in *BLh76, ff. 134v-5, 137v; and Albertus Magnus *Minerals*, Bk. 2, tr. 2; pp. 89-90, 106 of Dorothy Wycoff edition (Oxford, 1967).

[7]*CUc 243, 13th c.?, ff. 31, Anony. Inc.: "Habete celi silentium et ingratitudinis immance scelus . . . ."

[8]From the lapidary of Alfonso X (el Sabio, 1221-1284) and reproduced in facsimile, *Lapidario del rey d. Alfonso X; Codice Original* (Madrid, 1881) and commented on by Joan Evans, *Magical Jewels of the Middle Ages and Renaissance* (Oxford, 1922), p. 44.

lapidary warns that the lapidary user must have knowledge in astronomy, mineralogy, medicine and, moreover, be of high intelligence.[8] Raymond Lull admits that many virtues of the stone *adamans* come from the "art of magic"[9] and Damigeron mentions the hypnotic effect (crystal-ball gazing?) of the stone *diadocus*.[10] Some lapidaries give more emphasis to medicinal qualities while others belong more to a popular class that stresses the supernatural.[11] Vincent of Beauvais explicitly separates the magical virtues of stones from the medicinal characteristics.[12] While the usual literary form for lapidaries is an alphabetical discussion of stones—their features and virtues—some lapidaries are actually written in the form of prescriptions.[13] These stones were meant to be used both as amulets and as internal and topical medicines.[14]

The study of manuscripts affords the best evidence that lapidaries were a part of medical literature. Numerous examples in prefaces, texts, or marginal notes support the contention that lapidaries, far from being a debased form of medieval literature, were an accepted aspect of medieval science.[15] For example some manuscripts are signed as being owned

---

9*BMs 2008, ff. 217v-8.

10*BLh 76, f. 133v (p. 200, Evans ed.).

11*BLr MS A. 273, 14th c.,ff. 64v-68v (see Evans' comments on this MS in *Magical Jewels*, p. 70).

12*Speculum Naturale*, Book 8 (1494 edition), chapters 3, 5, 10, 21 etc.

13e.g. *BLas 1471, late 14th c., ff. 56-64. Inc.: "Distinccio ad Tingendum cristallum viridem. . . ." The work ascribed to Albertus Magnus called the *Liber aggregationis* or *Experiments* or *Secrets of Albert* discusses about forty-five stones, and each is written as receipe, typically as follows: "Si vis vt sol appareat se sanguinens. accipe lapide que clotopis vocatur. . . ." as found on f. 31v, *BL 177, late 14th c., ff. 31-2. Other manuscripts of this work are: *BMs 3281, late 13th-early 14th c., ff. 17-21v; *BMe 2852 f. 67- ;BMar 251, 14th c., ff. 25-36v; BMad 32622, 14th c.. ff. 84v- ;CUt 1351, late 15th c., ff. 33-9; *BLd 37, 14th c., ff. 46-55; *BLd 147, 14th c., ff. 107-13v; BLd 153, 14th c., ff. 176-9; BL 177, late 14th c., ff. 31-2; (?) Clermont-Ferrand 171, 13th c., ff. 116-(9?) ; VE L.VI. LIX, 15th c.; BE 968, 14th c. f. 299 - ; CLM 444, 15th c., f. 197 - ;'''Er 550, 15th c., ff. 256v-61; '''Zürich, Zentral-bibl. C101, 15th c., ff. 117v - 26. For general discussion of the *Experimenta* see chapter 63 of Lynn Thorndike, *History of Magic and Experimental Sciences*, (New York, c. 1923), vol. 2, 720-30.

14Additionally, there are numerous examples in the traditionally recognized medical literature to support the wide use of stones in medicine. For instance Bruno in his *Surgery* speaks of cures by antracite and the ruby (*VE 2301, 14th c., f. 23); John of Gadesden (*Rosa Anglica*, as cited by Evans, *Magical Jewels* [1922], p. 112) prescribes a lodestone and coral necklace assist in childbirth; and Bernard Gordon (*Lilium Medicinae*, 2. 25; Evans, p. 126) advised the use of stone charms against epilepsy. Numerous other examples are scattered in Evans (*Magical Jewels*) and L. Thorndike (*History of Magic and Experimental Science*).

15e.g. The excipit to *CUj Q. D.2 (44), 12th - 13th c., f. 158: "Dirrund cil qui ves convisterunt . . . mais sil se volunt prepenser et les peres espermenter. lur creatur auresunt. pur les miracles quo il verrunt. Oue il prosa pur tote gent. as peres medicinement. En surque tut quatre maneres mustrat medicine des peres. . . " And with marginal notes of a medical nature *BMs 340, 14th c., ff. 1-3v; VA lat. 4251, 14th c.?, ff. 93-104; *BN lat 8454, 13th c., ff. 40v-54v; *VA lat. 10046, 16th c., ff. 1-12v. *BLd 13, f.5; *BN fr. 14969, 13th c., f. 74: "Li mirei trovent grant succors, Cil ki conoissient lur valurs. A fere medecinement." Aristotle in '''Mon MS 277, 15th c., f. 127v (p. 385, Rose ed.) has under pearl: "Et propter hoc medici commiscent cum eis alias species quam plurimas, ut non Iedanti."

or written by doctors of medicine.[16] Lapidary texts are frequently found in manuscript codices along with other medical treatises, all written in the same hand. Some eighteen manuscripts of Marbode of Rennes' (1035-1123) *De lapidibus* were found conjoined with Macer's *De herbis*.[17] An association between lapidaries and herbals is common. At least twenty-three medical manuscripts include lapidaries.[18] The frequent beginning of Damigeron and Marbode manuscripts is: "Here is contained [the treatise] on the names of stones which are used in the art of medicine."[19]

The connection between lapidaries and the art of medicine seems to be principally a late eleventh-century development. Antiquity had produced such lapidarists and commentators on stones as Theophrastos, Kyrannides, Pliny, Dioscorides, and Solinus; but the early Middle Ages, excepting Isidore, paid scant attention to lapidaries other than to the Christian symbolic variety.[20] Bede and Hrabanus Maurus each wrote commentaries on the Christian stones but typically the discussions are more symbolic than medical.[21] The substance of the Christian lapidaries was later integrated into the

---

[16]Examples of medical men writing a lapidary are: *VA lat. 10046, 16th c., p. 15 (owned by a *medicus*) *Glascow 468, 14-15th c., f.5 (signature in late 16th or 17th c. hand); *FLa 1520, 14th c. (one, containing Kyrannides, Marbode, and two other lapidaries, was owned by Mizaldus, a medical man and mathematician [at Montpellier?]).

[17]*CU, Ff. VI.53, 14th c., ff. 189-204v; *CU Kk. IV 25, 13th c., ff. 106-112; Douai 217, 13th c., ff. 120v - (126?) mEa 0 62b, 13th c., ff. 78-90v; BMh 3353, ff. 39-48v; *BMs 231, 14th c., ff. 24-32v; *London Wellcome 531, 15th c., (abbr. Italian prose version); mMon 277, 15th c., ff. 112-116v; mCLM 23479, 11th c., f.4v; *BLd 13, 12th c., ff. 1-17; *BN 5009, 13th c., ff. 98-109; *BN 8454, 13th c., ff. 40v-54v; BN 11210, 15th c., ff. 64-82; *BN 16702, 13th c., ff. 1-6v; Prague 1375 (VII.G. 25), 12-13th c., ff. 1v-13; Savignamo 26, 15th c., ff. 36-39?; Tours 892, late 12th early 13th c., ff. 47v - 64v; VA lat 10046, 16th c., ff. 1 - 12v. References are to folios of Marbode and not of Macer.

[18]Bern Stadbibl. A. 91.11, 12th c., f. 1v; *CUj Q.D.2, 12th - 13th c., ff. 148 - 158v; EA F. 303, anno 1328-1341, f. 93; BMad 16566, 14 - 15th c.; BMar 342, 14th c.; Mon 503, 14th c., ff. 57v - ; *CLM lat 14851, 13th c., ff. 37 - 39v; CLM lat 18444, 15th c. ff. 202 - (3?); *BLas 1471, 14th c.; Oe 35, 14th c., ff. 230 - 235v; Paris Arsenal 3174, 15th c.; *BM lat 10448, 13th c., f. 152; Paris St. Geneviève 2261, 15th c.; Prague 839 (v.B.22), 13-14th c., ff. 77-78v; *VA Barb.343, 15th c., ff. 33-7v; *Va 10046, 16th c., ff. 15-78; VE L.VI.LIX, 15th c.; *VI 2301, 14th c., ff. 62-64v, 81-2; *VI 2898, 15th c., ff. 92 - 5v; *VI 5512, 15th c., ff. 350 - 1v; *VI 11235, 16th c., ff. 89 - 97v; *VI 12901, 13th - 14th c., ff. 94 - 125v.

[19]e.g. *BLh 76, early 12th c., f. 131: "Hic continentur epistolæ due. quas Euax. Arabie rex misit Tiberio imperatori. De nominibus et virtutibus lapidum qui in arte medicine recipiuntur." Also *VA lat. 2403, 14th c.?, f. 87 and Saint-Omer 142, 12th c.

[20]This conclusion was suggested for early English lapidaries by R. M. Garrett, *Precious Stones in Old English Literature* (Leipzig, 1909), p. 6, who notes that (with few exceptions) they are limited to a discussion of stones in the Bible. To be certain Solinus, Isidore, and Pliny existed through the early Western Middle Ages. I have found a text edited from Solinus and only from his discussion of stones in an unidentified Ninth Century MS, *VE 15269, 2 folios. Isidore's discussion on stones is occasionally found as a separate lapidary as in *BN 7418, 14th c.?, ff. 109v - 115 (?) and mEa F. 346. early 14th c., ff. 5v - 6 (extracts). The Christian lapidaries are studied by Lynn Thorndike, "De lapidibus," *Ambix*, 8 (1960), 6 - 23 and (with errors) Léon Baisier, *The Lapidaire Chrétien, Its Composition, Its Influences, Its Sources* (Disser., Washington: Catholic U. P., 1936).

[21]Bede *Explanation Apocalypsis*, 3, (Migne, *P. L.*, cols. 197-203); Hrabanus Maurus, *De Universo*, 17 (Migne, *P.L.*, 110, col. 541 *and passim.*) In one manuscript Bede's comments on stones were extracted for a separate treatise in CUj 51, 12th c.

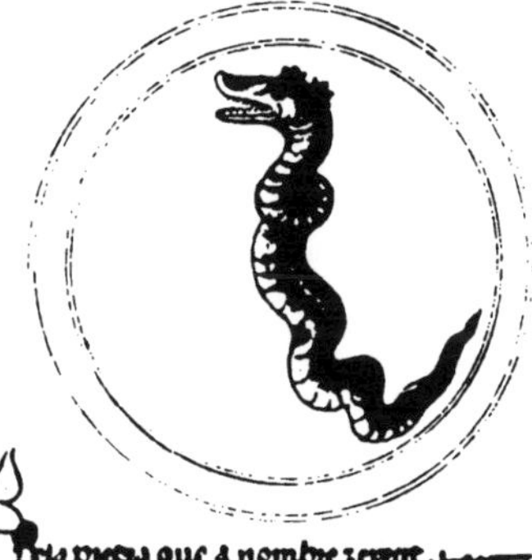

Excerpt from one of the medieval lapidary manuscripts. The reproduction is from Alfonso's Lapidary (folio 35 v), which depicts in the miniature at left the gathering of moonstone, called "Scopetina of the Moon" because it supposedly could be found only in full moonlight. The drawing on the right shows the stone zexegt. The two miniatures within circles are the zodiac sign for each.

This beautifully colored manuscript is in the Escorial collection of Spain and was translated for Alfonso X, el Sabio, King of Castile and Leon (1221-1284).

Reproduced in facsimile as Lapidario del rey d. Alfonso X (Madrid, 1881).

scientific lapidaries.[22] About 1090 Marbode of Rennes wrote *De lapidibus,* which inspired numerous copies.[23] I have found 137 manuscripts of *De lapidibus* alone. The connection between lapidaries and medicine is well represented by Marbode, but this connection was not produced by him. Contemporary with Marbode, other examples of medical lapidaries were being written dating from the eleventh century.

In the next few centuries so many lapidaries were formulated, both by well-known authors and by anonymous ones, that treatises on stones became one of the more popular types of medieval scientific literature. Albertus Magnus wrote the *Book of Minerals,* which includes a lengthy discussion of individual stones, sometimes copied by scribes as an independent treatise. I have found forty-seven manuscripts of this work alone.[24] Aristotle's lapidary (or pseudo-Aristotle) was translated from the Arabic or Hebrew by two separate people, one of whom was Gerard of Cremona, and these two translations are very different one from the other.[25] Kyrannides' treatise, originally in Greek, was translated into Latin. Kyrannides discusses the medical virtues of a stone, a bird, a plant, and a fish, each with the same initial letter from Alpha to Omega.[26] The Encyclopædists, Arnold of Saxony, Bartholomew the Englishman, Vincent of Beauvais, and Thomas of Centimpré, added many more texts of elaborate discussions of stones.[27]

Excepting Alfonso's lapidary which never enjoyed circulation

---

[22]Vincent of Beauvais *Spec. Nat.,* Bk. 8 (1494 ed.) frequently cites Bede and Hrabanus as authorities on stones.

[23]Léon Ernault, *Marbode évêque de Rennes* (Rennes, 1890). The dating of Marbode's work is my own. Studies of Marbode in the vernacular, especially include Paul Studer and Joan Evans, *Anglo-Norman Lapidaries* (Paris, 1924); and Léopold Pannier, *Les Lapidaires français des de tables et d'un glossaire* (Paris, 1882).

[24]The list is too long to be included here but it will be the subject of a separate study.

[25][m]Liege 77, 14th c., ff. 146v-152v, translated by Gerard and published by V. Rose, "Aristotles de Lapidibus and Arnoldus Saxo," *Zeitschrift für deutsches Altertum,* vol 18 (1875, new series), 349-82; and [m]Mon 277, 15th c., ff. 127-35 (*Ibid.,* 384-97).

[26]Evans (*Magical Jewels,* p. 18) writes, "The *Kyranides* is essentially a medical book, but its medicine is hidden behind an elaborate facade of alliteration." G. Sarton (*Introduction to the History of Science,* Vol. I, 347) reports Paschal as the Latin Translator in 1169 while *BMs 284, 15th c., ff. 88-125v says the translator was Gerard of Cremona. Also see, Thorndike, *History,* vol. 2, 229-35 and P. Tannery, "Les Cyranides." *Congress international d'histoire des sciences,* Geneva, 1904. I have found the following MSS of Kyrannides: *London Wellcome 116, mid 14th c., ff. 37-72v; *BMs 284; *BMar 342, 14th c., f.1 - ?; BLas 1471, 14th c., ff. 143-51, 159-67v; [m]Mon 277, 14th - 15th c., ff. 41-60 (Books 1-4); *FLa 1520, 14th c., ff. 1-(16v?); VE 37.A. 220, 16th c., ff. 11-73; Ea Q. 217 (as reported in Thorndike, *History,* 2, 233 but not in Schum's catalogue of Erfurt); Kraków 817 (CC VIII 65), 15th c., f.1-?. The Greek text is published by F. de Mély, *Les lapidaires de l'antiquité et du moyen âge* (vols. 2 & 3, Paris 1898-1902).

[27]I have used the following MSS and published texts: (1) Arnold of Saxony: Published from [m]Ea 0 77, 13-14th c., ff. 35-40 by Emil Stange, *Die Encyklopädie des Arnoldus Saxo. . . .* (Disser., Erfurt, 1905) and V. Rose, "Aristotles. . . ." *Z.f. d. Altertums,* 18 (1875), 424-55. I have seen and identified more Arnold manuscripts: *Bn 7475, 13th c., ff. 125-140v; *VA lat. 4482, anno 1448, ff. 79-89v; [m]Erlangen 423, 14th c., ff. 147-54v (known to Rose); and [m]Prague 2027 (XI, C.2), 15th c., ff. 238v-48v. (2) Bartholomew The Englishman *De proprietatibus rerum* (1491 edition) and *VA lat. 707, 14th c., ff. 116-28 (section on stones),

outside Spain,[28] the most elaborate lapidary is an alphabetical discourse on 130 stones, gems and minerals. This particular work is known in six unstudied and unpublished manuscripts ranging from the thirteenth through the fifteenth century. Two manuscripts ascribe the authorship to Bartholomæus de Ripa Romea.[29]

A lapidarist of sculptured gems, known as Zæl or Thetel, also was popular, judging from the existence of some twenty-two manuscripts.[30] Although there is no modern recognition that a particular image or Zodiac sign might affect the powers of a gem, medieval belief in sculptured gems probably was widespread, as exemplified by Zæl's popularity and the frequency with which he was quoted.[31]

Anonymous lapidaries are more frequently medical manuscripts than are those by well-known authors like Aristotle, Albertus Magnus, Zæl and others. These lapidaries have remarkable individual-

(3) Vincent of Beauvais *Speculum Naturale* (1494 edition) (4) For Thomas A. Contimpré, I have used only MS copies. Since Zael was copied by Thomas in a section of his work it is possible that there is confusion between the works of Zael and Thomas. Some folios refer only to the section on stones. *BN lat. 523a, 13th c., f. 12-?; Brux 8902, 15th c., ff. 209-67; *VA 724, 14th c., ff. 67-74 (on stones only); *BMe 1984, 13th c., ff. 34-145; BMs 2428, 13th c., f.2 - ? *VA 822, 14th c., ff. 23-58v; *VAp 1144, ff. 154-64v (stones only); CLM lat. 13582, 14th c.; *VE 2317, 14th c., ff. 49-53v; *VE 2442, 13th c., ff. 1-4v (maybe Zael); Graz 1249, 13th c. (ref. by Thorndike in *Ambix* 8 [1960], p. 14); [m]Erlangen 434, 13-14th c., ff. 152-6 (frag.); [m]Brno Mk. 46, 15th c., ff. 81v (excerpts); BMar 164, 15th c., (Thorndike, *History*, II, 372 ff.); *BMar 323, 13th c., ff. 1-98.

[28]See John E. Keller, "The Lapidary of the Learned King." *Gems and Gemology*, vol. 9 (1957-8), 105.

[29]*London Wellcome. MSS 116 and 117.

[30]The list of Zael MSS is too long to be included here but a preliminary study of this writing was made by Thorndike, *History*, Vol. 2, pp. 390, 399-400, who identifies the author as Sahl ben Bist ben Habib, of the Ninth Century. The texts I have found show remarkable variation. One text from BLd 79, 13th c., ff. 178v - 180 is published as Appendix E by Evans, *Magical Jewels* (1922), pp. 235-8. I have found many more texts than previously identified.

[31]e.g. VI 2442, 13th c., which is a version of Thomas of Cantimpré on f.4v: "Nota de lapidibus. Sequitur relatio antiquorum scripturatum de sculpturis lapidu(m) nec app(ro)bante multum nec penitus refutante. huic autem sciendum et secundum figuris que abantiquis sculpebant in gemmis. virtus lapis monstrabatur unde Thechel phylosophus quidem ideorum scripsit libellum de lapidibus sculptis a filus israel indesco quem nos transtalimus in latinum. De sculpturis lapidum. In quocumquam lapide sculptum invenis gemmos vel aquariam sanat a febribus quartanis et paralisi gratum facit gestantem." Another lapidary of engraved gems with medical value is the Lapidary of King Ptolomy which was noted by L. Thorndike ("Traditional Medieval Tracts Concerning Engraved Astrological Images," *Mélanges Auguste Pelzer*, Louvain, 1947, pp. 260-1). This lapidary of uncertain origin begins in VI 5311, 14-15th c., f. 35, rubric: "Regi Ptolomeo Rex Azarius de lapidibus sanctificatos scripsit. et in templo apollinus scripsit et posiut autem fundamenta subusa in egipta manet. . . ." It continues by giving the signs, e.g. *Pegasus, Andomeda, Cassipia, Lepus* etc., and says what virtues stones with these images engraved on them have. It is especially concerned with medical items. The first part always says stones (lapides) without mentioning any certain type. Then (f. 35v) it mentions variously colored stones and how they should be mounted and engraved. Finally (f.35v) it mentions specific stones and how they should be engraved. The Ptolomy lapidary is also found in *BLas 1471 14th c. ff. 64v-5v and BN fr. 2009, f. 64v (in Latin) and quoted in *VI 11235, 16th c., f. 89 r and v. There is yet another major lapidary text of engraved gems, attributed to Marbode, but my investigation does not support this as an authentic Marbode work. It begins: "In quocunque lapide inveneris Arietem Leonem. . . ."; and it is found: [m]Bern 410, 14th c., ff. 72-4v; CUt 1122, 15th c., ff. 173v-6v; *BMad 18210, 13th c., ff. 103v-5; BLd 193, 14th c., ff. 28-30; *Oc 221, 14th c. ff. 54-5; BN lat. 6755, 15th c., ff. 34v-6; Prag. 629 (IV. C. 2). 15th c., ff. 22v-5v; VI 3408, 14-15th c., ff. 4v-5v.

ity, given the medieval practice of relying on authority. They range, for instance, from one short medical lapidary of the twelfth century, which has ten stones, to two large and different lapidaries of the fifteenth century with 106 and 108 stones described.[32]

That lapidaries were not a static form of medieval literature can be illustrated by a case study of the information conveyed in manuscripts concerning a single stone and how this was transmitted and changed, with additions and deletions. The stone selected is *smaragdus,* which came to mean emerald; but in antiquity the name means a variety of green stones ranging from transparent, deep green beryl to green marble, serpentine and alabaster. The present purpose does not include a definitive attempt at identification; rather our method is to examine briefly the ancient authorities on whom medieval writers based their accounts.

Pliny (N.H. 37, 16-19, 62-75) and Theophrastus (*De Lap.* 23-7), on whom Pliny based most of his account, describe a variety of green stones. The only virtue attributed to *Smaragdus* by Pliny and Theophrastus is that it refreshes strained eyesight when one looks at or through this stone. Since Pliny says engravers produced this effect and Nero watched gladiatorial shows through smaragdus (*in smaragdo*), a probable conjecture is that the stone was cut as a lens and used as a sunglass.[33] Medieval evidence appears to substantiate this hyothesis. Damigeron, a lapidarist of the second century(?), stated:

"Smaragdus is the most beautiful and strongest stone to all divine acquatarians. Carried, it increases one's substance, makes one pure, and helps one's speech. To a great extent it averts harm in storms. It is perfected thus: a scarab ought to be sculptured on it, then on the underside an image of Isis standing, and afterwards bore a hole lengthwise, next string a golden thread through the opening, consecrate it, and put in a good location to ornament and to confer other

---

[32]*BN lat. nov. acq. 873, 15th c., f. 189; Inc.: "Lapis saphiri virtus est ut ubicumque fuerit demon illic pervalere non portit. Lapis contra fulgura. . . ." It also discusses, *sardius, crisolitus, smaragdus, ametistes, topazius, amandnus, berillus,* and *onichilum.* VAb lat. 343, 15th c., ff. 33-7v: 106 stones with medical virtues. Inc.: "Adamas est lapis preciosus obscurior cristallo. . ." *BLas 1475, 15th c., pp. 519-40. Inc.: "Et si negociis non paucis cum infirmorum tum lanquidorum satis superque satis detentus fuerim. . . ." Writers most often cited are Serapion: *Aggregatus,* "Albertus in Lapidaris," "Evax" [Marbode or Damigeron], Galen, Johannes Mesue, Ysaac Benjamin, and Avicenna. Generally each entry begins with the stone's name in Latin, then the unknown author gives the Arabic name in Latin alphabet and sometimes the Greek word. For instance, (p. 521) "Lapis Margarite latins: Arabico bagar allulo sive albalo margarita."

[33]According to E. Rosen, "The Invention of Eyeglasses," *Journal of the History of Medicine,* vol. 11 (1956), 13-46, 183-218, eyeglasses were invented in the Pisa-Lucca region, possibly in Venice, shortly after 1286. The German word for spectacles which seems to come from the stone beryl (German, *Berille = eyeglasses*) points to the connection between sculptured concave lens from transparent stones. The lapidary evidence points to a conclusion that the conception of eyeglasses was continuously present during the Middle Ages with antecedents in Antiquity. Rosen's evidence (p. 34) comes partly from a sermon preached by Giordano of Pisa who gives us the approximate date of the invention. But this sermon contains the line: "Up there in Paris is a great art of carving and cutting precious stones, which is a great art there." Marbode and Raymond Lull both speak of glass substitutes for natural stones. Venetian guild regulations of crystal workers (*Ibid.* pp. 211-7) speak of *lapides ad legendum* or "stones for reading" and advocates selling glass for glass and presumably not as for precious stones. It seems apparent the spectacles were carved from precious stones and from there came the natural substitution of glass.

good things, for then you will see glory from the stone which God bestows on it."[34]

While Dioscorides[35] and Galen are silent about *smaragdus,* Isidore of Seville condenses Pliny, stating that there are twelve kinds and that it is pleasing to the eyes.[36] Using a geographical framework for his discussion, Solinus speaks of *smaragdus* in juxtaposition to the animals called griffins which mine gold. Solinus also tells of the sculpturing of lenses from this stone.[37]

This is the information about *smaragdus* transmitted to the Western Middle Ages, exclusive of Islamic writers. To show the wide variation in medieval lapidaries, we have attempted to integrate into a single text (given in the paragraphs that follow) the various entries about *smaragdus.* The authors, and the manuscripts and publications of their works utilized, are linked to specific information in the text by the abbreviations given in parentheses (and explained in the accompanying tables of abbreviations. *See page 48*).

"*Smaragdus* is green (PsAlb, R, Eg), very green (VAb, VE BRR, Alb, A), so green that it tinges the air (by looking through it?) (Alb, VB, VA_{r2}, HB, BRR, M_1, C, A_1), clear (Ar), very transparent (Ar, AS-2, PsAlb, M_1, A_1,), of various colors (AS-1), the greenest of all stones (M, A_3, BLau, BLcl, BLd, Va_{r1}, 12 VA, BA, M_1), greener than all tree leaves and plants (A_3, 12 VA_r, 12VA, BA, VB, VA_{r2}, TC, Pe), the greenest thing in the world (CLM, 12VAr, HB, X, P). It is a valuable and precious gem (Alb, VE, Pe, A, A_1, and rare (VE_1), but not rare (Alb). In its center one can see his image (C) and it does not change its beauty because of sunshine or clarity (M_2, A_1, A_3). If the stone is hollow it can do great good (A_2?).

There are many varieties (BRR, VAr2, VB,PsAlb) twelve kinds (M, TC, BLd, VAb, CLM, As-1, C), six kinds (M_1), or five kinds (A). One variety is from Scythia (M, CU, M_1, C, A_1, A_2, A_3), which is the best (TC, Alb, Bld, VAb, VAr2, VB, AS-1), from Sicily (12VAr), Bactria (M, M_1, VB. C, A, A_1, A_3), Syria (CUp, P, Eg), Egypt (BLd, VAr2, VB, A_3), the Nile (M, Alb, AS-1, A, C, M_1, A_1), Britain (Alb, VAb, AS-1, A), Cyprus (BLd, A), *Kiciati?* (VAb), Paradise (P, Eg, M_1, A, A_1), a river in Paradise (A_2), Tyre from water out of Paradise (Pe, M_1, A_1), and, finally, Ethiopia but this kind is not valuable (A). Some varieties are bad (C). The Scythian kind is taken by the Arimaspians from the nests of griffins who guard it with great ferocity (variously told in M, A_1, M_1, A_2, A_3, TC, Alb, CU, VAv, 12 VAr, VB, AS-1, A, C). The Arimaspians have no head or neck but an eye in the middle of their chests (VB, C), or some say its one eye is in the middle of their foreheads (P, Pe). Some say griffins have four feet (CU, 12VAr), two wings (Pe), and are similar to a lion's body (Pe, CU, VB) while some look like goats and others eagles (CU, VB).

A traveller from Greece, a truthful man and a careful observer, said that this stone occurs in submarine ledges of rock (Alb). It is found in earth under the sea and is a type of metal (C). It is found in rare metals (BLd). Cæsar (Pe) or Nero (M) watched gladiatorial shows through this stone (M,C). Anyone can do this (Bld). Through it Nero saw

---

[34]Translated by me from *BLh 76, early 12th c., f. 139 (published by Evans, *Magical Jewels* [1922], p. 212) and *BN 1 at 7418, 14th c. (published by E. Abel, *Orphei Lithica* [Berlin, 1881] p. 168). The text varies considerably. Damigeron is an obscure writer in Greek and known mostly through some fragments in Aetius of Amida. See V. Rose, "Damigeron de Lapidibus," *Hermes,* vol. 9 (1875), 471-91; F. de Mély, *Les Lapidaires. . .,* (1898), vol. 2, p. xiii.

[35]It is not in the printed Greek text by M. Wellman (Berlin, 3 vols. 1958 reprint) and the old Latin translation of Dioscorides in *CLM 337, 8th c., has a lacunæ where this stone might appear but the Alphabetical Dioscorides, probably edited by Constantine, has the same text as Damigeron *(CUj Q.D.2 [44], 12-13th c., f. 92v).

[36]*Ety.* 16.7. 1-15. (1): "Sculpentibus quoque gemmas nulla gratior oculorum refectio est. Cuius corpus si extentum est, sicut speculum ita imagines reddit, Quippe Nero Cæsar gladiatorum pugnas in smaragdo spectabat."

[37]Solinus 15. 22-8 (pp. 86-9, T. Mommsen ed.).

III

Key to Abbreviations

I. Known Writers:

M = Marbode's lapidary in Latin as publ. *P. L.* col. 171, vols. 1744-5 (Pagination given only to entries on smaragdus for all citations.).
VB = Bede's *Expl. Apocalypsis* (*P. L.*, cols. 189-9).
BA = Bartholomæus Anglicus, Bk. 16, chap. 88, 1491 ed.
HB = Lapidary of Hildegard of Bingen (as publ. *P. L.*, 197, col. 1249-50).
Ar = Aristotle's lapidary (*Mon 277, p. 127v, p. 285, Rose ed.)
CL = Costa ben Lucca in *BN lat. 7337, 14th c., p. 115.
AS-1 = version 1 of Arnold of Saxony, *BN 7475, ff. 135v - 6.
AS-2 = version 2 of Arnold of Saxony, *VA 4482, f. 85.
RL = Raymond Lull in *BMs 2008, ff. 214-5.
TC = Thomas of Cantimpré, *BMe 1984, f. 135.
Pt = Lapidary of King Ptolemy, *BLas 1471, f. 65v.
AIG. = Albertus Magnus *Book of Minerals*, *Wellcome 14, f. 31; also Bk. 2, Tr. 2 (pp. 118-20, Wyckoff ed.)
PsAlb = Pseudo Albertus Magnus *De Virtutibus Lapidibus*, pp. 141-2, 1740 ed.
BRR = Bartholamæus de Ripa Romea, Wellcome 116, pp. 9-10.

II. Anonymous MSS:

*CUp = MS 111, 17th c., f. 207.
*CU = Kk. 4.25, 15th c., f. 125.
*BLau = MS d.4.15, 12th c., f. 119v.
*BLcl = MS 178, 15th c., f. 131v.
*BLd = MS 13, 12th c., f. 23.
*BN = MS 14470, 12th c., f. 38; and *BN Nouv. Acq, 873, 12th c., f. 187v.
*VAb = MS lat. 343, 15th c., f. 37.
*VAr1 = MS lat. 45, 12th c., f. 117v.
*VAr2 = MS lat. 21, 11-13th c., f. 24.
*VE_1 = MS 2378, ff. 49v - 50.
*CE_2 = MS 1365, 14th c., f. 81v.
*CLM = MS lat. 14,851, 13th c., ff. 38v-9.

III. Lapidaries of 12 stones:

*12VAr = MS 258, early 13th c., f. 43.
*12VA = lat. 3267, 15th c.?, f. 59v.

IV. Published vernacular lapidaries:[38]

M_1 = First French Version of Marbode in *BN lat. 14470; BN fr. 24870; VAmscl. 145, Arm. XV; Paris St. Genev. 2200 — published by Studer & Evans, *Anglo-Norman Lapidaries* (Paris, 1924), pp. 36-8.
A = Anglo-Norman Verse Adaption in BN fr. 14969 & CUp 87, publ. *Ibid.*, pp. 87-8.
A_1 = First Anglo-Norman Prose Lapidary in *BN. n.a. lat. 873, *BMr 12 F XIII, and *BLd13, *Ibid.*, 98-9.
A_2 = Second Anglo-Norman Prose Lapidary in CUpem 87, CUpemIII, BN fr. 1097, BN fr. 2063, FNcs C.7.612, Paris Arsenal 3516, see *Ibid.*, pp. 121
A_3 = Third Anglo-Norman Prose Lapidary in BN fr. 25247, *Ibid.*, p. 141.
C = Cambridge Version of Marbode in *CUp 235, *Ibid.*, p. 163-4.
X = Apocalyptic Lapidary in CUp 87 and in a MS possessed in private by Lord Bath, *Ibid.*, p. 268.
P = BLad MS A 106 published in J. Evans & M. Serjeantson, *English Mediaeval Lapidaries* (Oxford, 1933), pp. 40-1.
R = Richardoune's Verses in BMad 34360, *Ibid.*, p. 61.
Pe = Peterborough Lapidary, MS 33, 15th c., *Ibid.*, pp., 85 ("Esmeraude"), 103 ("Smaragdus").
Eg = English Translation of Second Anglo-Norman Prose Lapidary in BMs 2628, *Ibid.*, 121.

---

[38]A study to show variations in the published French lapidaries is in an unpublished master's thesis by Caroline Vogler Diehl, "An Analysis of the Medieval French Lapidaires," (Chapel Hill, 1938).

what he wished to see (P) and could learn what he wished to know (A_2). Nero loved this stone (M_1, A); he had a mirror made of it (Pe, M_1, C, A, A_1, A_3); both Cæsar and Nero used the stone in battle to bring victory (A_3). It foretells the future (M, AS-2, PsAlb, BRR, BLsu, BN) and makes things known in water (M_1, A, A_1). Worn with reverence (M), it bestows wealth (M, CUp, Alb, P, Pe, Eg, M_1, C, A, A_1, A_2, A_3). It makes ones speech eloquent (M, BRR, Alb, AS-1), dreadful (Pe), and verbose (M_1). This quality helps to make business deals (TC, CLM, BN, M_2), especially from men in the city (CLM). Worn around the neck it enables one to answer his friends (C).

Smaragdus has great use as a medicine (R). Worn around the neck (Alb, BLcl, VAv, BN, CL, Ar, AS-1), or on the finger (CL, Ar), put in the mouth (PsAlb) or even carried (TC, RL), it cures those with epilepsy, (M, TC, BRR, Alb, BLcl, VAv, VE_1, CLM, RL, BN, PsAlb, CL, Ar, As-1, Pe). For one struck with an epileptic seizure, put this stone in the mouth so that his spirits are revived. Afterwards keep the stone in the mouth and have the patient say nine times in the morning, "Just as the spirit of the Lord replenished the world so does this pleasing thing revive the home of my body so that nothing can prevail against it." Thus the epileptic is cured but the stone should be kept daily near one so that he may say these words in the morning and health is preserved (HB). It was prescribed for King Robert when he had a seizure (RL).

Medicinally it is cold and dry (AS-1) but in milk it is given for the heart or stomach ailments because of its warming effect on the body (HB). Hung around the neck (M, Alb, A_1, A_2, A_3), it keeps one from semi-tertian fever (M, A_1, A, M_1, A_2, TC, BRR, Alb, VE_1, CLM, Pe). Similarly worn it protects infants or boys (BN, CL, Ar). He who wished to be cured in the head ought to put the stone in his mouth. The stone warms him if it has a hole bored in it and if it is soaked. When wet, rub it on the forehead, and replace in the mouth for a few hours. When more phlegm and saliva are produced, put it in a piece of linen cloth over a small vessel with warm wine in it and strain the wine through the cloth. Then prepare a lye solution by putting the wine with crushed beans. Drink this and the brain will be purified and phlegm and saliva become diminished (HB). *Smaragdus* strengthens eyesight (VAb, VE_1, BLcl, AS-2, CLM, Ar, M_1, C, A, A_1, A_3) because of its soothing green luster (M, BRR, Alb). Wash the stone in olive oil first for this helps the eyes (TC, CLM). For this it ought to be sculptured into concave lens (BRR). Moreover, this wonderful stone cures gout (Pe, M_1, A_1, A_3), and hemorrhoids (BLcl), and it stauches a blood flow (BA, Pe). All poisons are checked by the stone, especially snake and scorpion bite (AS-2, VAb). If you take poison orally, put *smaragdus* over a linen cloth, lay on small pieces of cloth and cook it so that the stone is warmed for three days. Follow this procedure (by putting the stone in your mouth), then the poison will be destroyed (HB). In fact, *smaragdus* cures all debilities and diseases of man (HB, R, BLcl) especially those of a cold nature (P). For such a cure as this stone produces, money should not be taken since in an act of charity all things have greater power (RL).

So many are the virtues. Generally it comforts one (AS-2). It prevents storms (TC, M, CUp, BRR, Alb, VAb, VE_1, CLM, A, A_1, A_2, RL, AS-1, P, R, Pe, M_1, C) lightning (P, A_3, C), and all disasters (Pe). If a plague is coming and one is unable to continue in the face of this disturbance, then put this stone in your mouth. This causes saliva which is warmed by the stone and thus the whole body is warmed thereby excluding the pests (germs) from the body. (HB). It makes one intelligent (AS-2, PsAlb), increases memory (AS-2, PsAlb, Alb, VAv, As-1) and hope (PsAlb, AS-1), inclines one toward chastity (Alb, P, X) and against lechery (Pe, Eg), gives patience (RL) and prevents fornication (A_3). Albertus says, "It has been found by experience in our own time that this stone, if it is good and genuine, will not endure sexual intercourse; because the present King of Hungary wore this stone on his finger when he had intercourse with his wife, and as a result it was broken into three pieces." (Alb) It keeps the seed of man in a woman's body so that the child's limbs shall not be misformed (Eg). The stone is pleasing to God (CUp, X, A_3), helps one to pray (12VAr), keeps one strong in faith (CU, 12VAr, 12VA, 12VArl, P) and acceptable to comrades (A_1, A_3). One who wears it should have his body clean and have love in his body and soul, thus he can perform good works (Pe). It acts against illusions, demonic phantasies, and demons (BLcl, VAb, RL, AS-1, R, Eg). As the third stone on Aaron's breastplate (P, Pe), it is a sign of the trinity (P). It makes fields fertile (HB) and is sought after by magicians (Alb).

The stone makes air next to it cold

but the sun warms it (HB) To keep its greenness it should be washed in olive oil (C, M, A_1, A_2, A_3) or in wine (A_3, M, C). Green ink can be made by soaking it in wine and oil (A. A_1). *Smaragdus* ought to be set in steel and worn on the left side (Eg) but some say only gold is a proper setting (A_2, A_3). It ought to be carried with a scarab sculptured on it (Pt) with the following inscription "+ 0 + N + if you want variety + SA + DA + YT" (VE_2) or an image of Christ (12VA).

One is immediately struck by the remarkable variations among the lapidaries in the information concerning what is presumably one stone. In fact, hardly any two lapidaries among the many hundreds are alike. Far from relying entirely on classical authorities, the lapidarists often felt obligated to relate their own experiences about the wonderful effects of stones. For instance, two stones, *hexecontalithos* and *pantheros*, have no virtues ascribed to them by Græco-Roman authors but medieval lapidaries cite many beneficial results.[39] Albertus Magnus adds his own observations on stones.[40] When one becomes aware of the large number of stones and the variations, sometimes contradictions, in information about them, it is obvious that the compiler of a lapidary exercised personal judgment of some kind in determining what to put into his particular text.

The medieval bestiary literature also played a part in the medical

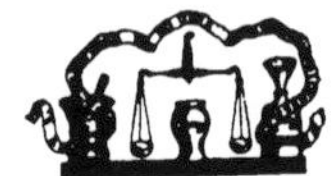

lore of the Middle Ages, as recently reported by Thomas R. Forbes.[41] This bestiary literature was, relative to the lapidaries, more static in "scientific" content. That is to say, the bestiaries were more a copying exercise and less a practical guide, as compared with lapidaries. While the bestiaries were permeated with Christian influence, the lapidaries remained relatively impervious to it until the late Middle Ages.[42] This is no mere curiosity, since we have come to expect magic, religion, and science to be inextricably connected in literature of the Middle Ages. The variations and individual character of the numerous lapidary texts suggest that the lapidarists were giving what they thought to be workable, pragmatic knowledge, whereas the bestiaries appear to be more concerned with traditional curiosity items on animal lore. Lapidaries are to be compared with herbals, with which they are associated in the codices, because they were a part of the medieval knowledge actually employed in pharmaceutical work and in therapeutics.

---

[39]*e.g.* Pe MS 33, 15th c., f. 3 (Evans & Serjeanston, *Eng. Med. Lap.*, p. 71) has medical effects while Pliny (37.60.167), Solinus (31.3) and Isidore (16.12.5) are silent on virtues. Under *Pantheros* or Panther stone Pliny (37.66.178), Solinus (no entry), and Isidore (16.12.1) have only a description but Pe MS 33, 15th c., ff. 13v, 16v (*Ibid.*, pp. 105, 117) say it is a cure for poisoning and evil and makes one bold and hardy while BMs 2628, 16th c., ff. 22v - 3 (*Ibid.*, p. 126) adds that it protects the fetus and mother, helps gnawing gout, and is a good jewel for women in childbirth.

[40]*e.g. Minerals* 2.2 (pp. 98-9, Wyckoff ed.) under *iris*.

[41]"Medical Lore in the Bestiaries," *Medical History*, vol. 12 (No. 3, 1968), 245-53.

[42]G. Sarton, *Introduction to the History of Science*, vol. 2, pt. 1, p. 48; Studer and Evans, *Anglo-Norman Lapidaries*, pp. xvi-ii.

IV

THE LATIN ALPHABETICAL DIOSCORIDES

Of all ancient writers on *materia medica* Dioscorides [204] (fl. A.D. 50-70) stands preeminent.[1] In his listing of the descriptions, habitats-locations, medicinal virtues and preparations of around 850 plants, animal products, and minerals, Dioscorides contributed in large measure to our knowledge of ancient pharmacy, mineralogy, botany, and, to a degree, ancient medicine and chemistry. The study of the transmission of his text is perhaps as important as an analysis of his actual writing. Both the Latin West and the Arabic East used Dioscorides' text to add their own experience with drugs he named and to contribute knowledge of new drugs by adding to his text.

Of the Dioscoridean Latin texts the version known as the Alphabetical Dioscorides was by far the most widely used between the early twelfth century and the late [205] fifteenth when the Greek text was printed. Little study has been made of this important family of manuscripts in order to determine such questions as: (1) Is the text truly based on Dioscorides? (2) If so, is it a new translation or a re-edited, older version? (3) If it is a new translation, was it made from the Greek, Arabic, or Hebrew? (4) Does the text include non-Dioscoridean insertions? By answering these questions, an important part of the history of medieval pharmacy will be better understood.

----

1. References to the original pagination are given in the margin.

A Latin translation was made in the late Roman or the early medieval period.[2] With only a few items omitted from the Greek text, this translation is a fairly accurate rendering into Latin. In five books, it follows the same classification system based on discussing in sections herbs, shrubs, animal products, and so forth. Extant copies of the full text are known in three manuscripts, two of the ninth century and one of the tenth.[3] Judging by the fact that there are no known manuscripts later than the tenth century and no identified use of this manuscript text by a later writer, the conclusion seems reasonable that the Alphabetical Dioscorides eclipsed the popularity of the older Latin version.

Fourteen manuscripts, dating from the twelfth through the fourteenth centuries, are extant of the complete Latin Alphabetical Dioscorides manuscript family

---

2. Charles Singer, "The Herbal in Antiquity and its Transmission to Later Ages," *Journal of Hellenic Studies* 47 (1927): 34-5, reports incorrectly that there were two early Latin translations in addition to the Pseudo-Dioscorides' *Ex herbis femininis* tradition. See my article on "Dioscorides", *Dictionary of Scientific Biography* 4 (1974): 119-23.

3. Munich, Bayerische Staatsbibliothek, Ms lat. 337, s. X, 160 fols.; Paris, Bibliothèque Nationale, Ms lat. 9332, s. IX, fols. 243-321v; Ms lat. 12,955, s. IX, fols. 1-197. K. Hoffman and T. M. Auracher began editing Munich 337 (*Römanischen Forschungen*, 1 [1882]: 49-105) and the project was continued by H. Stadler (*ibid.* 10 [1897]: 181-247, 369-446; 11 [1899]: 1-121; 13 [1902]: 161-243; 14 [1903]: 601-636). Stadler used also BN 9332 for editing books 2-5. Book One, using BN 9332, is reedited by H. Miheuscu, *Dioscoride Latine Materia Medicina libro primo* (Iasi, Romania, 1938). Paris, BN lat. 12,995 was not known to any editor, yet it has the most complete text of *De materia medica*. In citing the Old Latin translation in this article I chose to use BN 12,995. There are manuscripts containing fragments of the Old Latin translation.

group.[4] Dioscorides' "Preface" to *De materia medica* is the same text in both the Old Latin translation and the Latin Alphabetical Group.[5] This "Preface" is included in a codex of miscellaneous medical texts found in Bamberg, Staatsbibliothek Ms Med. 6, s. XIII, fols. 28v-9.[6] The incipit reads "Incipit prologus sequentis libri per alfabetum transpositi secundum constantinum". According to the records of the Bamberger Staatsbibliothek, Karl Sudhoff saw this manuscript in March, 1915, and, apparently on the basis of Sudhoff's notes, Henry E. Sigerist reported that this version was by Constantine the African [206]
(d. c. 1085) who is most likely the one to whom the Alphabetical editorship is ascribed. In any case, Sigerist says, it indicated that the author of the incipit expected such a work to come from the Salerno region.[7] Modern writers, however, have not included the Alphabetical Dioscorides among those works attributed to Constantine the African.[8]

There are approximately 696 entries in the Alphabetical Group, the exact number depending on the accounting procedures. In comparison, the Old Latin translation has

---

4. A complete list is forthcoming in the *Catalogus Translationum et Commentariorum* series.

5. A critical text of the "Preface" was prepared by Hermann Stadler, "Die Vorrede des lateinischen Dioskorides," *Archiv für lateinischen Lexicographie und Grammatik*, 12 (1902): 11-20.

6. A full description of the Ms is given by F. Leitschuh and H. Fischer, *Katalog der Handschriften der kgl. Bibliothek zu Bamberg* (Bamberg, 1887-1912), 1, pt. 2, 433-5. I have seen this manuscript.

7. Henry Sigerist, "Materia Medica in the Middle Ages," *Bulletin of the History of Medicine*, 7 (1939): 420-1.

8. e.g., Heinrich Schipperges, *Die Assimilation der arabischen Medizin durch das lateinische Mittelalter* (Wiesbaden, 1964), pp. 26-7; Rud. Creutz,"Der Arzt Constantinus Africanus von Montekassino..." *Studien und Mitteilungen zur Geschichte des Benektiner Ordens und seiner Zweige*, n.s. 19 (1929): 11-24.

831 chapter entries and the Greek text by Max Wellmann has 827. However, a comparison of the items in the Alphabetical Dioscorides reveals that the Alphabetical Dioscorides has excluded many more entries than the statistics suggest because it includes entries on many new drugs, some with Arabic names, not in the Greek Dioscorides. Among the 96 items beginning with the letter "A", some fifteen are not found in Dioscorides' Greek text. Further a line by line comparison of those entries found in the Greek Dioscorides text and the Old Latin translation, reveals that the editor was copying directly from the Old Latin translation.[9] The so-called Latin Alphabetical Dioscorides was not a new Latin translation from the Greek, Arabic, or Hebrew but a new pharmaceutical treatise based directly on Dioscorides. It contains a significant preponderance of new information on old drugs as well as a listing of new drugs and their virtues. A majority of the entries, some fifty-four of the ninety-six "A's", for instance, take the Old Latin translation as the framework and add to the commentary.

An estimated thirty per-cent of the text is from entirely new sources. What the extra source or sources were is determined. In 1874, Valentin Rose observed (in a brief note) that the editor was familiar with Pseudo-Oribasius, Isidore of Seville, Evax-Damigeron, and Galen's *De simplicium medicamentorum*, but he did not observe that Arabic sources were used either directly or
[207] indirectly.[10] Some of the new information about old and new drugs bears some resemblance to Constantine's *De gradibus* and Isaac Judaeus' *Practica*, but these sources do not appear to be the only authorities. The only authors named are classical, namely, Galen, Hippocrates,

---

9. For an example, compare the entry *alimus* in the Old Latin translation, represented by Paris, Bibliothèque nationale, Ms lat. 12,995, fol. 26v, with the alphabetical version, represented by Cambridge, Jesus College, MS Q. D. 2, s. XII-XIII, fol. 19v.

10. Valentin Rose, "Über die *medicina plinii*," *Hermes*, 8 (1874): 38n.

and Cato.[11] It is conjectural whether or not Constantine the African is the author-editor of the alphabetical version. Normally, as an author, he was concerned with translations from the Arabic, but, in this case, he, or the author, merely added to the old text new authorities some of whom wrote originally in Arabic.

About 1300, Pietro d'Abano wrote a gloss on the Alphabetical Dioscorides.[12] His commentary is preserved in only one manuscript, Paris, B.N. lat. 6820, s. XIV-XV, which adds still more items to the listing of materia medica and more information about older drugs. When the text of the Latin Alphabetical Dioscorides was first published in Colle de Val d'Elsa, Italy, in 1478 and again in Lyons in 1512, the printers took the text of Paris B.N. lat. 6820 as their basic text. Included in the Latin text ascribed to Dioscorides, are many of Pietro d'Abano's comments which the printer did not distinguish from Dioscorides. Only a portion of the printed text is actually related to Dioscorides' original work.

A great need exists for a critical text of the entire Latin Alphabetical Dioscorides. It is important because Dioscorides' transmission is a veritable history of the knowledge of Western pharmacy during the Middle Ages. Medieval editors of the text and copyists of individual manuscripts added to Dioscorides' writing as a means of contributing their experiences with various drugs in the context of their needs. On the basis of

---

11. Cambridge, Jesus College, Ms Q. D. 2, fols. 45 r&v, 48, 100.

12. Lynn Thorndike, "Manuscripts of the Writings of Peter of Abano," *Bulletin of the History of Medicine*, 15 (1944): 216; Leo Norpoth, "Zur Bio-, Bibliographie und Wissenschaftlehre des Pietro d'Abano...," *Kyklos* 3 (1930): 306; and S. Ferrari, "Per la biografia e per scritti di Pietro d'Abano," *Atti della R. Accademia dei Lincei Anno CCCXII*, 15 (1915): 682-683. All three authors report that Paris, B.N. lat 6819, is also of Pietro d'Abano's commentary but the Ms is merely of the Latin Alphabetical Dioscorides.

this preliminary study, it seems likely that the Alphabetical version was authored by Constantine the African
or, at least, it was certainly a product of the School of
Salerno. At this point it can be said that the Alphabet-
[208] ical Dioscorides was based on the Old Latin translation
with a significant portion of its total information added
by the author/editor in the late eleventh or early
twelfth century in order to bring Dioscorides up to-date.

V

AMBER IN ANCIENT PHARMACY*

The Transmission of Information About a Single Drug:
A Case Study

MILLIONS of years ago forests grew near the present shores of Denmark and Germany. The coniferous trees secreted large amounts of resin. In the geological ages which followed, many of the trees became victims of a creeping ocean. Time and the sea hardened the resin into a fossil called amber. When man evolved, he learned to use amber as an ornament, as a medicine, and, because of its peculiar electrostatic qualities, as a magic amulet. This electrical attraction of amber captured the imagination of ancient authors who seem never to have tired of drawing moral inferences from the result of rubbing this diamond of the earth with wool.[1] By a circuitous route a Greek word for amber, *electron*, came to mean "electricity." Amber was to the ancients a stone: It was a beautiful stone that strangely burned with a pleasant odor. Little wonder then that primitive man associated amber and magic.[2]

The ruins of Troy, Mycenae, and Babylon and graves before the tenth century B.C. in Italy preserved amulets and necklaces of amber from northern Europe.[3] Seals, statues, and ornaments for dress were commonly made from this vegetable resin.[4] A figurine of amber is said to have sold for more than a number of human beings (Pliny *N.H.* 37. 12. 49). It is not strange that sooner or later a definite pharmacologic action of amber would be inferred by the trial and error method of folk medicine. From antiquity to modern times amber is recognized as useful in materia medica. For instance, in the first century A.D. Pliny writes, "Amber is not without its utility in medicine; but it is not for this reason that women like it. It is beneficial for infants when it is

*Presented to the American Institute of the History of Pharmacy, Section on Contributed Papers.

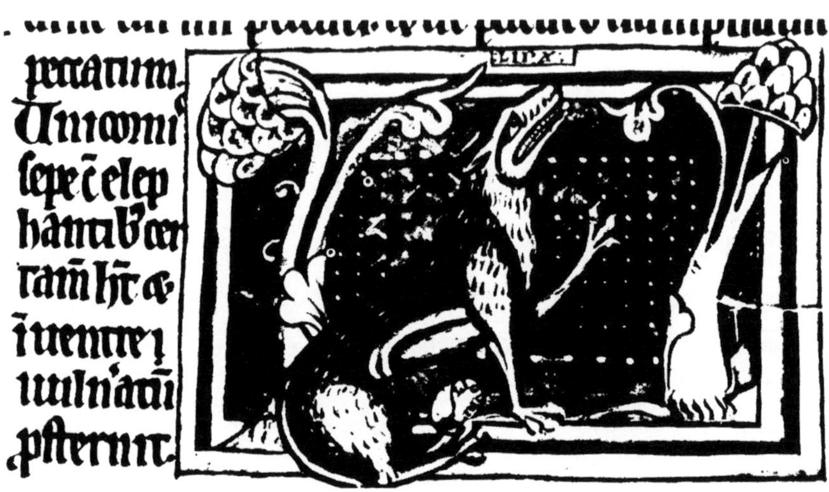

The "lynx-stone" or lyngourion is shown under a lynx in this late twelfth-century bestiary, which includes the old Greek story of amber originating from the urine of lynx. (Oxford, Bodleian Library Ms 764, fol. 11)

attached to them in the form of an amulet."[5] A physician in a respected journal of the nineteenth century reports without disapproval that women hang necklaces of amber on the necks of infants in order to protect them from the convulsions of their first teeth.[6]

Present translations of Egyptian, Babylonian, Sumerian, and Assyrian texts on drugs reveal no indication of the use of amber in the wide range of materia medica of these peoples. The Ebers, Ani and Edwin Smith papyri say nothing of amber.[7] Similarly amber has not yet been identified in Sumerian and Assyrian texts.[8] More modern scholarship needs to be invested in the area of the pharmacy of the ancient Near East. It is extremely difficult, if not at times impossible, to identify obscure nouns in ancient Near Eastern texts without an ample supply of references to these terms in different contexts. So we must leave open the question of whether amber actually is mentioned in Egyptian, Hebrew, Sumerian and Assyrian literature.

The problems involved in research of amber in ancient materia medica are compounded by imprecise nomenclature and by several philological problems. The Greek language has at least two words which mean amber, both of which were adapted by the Romans into Latin. Plato (*Timaeus* 80. b-c), Plutarch (*Platonic Questions* 7.7), and Diodorus of Sicily (*Library* 5. 23. 1-4) employ the word *elektron* when referring unquestionably to amber; but Strabo (*Geography* 3. 2. 8), Pliny (*Natural History* 33. 23. 80-1) and Pausanias (*Periegesis of Greece* 1. 12. 7) speak of a residuum or alloy of gold and silver which is also called *elektron*. The earliest known use of that word is in the *Odyssey* (4. 73; 15. 460; 18. 296), where the context points to the translation "amber," not to the metal alloy (in at least two places: 18. 296, and 15. 460).[9] At all times care must be exercised in identifying amber in Greek texts.

The Greek word *liggourion* or *lyngourion*, variously spelled in both Latin and Greek, probably means amber and has no double meanings. Theophrastus (*On stones* 28) describes its as follows: "Lyngourion . . . is remarkable in its power . . . seals are cut from this, too, and it is very hard, like a real stone." He further states that it has the power of attraction, just as *elektron*.[10] Strabo (*Geog.* 4. 6. 2) explains the situation more definitely: "And they also have in their country excessive quantities of *lyngourion* which by some is called *elektron*."

Theophrastus (*On stones* 28) says that "amber is said to be the urine of wild animals, who, jealous of their excretion, bury it, and it subsequently hardens into the stone *lyngourion*. Pliny (N.H. 37. 12. 52-3), Dioscorides (*Materia Medica* 2. 81), Ovid (*Metamorphosis* 15. 412-5), Aelian (*On animals* 4. 17), Isidore (*Etymologies* 16. 8. 6-8) and Claudius (*Epis. ad Serenam* 31. 7) specify that the animal whose urine is valuable is the lynx. Curiously, Jerome (translating Exodus 28: 19 with its description of the high priests' costume jewels) wrote in a letter (*Epis.* 64. 16) that he could find no information about *ligurius* (without doubt, *lyngourion*) in books on stones.

The Greek derivation seems clear: from λύγξ for "lynx; and οὖρον for "urine."[11] Theophrastus (*On stones* 16), Strabo (*Geog.* 4. 6. 2), and Pliny (*N.H.* 37. 11. 35) connect amber with the Ligurians. The results of the J. M. DeNavarro study on ancient amber trade routes show that an amber route had as its Mediterranean terminis the ancient port of Massilia, the area of the Ligurians.[12] Since the Phoenicians traded with the Ligurians, it can be reasonably conjectured that the Phoenicians, and those to whom they delivered the product, attached to it the ethnic name *ligurion*. An amber necklace in the *Odyssey* (15. 460) came from a Phoenician trader. The Greeks, wanting an explanation for all, must have wondered why amber was called *lyngourion* and, hence, there developed the strange story of "lynx-urine," for that is what *lyngourion* sounds like![13]

Unlike Greek literature, at least one Roman writer offered detailed data on amber. Pliny the Elder admits no uncertainty concerning the Latin *sucinum* for amber. He writes:

> It is well established that amber is a product of islands in the Northern Ocean, that it is known to the Germans as 'glaesum,' . . . To resume, amber is formed of a liquid seeping from the interior of a species of pine, just as the gum in a cherry tree or the resin in a pine bursts forth when the liquid is excessively abundant. The exudation is hardened by frost or perhaps by moderate heat, or else by the sea, after a spring tide has carried off the pieces from the islands. At all events, the amber is washed up on the shores of the mainland, being swept along so easily that it seems to hover in the water without settling on the sea-bed. Even our forebears believed it to be a 'sucus,' or exudation, from a tree, and so named it 'sucinum.' That the tree to which it belongs is a species of pine is shown by the fact that it smells like a pine when it is rubbed, and burns like a pine torch, with the same strongly scented smoke, when it is kindled . . . That amber originates as a liquid exudation is shown by the presence of certain objects, such as ants, gnats and lizards, that are visible inside it. These must certainly have stuck to the fresh sap and have remained trapped inside it as it hardened.[14]

Pliny quotes various theories of amber's origin in Greek writings and concludes: "We can forgive them all the more readily for knowing nothing about amber when they betray such monstrous ignorance of geography."[15]

The earliest Greek writings involving extensive knowledge and use of materia medica are the so-called Hippocratic collection edited by E. Littré.[16] From these texts modern experts have constructed a list of between three and four hundred substances, but amber is not among them.[17] Once the Hippocratic works use the term *elektrodes* as an adjective meaning "amber-like" and referring to the color amber.[18]

According to Theophrastus, Diokles of Karystos, a Greek physician and author around 350 B.C. of a Greek herbal, wrote about amber (*lyngourion*).[19] D. E. Eichholz believes that Diokles remarks on *lyngourion* occurred in his discussions of the kidneys and the urinary tract.[20] Diokles provides the first identified recorded mention of amber in medicine. But inclusion of amber in his lists of materia medica and his medical treatise probably merely reflects a much older practice.

The herbal in antiquity is a list of various substances, for the most part of vegetable origin, employed as materia medica. Dioscorides in the first century compiled an herbal of some five hundred items, 130 of which are in the Hippocratic works edited by Littré.[21] *Lyngourion* or *elektron pteruyophoron*, as Dioscorides notes, is the urine of the lynx hardened into stone and called by this name "because it draws feathers to it." When drunk with water, lyngourion benefits the stomach and intestines affected by the flux (diarrhea?).[22]

Elsewhere in his work Dioscorides confused amber with the sap of the black poplar, thereby either originating or giving impetus to an error that caused difficulties in later Islamic and Western medieval medicine. Under the entry *aigeiros* Dioscorides identifies the sap of the black poplar as tears from trees growing by the river Padus.[23] Here Dioscorides is referring to a Greek myth about amber's origin.[24] According to legend, the youth Phaethon, the son of Helios, desired to follow in the same profession as his father. But when he persuaded Helios to allow him to drive the four-horse sun-chariot across the sky, the task proved too difficult. Traversing the heavens in an erratic manner, he set the sky afire, producing the Milky Way. Zeus immediately smote Phaethon from the sky with a thunderbolt. Phaethon fell from the sky and landed at the mouth of the river Padus (Po) where his body was committed to the lapping waters. Phaethon's sisters, competing one with another in grief, stood dripping tears on the bank of the Padus. For one, two, three seasons they continued mourning until they underwent a metamorphosis, becoming poplar trees. In this form, the sisters of Phaethon, at the same time each year, drip tears into the waters of the river. When the tears harden in the cold water, they become amber. All accounts of this story employ the word *elektron* for amber, never *lyngourion*. The Greek term *aigeiros* (Latin, *populus nigra*) means "black poplar."

By some, Dioscorides observes, *aigeiros* is called *elektron* and by others *chrysophoron* because it yields upon rubbing a sweet smell and has a golden color. The leaves of the black poplar tree are mixed with vinegar to abate gout pains and the seed is an emollient. Ground into a powder, the sap is consumed for stomach and intestinal pains resulting from the flux.[25] Thus Dioscorides makes black poplar and amber synonymous by statement, by usage, and by connection with the Phaethon legend.

Galen's treatise *On Simple Medicines by Temperament and Powers* has a full entry and description of the medicinal uses of black poplar (*aigeiros*), but there is no suggestion that this may be amber (either *lyngourion* or *elektron*).[26] In his study of plants Theophrastus makes repeated references to black poplar without hint of a connection with amber.[27] Apart from the Phaethon legend in literary usage and Dioscorides' entry for *aigeiros*, no relation can be seen between black poplar and amber.[28] The apparent fault lies with Dioscorides though he was probably relying on some source unknown and unavailable to us. The error thus probably did not originate with Dioscorides but the confusion between amber (*elektron*) and black poplar (*aigeiros*), and their respective uses as drugs, can be directly traced to him. Possibly Dioscorides' source distinguished between old hardened pine resin and genuine amber as did the early Chinese writers, but Dioscorides in his zeal to simplify and to catalogue dropped the qualifying distinctions.[29] Though not as credulous as many authors, Dioscorides, according to Charles Singer, "exhibits no critical powers and little genuine scientific interest or capacity."[30]

In the legacy of ancient medicine only the reputation of Galen can be compared to the towering image of Hippocrates. As court physician to the Emperor Marcus Aurelius, Galen amassed a prodigious display of medical works in both theory and practice. He stressed the use of drugs, or at least considerably added to the number and use of drugs compared to the relatively few drugs found in the Hippocratic collection. In his treatise *The Composition of Medicines According to the Parts of the Body* (Bk. 7) Galen gives a recipe for a "lozenge of amber (*elektron*)" which reads:

> "Lozenge of amber. It is made for hemoptysis, coughing both protracted and fresh, consumption, spitting up of humors, suppuration, suffering in the bowels, dysentery, and flatulency. It is also good for the ear. R_x: Clean flea-wort plant 45 drachmae, Illyrian iris, mastic, filings of amber, saffron, of separate ones, 30 drachmae, opium 15 drachmae. [Put] the beatened flea-wort plant in warm water for soaking and when this is viscous and gluey, it shall be put in water [again]. Force out to a liquid. Prepare the medicament with this. Shape this into a lozenge. Give three obols when one is going to sleep. . . ."[31]

Also prescribed is a "Neapolian lozenge" containing amber filings (*elektron*) for hemoptysis, suppuration, consumption, and rheumatic afflictions (literally, "running" or "flux")[32] Elsewhere in the same treatise a prescription which includes amber is given for consumption and flatulency.[33] On the authority of Antipater, Galen discusses remedies for diseases of the mouth (*stomatikos*) which include amber.[34] Likewise, Galen says Nikostratos prescribes amber for disorders in the stomach but he cautions against administering only "pure amber (*katharon elektron*)"[35] Amber is not mentioned in Galen's treatise *On Simple Medicines by Temperament and Powers* nor in the treatise *On the Composition of Medicines by Family.*

Galen's contemporary, Rufus of Ephesus, recommends amber (*elektron*) among the "approved" drugs according to Aetios of Amida,[36] but this is his only reference to amber, outside of a highly doubtful fragment found in Rhazes, an Islamic writer.[37] Our knowledge of this excellent Greek anatomist and physician is much too scant, however, to allow definite opinions of his use of amber.

Among the extant ancient authors, Pliny the Elder is the leading expert on amber, and yet few others include more misleading information. Pliny devotes two chapters, one very long, to the origins, composition, and usages of amber and methodically quotes some twenty-six writers, many of whom are known today only through his mention.[38] Pliny stated that amber has utility in medicine, as previously observed, though it was not for this reason that women liked it. Peasant women in the lands north of the Po River, he reports, wear amber necklaces to prevent afflictions of tonsillary glands and fauces.[39] Amber amulets also benefit infants.[40]

Callistratus, otherwise an unknown writer,[41] is cited by Pliny as an authority on the medicinal uses of amber. Being of benefit to people of all ages, amber can be either worn as an amulet or drunk (presumably in a powdered solution) as a preventive of delirium and as a cure for strangury.[42] Pliny writes:

> According to Callistratus, this kind of amber cures fevers and diseases when worn as an amulet on a necklace, affections of the ears when powdered and mixed with honey and rose oil, as well as weak sight if it is powdered and blended with Attic honey, and affections even of the stomach if it is either taken as a fine powder by itself or swallowed in water with mastic.[43]

It is regrettable that Pliny did not specify which diseases. But Pliny was no physician, although often cited in the Middle Ages as a medical authority.

In a subsequent chapter Pliny reluctantly includes a discussion of *lyncurium* (from Greek, *lyngourion*). His inclusion of *lyncurium*, he says, was forced by authors who maintain its reality. After relating the so-called details of *lyncurium's* original state, lynx's urine, Pliny expresses profound doubt about the truth of such a story and outright disbelief that *lyncurium* exists in his own day. Simultaneously then, Pliny posits, its alleged medicinal properties are equally false; for example, there are those who assert that *lyncurium* taken orally in a solution disperses urinary calculi. Taken in wine or only looked upon, *lyncurium* cures jaundice.[44] In fact, in his section on animal materia medica, Pliny states without qualification that "the urine of the lynx" is remedial for strangury and pains in the throat.[45] Theophrastus, on the authority of Diokles, is the only source that Pliny acknowledges for his discussion of *lyncurium*.[46] Max Wellmann believes that Pliny's information on *lyncurium* was based, in part at least, on Juba, whose books are now lost but who is known to be a major source for the *Natural History*. Pliny's doubt about *lyncurium*, Wellmann believes, came not from Juba but from Xenocrates of Aphrodisias, a Greek physician of the first century, A.D.[47] Whoever was his source and whatever his personal opinion on the matter, Pliny does record that *lyncurium* or amber was a cure for urinary calculus, jaundice, strangury, and pains in the throat.

Amber (*elektron*) is also mentioned by Aretaeus of Cappacodia (2nd century A.D.) as a lozenge for "bringing up the blood."[48] Aretaeus, a member of the pneumatic school of medicine,[49] says that internal remedies are more important than external remedies for one who is bleeding, because medications drunk or swallowed come nearest the injured parts. There are three kinds of internal remedies: "either they are calculated by the contraction or compression of the vessels to bind the passages of the flux; or to incrassate and coagulate the fluid, so that it may not flow, even if the passages were in a state to convey it; or to dry up the outlets, by retaining the blood in its pristine state, so that the parts may not thus remain emptied by the flux, but may regurgitate where the effusion is."[50] Aretaeus prescribes a compound medicine of tried efficacy, a lozenge of amber which, from Aretaeus' context, presumably means that it will induce coagulation.[51] This is probably the same lozenge that Galen prescribed.

About 410 A.D., Marcellus Empiricus, a Gallo-Roman, compiled a book of medicaments combining Celtic medicine, rank superstition, and traditional knowledge.[52] Marcellus' use of amber is extensive. Like Galen and Aretaeus, Marcellus recommends the lozenge of amber (Latinized for, *dielectrum*) for stopping the blood (hemoptysis).[53] Saffron, amber, Chire mastic gum, Illyrian iris, opium, and psyllium plant comprise the formula. These are exactly the same ingredients that Galen prescribed, but Galen attributed more benefits from the lozenge than just for hemoptysis.[54]

For colic, Marcelus writes, "you pulverize amber (*sucinum*) and out of its powder you take two measures to be drunk in lukewarm water for three days."[55] For those afflicted with the stone there is a liquid preparation of amber (*sucinum*), Italian catnip, seselis, pepper, saxifrage (literally, stonebreaker), rock-parsley, cyperos, and ginger. Taken as directed, this remedy condenses the stone and thus permits its passage through urine as waste.[56] For goitre, "true amber (*sucinum verum*)" is placed in a fresh pot, boiled down half way, removed and incinerated and finally rubbed to ashes.[57] For a palpitating heart place "true amber" in boiling water and drink the solution over a period of three days.[58]

Oribasios (b. c. 325 at Pergamum) quotes accurately Galen's prescription for the amber lozenge.[59] A friend and physician of Julian the Apostate, Oribasios is credited by George Sarton as a courageous fighter against the tide of superstition.[60] Elsewhere in his vast medical encyclopaedia, Oribasios recommends amber (*elektron*) among other medicines for stopping bleeding.[61] In the discussion of suffering in the bowels (*koiliakos*) ascribed to Oribasios, he refers to "the amber lozenge for dysentery" and adds that it is also excellent for hemoptysis and that it works for stomatic disorders, consumption, coughing, suppuration, running of the bladder, and suffering in the bowels.[62] Though the ingredients are much the same as in Galen's amber lozenge, nonetheless this reference in Oribasios is no mere copying of Galen's text. Modifications were made with some ailments deleted, namely flatulency and ear trouble, and some added, namely, running of the bladder. Though Latin translations of Oribasios existed during the middle ages, amber has not been found in the Latin texts.[63]

In his discussion of coagulating a blood flow by internal medications, Caelius Aurelianus (fl. ca. 430 A.D.) mentions the lozenge of amber.[64] Caelius is the Latin translator and commentator of Soranus, a prolific Greek author of the second century A.D. Apparently the amber lozenge prescribed in Caelius' *Chronic Diseases* (five books) was taken from Soranus' *Chronic Diseases* (also in five books). Though Caelius' version may vary from Soranus' text through added comments or deletions, we may hypothesize that Soranus advocated amber internally for bleeding.[65] The form "*trochiscos . . . dielectru*," used in Caelius' text, was the same as appears in Marcellus' prescription for an amber lozenge for stopping a blood flow. Possibly Marcellus' source was also Soranus since Galen's amber lozenge was not only for hemorrhaging but for a variety of other ailments.

Paul of Aegina, a Greek physician of the sixth century A.D., writes in his book of *Simples*:

> Amber *(elektron)*; they say that it is the tears of the black poplar *(aigeirou)*, which are discharged into the Po River and are solidified into a substance like gold. This, being pulverized and drunk, prevents the flux of the stomach and bowels [probably, dysentery] and stops bleeding.[66]

Paul has a separate entry for black poplar (*aigeiros*) but the text contains no hint of a relation to amber.[67] Certain Latin manuscripts, the earliest dating from the eleventh century, purport to be Paul's Third Book. This alleged Latin version of Paul's work mentions the lozenge for amber (*de electro trociscus*) and a preparation, for ailments of the heart (*De cordis passionibus*), containing amber (*electrum*) among other igredients.[68] The fact that the Greek and not the Latin word for amber is employed suggests the possibility that the Latin manuscript might have been based on an original Greek text.

Aetius of Amida was a Mesopotamian physician and court physician to Emperor Justinian I. Examination of Aetius' medical encyclopedia, *The Book of Medicine*, proves that it is based chiefly on Galen and Archigenes.[69] Aetius warns the reader before his discussion of amber that *elektron* is also called *soukinon* and *liggourion*. Amber is taken, he advises, for strangury and disorders of the stomach, and golden amber (*chryselektron*) with mastic gum cures pains of the stomach.[70] It is doubtful if Aetius influenced the Latin middle ages as there is no known Latin translation until the so-called Renaissance.[71]

The negative aspects of any investigation often prove as informative as the positive results cited above. Many notable medical writers in antiquity and the early middle ages fail to include amber among their recommended drugs. For instance, Celsus (1st c. A.D.) makes no mention of amber despite the extensive materia medica in his work[72] Even writers like Galen, Oribasios, and Paul mention amber only infrequently, as compared with the attention given to many other drugs. Theodore Priscian (5th c. A.D.), Cassius Felix (1st c. A.D.), Adamantius (4th c. A.D.), Gargilius Martialis (3rd c. A.D.), Alexander of Tralles (6th c. A.D.), Sextus Papyriensis Placitus (4th c. A.D.), and Scribonius Largus (1st c. A.D.),[73] all outstanding medical commentators, leave no record of employing amber in their prescriptions. Similarly the herbal of pseudo-Apuleius (from the late fourth or early fifth century) omits reference to amber despite the fact that amber had been included in Dioscorides' famous herbal.[74] Probably Greek in its original composition, pseudo-Apuleius' herbal became the most widely read of late classical medical works.[75] The *Glossae Medicinales*, compiled around 700 A.D. on the basis of Galen and Hippocrates, likewise do not include amber in the list of drugs and other therapeutic items.[76] Amber also does not appear in the works of the early medieval medical writer Benedetto Crespo (8th c. A.D.).[77] Amber was, therefore, not extremely employed in early medieval materia medica.

Even when reading an ancient text on amber, one can never be certain that what we call amber is what was meant in antiquity. At least a few ancients pointed to ignorance and errors in the written word about amber.[78] Natural amber varies in color according to the amount of impurity.[79] In antiquity these variations were viewed as different varieties of amber. Demostratus, on the authority of Pliny (*N.H.* 37. 11. 34), says the *lyncurion* voided by a male lynx is fiery red, whereas by a female it is white or at least less pronounced in color.[80] Philemon, also quoted by Pliny (*N.H.* 37. 12. 47), mentions that there are three actual varieties: (1) a white amber that "has the finest scent, but, like the waxy kind, it has no value"; (2) a red and more highly valued amber, especially if it is transparent but not too brilliant; (3) and a Falernian amber, named after Falernian wine because of its soft transparent hue. Pliny concludes that amber may be found in any shade because in his day it was tinted artificially as desired.

Other substances, such as ambergris, might have been identified as a variety of amber. Pliny and Philemon observed that there is a white, waxen amber and Pliny distinguished between two varieties, a white amber and waxen amber. The latter would fall into none of Pliny's own categories, previously stated. Pliny (*N.H.* 37. 11. 36) noted that in India amber (*sucinum*) was a preferable substitute for frankincense. This strong aromatic quality is more suggestive of ambergris than amber. Obviously, ambergris washed up on ancient shores just as it does today. A white amber, produced because of lime impurity, is rare but possible in nature.[81] It is unlikely, however, that the adjective "waxen" could describe any amber accurately. Since this adjective is applied in modern descriptions of ambergris, ambergris may well have been mistaken in antiquity for amber and merely called the "white, waxen amber." If it were so mistaken, it would not have analogous pharmacologic properties which would explain Pliny's assertion that it had no value. Further the Greek and Latin languages possess no word for ambergris, so this leaves open the possibility that it might have found a utility and confused identity under other terms. Interestingly there is no mention of ambergris or amber as a trade item around the Red Sea, where ambergris is most often washed ashore the same way amber is washed ashore along the Baltic and North Sea. *The Periplus of the Erythraean Sea,* which is an ancient guide for sailors trading along the Red Sea and Indian Ocean (ca. 1st c. A.D.), does not mention any item resembling either amber or ambergris.[82] The question must be opened as to whether the ancients confused amber and ambergris in a different way from the late medieval confusion of terms.

Let us summarize the attempt by ancient writers to relate information about amber's properties. Dioscorides and Aetius, for instance, knew that *elektron* and *lyngourion* were the same, but Pliny did not know for sure. Dioscorides, nonetheless, confused amber and the sap of the black poplar. Galen, Paul, and Aretaeus used the Greek term, *elektron,* without any synonyms to aid the reader. The Latin writers Marcellus and Caelius Aurelianus borrowed from

Galen the Greek form, *dielectrum.* Curiously for in his other references to amber Marcellus employs the Latin word, *sucinum.* Aetius recommends, "*elektron* or *lyngourion* or *soukinon*" for strangury and stomach disorders, but for pains in the stomach he specifies *chryselektron.*[83] Pliny says Callistratus coined a new word for amber, *chryslectrum,* "goldenamber."[84] In recording one prescription Marcellus prescribes the use of *sucinum verum,* "true amber," and Galen refers to *katharon elektron,* "pure amber." Despite these attempts by Aetius, Marcellus, and Galen to be more precise, the nomenclature remains very confused within the works of ancient medieval writers.

Why should there be confusion of this sort? Perhaps because the remedial effects attributed to amber were first discovered in folk medicine and later described by medical writers. When a writer discovered a folk remedy, he recorded it in the term by which it was introduced to him. This would explain why Pliny would have different medicinal uses for *sucinum* and *lyncurium,* but, admittedly, Pliny was an encyclopedist. Marcellus, a medical writer, had different uses for *dielectrum* and *sucinum,* although both terms mean amber. If there had been empirical therapeutic checks, presumably the ambiguous words *elektron* and *lyngourion,* to say nothing of *aigeros,* would have been deleted by medical authorities from their writings in favor of *sucinum,* which is unambiguous.[85] Such was not the case with ancient writers, at least in regard to amber.

This curious substance that we call amber thus provides a useful case-study of the linguistic problems involved with one substance, and the efforts by the ancients, working within their cultural context, to find and transmit pharmaceutical knowledge.

Notes and References

1. Many ancients saw a "spirit" or "soul" in inanimate objects and, from this property, they drew moral inferences. On amber and magic, see Plato *Timaeus* 80. b-c; Thales in Diogenes Laertius *Lives* 1. 24; Demokritos *Frag.* A 165, Diels V, ed. and Plutarch *Platonic Questions* 7. 7.
2. Wolfgang LaBaume, "Die Bedeutung des Bernsteins im vorgeschichtlichen Volksglauben," *Mitteilungen des Westpreussischen Geschichtsvereins,* vol. 33 (1934),73; Karl Andrée, *Der Bernstein: Das Bersteinland und sein Leben* (Stuttgart, 1951), p. 92.
3. Karl Schuchhardt, *Schliemann's Excavations. An Archaeological and Historical Study.* Translated . . . by Eugénie Sellers (London, 1891), pp. 62, 196; Eric Ebeling and Bruno Meissner, eds., *Reallexikon der Assyriologie unter Mitwirkung zahlreicher Fachgelehrter* (Berlin, 1938), vol. 2, 1; David Randall-MacIver, *Italy before the Romans* (Oxford, 1928), pp. 59-60. According to Randall-MacIver, amber is found in great abundance in the graves of the Second Benacci period at Bologna (ca. 9th c. B.C.).
4. *Scriptores Historiae Augustae. Tyr. Trig.* 14. 5; Theophrastus *On Stones* 28; Pausanias *Periegesis of Greece* 5. 1. 12. 7; Dio Chrys. *Orations* 13. (434 R), Dindorf, ed.; Josephus *Antiquities* 3. 7. 5 (168); and possibly the stones in the priest's breastplate in *Exodus* 28: 19. For a study of amber art objects, many dating from the Roman Empire, see Otto Pelka, *Bernstein* (Berlin, 1920), pp. 27 ff. Recent developments in chemical analysis, especially infrared spectra analysis, conducted notably by Professor Curt Beck of Vassar College, have effected means to identify Baltic amber found in southern European archaeological sites as distinguished from non-Baltic amber, especially Sicilian amber. For example, see, C. Beck, E. Wilbur, S.

Meret, D. Kossove and K. Kermani, "The infrared spectra of amber and the identification of Baltic amber," *Archaeometry*, vol. 8 (1965), 96-109.

5. Pliny *N.H.* 37. 12. 50: Usus tamen aliquis sucinorum invenitur in medicina sed non ob hoc feminis placent. Infantibus adalligari amuleti ratione prodest.
6. Alexandre Gérard, "Observations et expériences sur la vertu de l'ambre jaune dans une maladie nerveuse de forme convulsive," *Journal des Connaissances Médico-Chirurgicales*, vol. 9 (1842), 15. But amber is not mentioned among drugs beneficial for infants cutting their teeth by Quintus Serenus, an early third century A.D. medical author (*Liber Medicinalis*, Vollmer ed.).
7. *Papyrus Ebers*, 2 volumes. Edited by G. M. Ebers (Leipzig, 1875); *The Papyrus of Ani. A reproduction in facsimile*, 2 vols. Edited, with hieroglyphic transcript, translation and introduction by E. A. Wallis-Budge (New York, 1913); *The Edwin Smith Surgical Papyrus*, 2 vols. Edited by James Henry Breasted (Chicago, 1930).

   In his study, *Die Pharmazie bei den alten Kulturvölkern. Historisch-Kritische Studien*, 2 vols. (Hildesheim, reprint, 1965), vol. 1, 58, Julius Berendes writes: "Diese berichten nämlich, dass von den Aegyptern Isis und Osiris als die Urheber der Medizin angesehen werden und dass die zwei und vierzig heiligen Bücher, von denen die sechs letzten, 'Ambre' genannt, über den Bau des Menschen, von seinen Krankheiten, von den Augenkrankheiten, von den chirurgischen Operationen, von den Frauenkrankheiten und den Arzneimitteln hendeln, dem Sohne des Menes, Athotis, dem zweiten Könige zugeschrieben werden." We have been unable to verify Berendes' sources, especially his mention of Manetho.
8. Sources checked: Martin Levey, *Chemistry and Chemical Technology in Ancient Mesopotamia* (Amsterdam, 1959), for Sumerian medical texts. Also Letter from Martin Levey, Department of History of Medicine, New Haven, December 13, 1961; R. Campbell Thompson, *A Dictionary of Assyrian Chemistry and Geology* (Oxford, 1936), pp. 166, 189; Campbell Thompson, *The Assyrian Herbal* (London, 1924); Campbell Thompson, *Assyrian Medical Texts* . . . (London, 1923); and Campbell Thompson, "Assyrian Prescriptions for the Head." *The American Journal of Semite Languages and Literatures* vol. 53 (1937), 217-38; vol. 54 (1937), 12-40.

   The Hebrew text of Ezekiel mentions *hašmal* in three verses (1:4, 27; 8:2). The Septuagint translated this as *elektron* and the Vulgate *electrum.* In the Syrian translation of the Hebrew version of Ezekiel there is no word for *hašmal.* Exodus (28:19), giving a description of the costume jewels to be worn by the priests, uses the Hebrew word *lešem* which the Greek Septuagint translated into and the Latin Vulgate into *ligurius.* In a letter, Jerome (*Letters* 64. 16), confesses concerning his translation: "Looking over the authors who write on the properties of stones and gems, I am not able to find out about *ligurius.*" Josephus (*Antiquities* 3. 7. 5) employs the word *ligurion* when referring to the vestments of the high priest. Dio Chrysostom(*Orations* 13 [434 R], Dindorf, ed.) writes of an "amber" costume (*i.e., elektron*). Elsewhere Dio (*Orat.* 79, Dindorf, ed.) specifies amber (*elektron*) in connection with the Celts whom he says traffic in it.

   George Williamson (*The Book of Amber*, London, 1932, p. 58) notes that amber is frequently found in the vicinity of Sidon. Jules Oppert (*L'Ambre Jaune chez les Assyrians*, 6) translates an Assyrian cuneiform inscription which, he feels, indicates the presence of amber from the Baltic and consequently very early commercial relations between Assyrian and northern Europe.
9. John M. Riddle, "Amber. An Historical - Etymological Problem," *Laudatores Temporis Acti. Studies in Memory of Wallace Everett Caldwell Professor of History at the University of North Carolina by His Friends and Students* (Chapel Hill, 1964), pp. 110-120.
10. See *Theophrastus: On Stones.* Translation by Earle R. Caley and John Richards (Columbus, Ohio, 1956), pp. 109-111. Caley and Richards point to various attempts to identify *lyngourion* as beleminte and hyacinth. Because Theophrastus, they suggest (p. 111), in referring to its hardness used the phrase "like-stone," his *lyngourion* is not a stone in the mineral sense. Caley and Richards conclude

V

that *lyngourion* is either amber or "a variety of amber." D. E. Eichholz's more recent commentary and translation of Theophrastus (*Theophrastus De Lapidibus* [Oxford, 1965] makes no attempt to identify *lyngourion*. The very definite statements by Pliny (*N.H.* 37, 13. 52-3) and Strabo (Geog. 4. 6. 2) leave no doubt that Theophrastus was wrong in making an implied distinction between *lyngourion* and *elektron*. Without doubt Theophrastus' *lyngourion* was amber.

11. Schmidt, "Aityron," *Zeitschrift für vergleichende Sprachforschung*, vol. 9 (1860), 399; Blümmer, "Bernstein," Pauly-Wissowa-Kroll, *Real-Encyclopädie* (Stuttgart, 1894), vol. 3, 300-1; and Hesychius' entry.
12. J. M. DeNavarro, "Prehistoric Routes between Northern Europe and Italy Defined by the Amber Trade," *The Geographical Journal*, vol. 66, (1925), 481 ff. A more recent study (but based on DeNavarro's research) is Arnolds Spekke, *The Ancient Amber Routes and the Geographical Discovery of the Eastern Baltic* (Stockholm, 1957). An earlier study, still valid on some points, is by William Pierson, *Elektron oder Ueber die Vorfahren, die Verwandtschaft und den Namen der alten Preussen* . . . (Berlin, 1869).
13. William Ridgeway, *The Origin of Metallic Currency and Weight Standards* (Cambridge, 1892), p. 110.
14. *N.H.* 37. 11. 42-6, Eichholz trans. in "Loeb Class. Lib."
15. *N.H.* 37. 11. 32.
16. Charles Singer, "The Herbal in Antiquity and its Transmission to Later Ages," *The Journal of Hellenic Studies*, vol. 47 (1927), 2.
17. Berendes, *Die Pharmacie bei den alten Kulturvölkern*, I, 175-235; and Singer, "The Herbal in Antiquity . . . ," *J. H. S.*, vol. 47 (1927), 2.
18. Hippocrates *Works* 4. 38 Littré, ed.: ἠλεκτρώδης
19. Theophrastus *On stones* 28; see also Singer, "The Herbal in Antiquity . . . ," *J. H. S.*, vol. 47 (1927), 2; Caley and Richards, *Theophrastus On Stones*, p. 113.
20. Eichholz, *Theophrastus De Lapidibus*, p. 108; Galen (*On the Natural Faculties*, 1. xiii [vol. 2, p. 30 Kühn, ed.] mentions Diocles as the author of such a treatise.
21. Singer, "The Herbal in Antiquity . . . ," *J. H. S.*, vol. 47 (1927), 19.
22. Dioscorides *Materia Medica* 2. 81 (vol. 1, 165, Wellmann, ed.):
τὸ δὲ τῆς λυγγός, ὃ δὴ λυγγούριον καλεῖται, ἅμα τῷ ἐξουρηθῆναι λιθοῦσθαι πεπίστευται· διὸ καὶ ματαίαν ἔχει τὴν ἱστορίαν. ἔστι γὰρ τὸ καλούμενον ὑπ' ἐνίων ἤλεκτρον πτερυγοφόρον, ὅπερ ποθὲν σὺν ὕδατι στομάχῳ καὶ ῥευματιζομένῃ κοιλίᾳ ἁρμόζει. ὄνου δὲ ουρὸν παραδέδοται πινόμενον νεφριτκοὺς ὑγιάζειν.
23. Dioscorides *Materia Medica* 1. 83 (vol. 1, 80, Wellmann, ed.).
24. For a complete list of sources for the Phaethon legend, see Riddle, "Amber in Antiquity. An Historical-Etymological Problem," *Laudatores Temporis Acti*, p. 114.
25. Dioscorides, *Materia Medica* 1. 83:
αἰγείρου τὰ φύλλα μετ' ὄξους καταπλαττόμενα ποδαγρικὰς ὀδύνας ὠφελεῖ. ἡ δὲ ἐξ αὐτῆς ῥητίνη μείγνυται μαλάγμασιν. ὁ δὲ καρπὸς μετ' ὄξους πινόμενος ἐπιληπτικοὺς ἱστορεῖται ὠφελεῖν. λέγεται δ' ὅτι τὸ ἐξ αὐτῶν δάκρυον κατὰ τὸν Ἠριδανὸν ποταμὸν καταχεόμενον πήγνυσθαι καὶ γίνεσθαι τὸ καλούμενον ἤλεκτρον, ὑπ' ἐνίων δὲ χρυσοφόρον, εὐῶδες ἐν τῇ παρατρίψει καὶ χρυσοειδὲς τῷ χρώματι, ὅπερ πινόμενον λεῖον στομάχου καὶ κοιλίας ῥεῦμα ἵστησι.
26. vol. 11, 816, Kühn, ed.
27. Theophrastus *On plants* 1. 2. 7; 1. 5. 2; 2. 2. 10; 3, 1. 1; 3. 3. 1; 3. 3, 4; 3. 4. 2; 3. 6, 1; 4. 1. 1; 4. 7. 4: 4. 4. 13. 2; 5. 9. 4.
28. e.g. Homer *Odyssey* 7. 106; 10, 510; 17. 208; *Iliad* 4. 482. Lucian *Astrology* 19: . . .
καὶ νῦν εἰσιν αἴγειροι καὶ τὸ ἤλεκτρον ἐπ' αυτῷ δάκρυον στάλαυσιν.
C. H. Oldfather, in the Loeb translation of Diodorus of Sicily (5.23). observes that the word *dakruon*. "tears", in the singular also means "sap."
29. Chinese materia medica, on the authority of Su Sang (11th c. A.D.). Wang Ts'ê-Ching, and Chang Yü-hsi (11th c. A.D.), makes a distinction between old hardened pine resin, *fu-ling*, and genuine amber, *hu p'o*. See, E. Bretschneider, *Botanicon Sinicum*, pt. 3: "Botanical investigations into the materia medica of the ancient Chinese," *J. N. China Brach. R. Asiat. Soc*, vol. 29 (1894-6), 534: Berthold Laufer, "Historical Jottings on Amber in Asia," *Mem. Am. anthrop. Ass.*, vol. 1 (1907), 224; Schott, "Skizze zu einer Topographie der Producte des Chinesischen Reiches," *Abh. d. k. Akad. Wiss. Berlin* (1842), 266-7.

30. Singer, "The Herbal in Antiquity . . ," *J. H. S.*, vol. 47 (1927), 19.
31. vol. 13, p. 86, Kühn, ed.:

    [Τροχίσκος ὁ δὶ ἠλέκτρου. ποιεῖ αἱμοπτυϊκοῖς, βήττουσι χρονίως καὶ προσφάτως, φθισικοῖς, ἀναφορικοῖς, ἐμπυϊκοῖς, κοιλιακοῖς, δυσεντερικοῖς, ἐμπνευματουμένοις. ἔστι δὲ καὶ ὠτικὴ ἀγαθή.]2 ψυλλίου καθαροῦ < μέ ἴρεως Ἰλλυρικῆς, μαστίχης, ἠλέκτρου ῥινήματος, κρόκου ἀνὰ < χ'. ὀπίου < ιέ. τὸ ψύλλιον βαλὼν εἰς θερμὸν ὕδωρ ἔα βρέχεσθαι καὶ ὅταν γλίσχρον καὶ κολλῶδες γένηται τὸ ὕδωρ, ἔκθλιβε τὸ ὑγρὸν ἐκ τούτου σκευάσας τὸ φάρμακον ἀναπλαττε τροχίσκους καὶ δίδου τριώβολον εις ὕπνον ἀπερχομένοις. ἔστω δὲ τοῦ ὕδατος ξε. γ'. ἐν ἄλλαις γραφαῖς ἐμβρέχεται τὸ ψύλλιον επὶ ἡμέρος γ'. εἶθ' ἕψεται ἕως ἀναβράσῃ τρὶς, εἶτα αἴρεται ἀπὸ τοῦ πυρὸς καὶ πάλιν ἐᾶται ἐπὶ τρεῖς ἡμέρας, καὶ τότε τὸ υγρὸν χωρίζεται πρὸς τὴν τοῦ φαρμάκου σκευασίαν.

32. vol. 13, pp. 86-7, Kühn, ed.
33. vol. 13, p. 94, Kühn, ed.
34. vol. 13, pp. 138-9, Kühn, ed.
35. vol. 13, p. 139, Kühn, ed.
36. Fragment from Book 11 of Aetios and collected in the edition, *Oeuvres de Rufus d'Ephèse* . . . Charles Daremberg and Ch. Emile Ruelle (Paris, 1879), p. 575.
37. Fragment from Rhazes *Continens* (*Oeuvres de Rufus d'Ephèse*, p. 494, Daremberg and Ruelle, eds.) reads in Latin edition: "Rufus: Medicamen conferens ad saltum cordis, ad angustiam et tristiam, et confortans cor. Recipe Buglossae aur. pon. x, carabae [i.e., Arabic for *amber*]. . . ." The use of amber for the heart is found in Islamic medicine and not to be found in ancient.
38. In an article, "Die Stein- und Gemmenbücher der Antike, "*Quell. Stud. Gesch. Naturw. Med.*, vol. 5 (1935), pp. 437-8, Max Wellmann writes: "Ohne Zweifel entfallen auf Xenokrates in dem Bernsteinkapitel abgesehen von den beiden in die Exzerpte aus Juba eingelegten Zitaten (37. 40) die Paragraphen 42-45 (über die richtige Gewinnung des Bernsteins auf Inseln des nordlichen Okeanos), ferner §47. 48 (über seine Arten Behandlung und Eigenschaften und §51 (über seine Verwendung in der Medizin nach Kallistratos), während in §46 ein weiteres Exzerpt aus Juba (Archelaos) vorliegt. Endlich gewinnen wir aus dem ersten Teil dieses Kapitels (§31f.) für Juba folgende Fachschriftsteller als Quellen: Sotakos, Zenothemis, Sudines, Mithridates, Metrodor) und Demostratos." See below, Wellmann's discussion of Pliny's sources for *lyngourion*.
39. *N.H.* 37. 11. 44: ". . . hodieque Transpadanorum agrestibus feminis monilium vice sucina gestatinbus, maxime decoris gratia, sed et medicinae; creditur quippe tonsillis resistere et faucium vitiis. . . ."
40. *N.H.* 37. 12. 51.
41. Kroll, "Kallistratos," (No. 41), Pauly-Wissowa-Kroll, *Real Encyclopädie* (Stuttgart, 1919), vol. 10, col. 1748.
42. *N.H.* 37, 12. 51.
43. *Ibid.*: "hoc collo adalligatum mederi febribus et morbis, tritum vero cum melle ac rosaceo aurium vitiis et, si cum melle Attico teratur, oculorum quoque obscuritati, stomachi etiam vitiis vel per se farina eius sumpta vel cum mastiche pota ex aqua." (D. E. Eichholz trans. in "Loeb").
44. *N.H.* 37. 13. 53: falsum et quod de medicina simul proditur, calculos vesicae poto eo eildi et morbo regio succurri, si ex vino bibatur aut spectetur etiam.
45. *N.H.* 28. 32. 122: Lynx's ". . . urina stillicidia vesicae. itaque eam protinus terra pedibus adgesta obruere traditur. eadem autem et iugulorum dolori monstratur in remedio.
46. *N.H.* 37. 13. 53.
47. Wellmann, "Die Stein' und Gemmenbücher der Antike," *Quell. Stud. Gesch. Naturw. Med.* vol. 5 (1935), 438-9.
48. Aretaeus *On the Causes and Indications of Acute Diseases* 6. 2. 16 (p. 124, Hude, ed.; Bk. 2, p. 178, Adams, ed.).
49. William David Ross, articles on "Archigenes" and "Aretaeus", *Ox. Class. Dict.* (1949), pp. 82, 86; Jerry Stannard, "Materia Medica and Philosophic Theory in Aretaeus," *Sudhoffs Archiv*, vol. 48 (1964), 27-53.
50. Translation by Francis Adams, *The Extant·Works of Aretaeus, the Cappadocian* (London, 1856), p. 424.
51. *On the Causes and Indications of Acute Diseases* 6. 2. 15 (p. 124, Hude, ed.) Bk. 2, p. 178, Adams, ed.).
52. George Sarton, *Introduction to the History of Science*, 3 vols. (Baltimore, 1927-48), I, 391.
53. *On Medicines* 16.94, Niedermann, ed.: "Trochiscus dielectru tantissimus ad aemoptoicos, id est sanguinem uel excreantes uel uomentes uel eos, qui maxime cum tussi sanguinem iactant."
54. cf. Galen *The Comp. of Med. accord-*

ing to Parts of the Body, vol. 13, 86, Kühn, ed.

55. *On Medicines* 29. 32, Niedermann, ed.: "Sucinum tundes et ex eius farina duo cocliaria cum aqua non nimium feruenti bibenda colico ieiuno per triduum dabis; efficaciter proderunt."
56. *Ibid.* 26. 114: "Calculos potio haec adsidue sumpta cum passo uel condito non sinit gigni eosque concrescentes confringit et per urinam harenae modo promit. Conficitur sic: Calaminthes, id est nepetae, — II, sil pictorium, piperis, sucini, saxifragae, petroselini, cyperi, zingiberis unicias singulas tundes et cribrabis et coclearium plenum cum uini mixta et calida potione ieiuno bibendum dabis."
57. *Ibid.* 15. 92: "Olei boni cyathum unum et sucinum uerum in ollem nouam mittes atque ad medias decoques, deinde sucinum tolles et combures et teres et puluerem eius in oleum supre scriptum mittes et una iterum diligenter teres atque inde tolibus, quotients opus fuerit, adpones; experieris magnum remedium."
58. *Ibid.* 21. 15: "Ad cordis pulsum siue salissationem sucinum uerum mittes in aquam feruentem et illic esse patieris atque inde per triduum laboranti singulos cyathos tepefactos, si nimium erit frigus, dabis bibendos. Hoc remendium et homini et animalibus prodest."
59. Oribasios *Synopsis ad Evstathivm* 3. 104 (p. 96, Raeder, ed.; vol. 5, p. 131, Bussemaker and Daremberg, eds.).
60. *Introduction to the History of Science*, vol. 1, 372-3.
61. *On Topical Remedies*, 10. 22 of *Works*, vol. 2, p. 430, Bussemaker and Daremberg, eds.
62. vol. 4, p. 568, Bussemaker and Daremberg, eds. The editors are uncertain whether to accept this treatise as Oribasios' work.
63. Lynn Thorndike, *A History of Magic and Experimental Science*, 8 vols. (New York, 1929), vol. 1, 571. We examined the following editions: Oribasios *Medicineium collectorum tomus tertius* . . . (no date); Oribasios. *XXI Veterum et clarorum medicorum Graecorum varia opuscula* (Moscow, 1808); Oribasios *Oribasii Sardiani Medici longe excellentissmi opera, quae extant omnia*, 3 volumes edited by I. B. Rasario (Basel, 1557).
64. Caelius Aurelianus *Chronic Diseases* 2. 166, Drabkin, ed. Caelius states that he had already given a description of the amber lozenge in a treatise entitled *Answers*.
65. *Gynaecia* is the only fully extant treatise of Soranus in Greek. Though this treatise contains considerable mention of materia medica, there is no mention of amber. See the edition of *Gynaecia* prepared by Owsei Temkin (Baltimore, 1956).
66. Paul of Aegina [Works] 7. 3, (p. 214, Heiberg, ed.).
67. *Ibid.* 7. 3 (p. 188, Heiberg): "Ηλεκτρον τὸ τῆς αἰγείρου δάκρυόν φασι κατὰ τὸν "Ηριδανον ποταμὸν ἀποχεόμενον καὶ πηγνύμενον χρυσοειδές ὅπερ πινόμενον λεῖον στομάχου καὶ κοιλίας ῥεῦμα καὶ αἷμα ἐπέχει.
68. Paul of Aegina, *The Third Book of Paul* 196 (p. 121, Heiberg, ed.). The context suggests that the amber lozenge was given for colic and diarrhea though the Latin text makes it uncertain.
69. Sarton, *Introduction*, I, 434.
70. *Books of Medicine* 2. 35 (Vol. I, p. 167, Oliviei, ed.): "Ηλεκτρον ἤ σούκινον ἢ λιγγούριον. Πινόμενον ἰᾶται δυσουρίαν λε καὶ στομαχικοὺς ὠφελεῖ, καὶ ὁ χρυσή·λεκτρος δὲ πινόμενος σὺν μαστίχῃ ἀλγήματα στομάχου ἰᾶται.
71. Lynn Thorndike, *Magic and Exp. Science*, vol. 1, 571. A Latin edition of Aetius' *Gynaecology and Obstetrics* translated by Janus Cornarius (Lyons, 1549) contains the word *ambra* in several of the later chapters, namely chapters 114 (col. 1026) and 122 (cols. 1028, 1029). The appearance of this Arabic word, especially coming toward the end of the purported Aetius' text and surrounded by other Arabic medical practices and drugs, makes it certain that Cornarius has either accepted an improper text or that he added new material to up-date Aetius' earlier work. The English translation of Aetius' *Gynaecology and Obstetrics* by James V. Ricci (Philadelphia and Toronto, 1950) is based on the Latin Edition of Cornarius, 1542, which we have not seen. However, since the 1542 and 1549 editions appear to be the same, we are confident that Aetius did not here mention amber, as Ricci translates *ambra*.
72. Celsus [*Opera quae supersunt*], Marx, ed.
73. Editions examined are: Theodore Priscian (pseudo) *Euporiston*, Rose, ed.; Cassius Felix *On medicine*, Rose ed.; Adamantius *On Flatulence*, Rose,

ed.; Gargilius Martialis *On Medicine*, Rose, ed.; Alexander of Tralles *On Epilepsy*, Puschmann, ed.; Sextus Papyriensis Placitus *On the Medicine of Animals* . . . (1539 ed.); and Scribonius Largus *Compositiones*, Helmreich, ed.

74. Apuleius *Herbal*, Hunger, ed.
75. Sarton, *Introduction to the History of Science*, vol. I, p. 392; Singer, "The Herbal in Antiquity . . ." *J. H. S.*, vol. 47 (1927), 37.
76. *Glossae Medicinales*, Heiberg, ed.
77. *Commentary on Medicine*, as published in *Patrologiae cursus completus*, vol. 89, Latin series, 369-76; and Jerry Stannard, "Benedictus Crispus, an Eighth Century Medical Poet," *J. Hist. Med.*, vol. 21 (1966), 24-46.
78. *e.g.*, Jerome *Letters* 64. 16; Diodorus *Library* 5. 23. 1-4.
79. George C. Williamson, *The Book of Amber* (London, 1932), p. 20 ff.
80. Also see Theophrastus *On Stones* 28.
81. Williamson, *The Book of Amber*, pp. 21-5.
82. H. J. Frish, Le Périple de la Mer Erythrée," *Göteborgs Högskolas Arsskrift* vol. 33 (1927), 1-145; Wilfred H. Schoff, *The Periplus of the Erythraean Sea* (New York, 1912). According to Schoff (p. 157, fn.), there is a date wine, called medicinal stomachic, mentioned by Strabo, Dioscorides, and Marco Polo. In a similar modern drink, Schoff says, aromatic spices including ambergris are added to the base of distilled date juice. There is no proof, however, that ambergris was an ingredient in the ancient drink.
83. *Book of Medicine* 2. 35.
84. Pliny *N.H.*, 37. 12. 51.
85. It will be recalled that the Greek writer Aetius did use the Latin *soukinon*. This same form ( ) was employed by Clement of Alexandria *Stromateis* 26 2, Stahlin-Fruchtel, eds.

VI

THEORY AND PRACTICE IN MEDIEVAL MEDICINE

If evidence were totally lacking, we might reasonably assume that medical practice, like language and customs, continued substantially unaltered from the late Roman period. Most historians of medicine, to the contrary, postulate a clear break between late Roman and early medieval medical practice.[1] The early medieval period is called the "Dark Ages" of medicine by Charles Singer;[2] other scholars bemoan "stagnant conventionalism"[3] and an era "restricted to literary pursuits in the shadow of the cloister."[4] Arturo Castiglioni's stan-

Portions of this paper were read at the American Historical Association (December 1969), Trent Society for the History of Medicine, Duke University (January 1970), and the American Association for the History of Medicine (April 1970). I am indebted to many friends and colleagues who have read the manuscript in various stages and have rendered invaluable assistance. Specifically I wish to thank: Professors Vern Bullough, Thomas Herndon, Phillip Thomas, Stanley Suval, Michael McVaugh, Edith Sylla, Ynez Violé O'Neill, and Lynn White, jr.

[1] For example, Max Neuburger, *History of Medicine*, 2 vols., trans. Ernest Playfair (London 1910) 1.276-298; Benjamin Lee Gordon, *Medieval and Renaissance Medicine* (New York 1959) 1ff.; E. T. Withington, *Medical History from the Earliest Times* (London 1894) 175-184. An example of the dominant view of early medieval medicine is seen by Charles Singer and E. Ashworth Underwood, *A Short History of Medicine*, ed. 2 (Oxford 1962) 68-69, who wrote, "Men lacked a motive for living [during the Middle Ages] . . . The curse of the science of medicine, as of all sciences, has always been the so-called practical man, who will consider only the immediate end of his art, without regard to the knowledge on which it is based. Monkish medicine had no thought save for the immediate relief of the patient. All theoretical knowledge was permitted to lapse."

[2] Charles and Dorothea Singer, "The Origin of the Medical School of Salerno, the First University: An Attempted Reconstruction," *Essays on the History of Medicine Presented to Karl Sudhoff* (Oxford 1924) 124; Charles Singer, "Medical Science in the Dark Ages," *Sidelights on the History of Medicine*, ed. Sir Zachary Cope (London 1957) 37-46, first read at a meeting in 1917.

[3] J. B. de C. M. Saunders, Review of Erwin H. Ackerknecht, *A Short History of Medicine*, *Isis* 48 (1957) 74.

[4] Arturo Castiglioni, "The School of Salerno," *Bulletin of the Institute of the History of Medicine* (BHM) 6 (1938) 884; see also Thomas C. Allbutt, *Science and Medieval Thought* (London 1901) 15; Paul Diepgen, "Zur tradition des Pseudo Apuleius," *Janus* 29 (1925) 160, cites the great manuscript curator at Berlin, Valentin Rose, as calling medieval medicine a "'reizvoll dunklen' Periode."

© 1974 by the Regents of the University of California. Reprinted from *Viator* Vol 5, 1974 pp. 157–84 by permission.

dard work, *A History of Medicine* (1,192 pages) devotes ten pages to the early Middle Ages, almost half the space given to prehistoric medicine.[5]

Protests against this view by A. Pazzini, Pierre Winter, C. Daremberg, and George Sarton[6] have succeeded only in reinforcing the notion of the Dark Ages by concentrating too often not on practice but on medical theory where the case for progressive changes is less clear. This disregard of practice and the emphasis instead on the more depraved theoretical medicine of the times is due in part to the influence of Karl Sudhoff, the father of the history of medicine, who had nothing but scorn for all that was not *Schulmedizin*. One of his students quotes him as saying, "All medicine practiced by laymen is only thievery from the All-Mother Medicine."[7]

Karl Sudhoff, Henry Sigerist, Charles Singer, and other pioneers of the history of medicine placed emphasis on finding and publishing early medical texts as well as determining their sources. The absence of theory in such documents was viewed as a degeneration of Graeco-Roman medicine, and the period's emphasis instead on simple recipes was considered unworthy of a vibrant medical profession. Moreover, doubt about the actual use of these recipes was expressed. In contrast to this bleak picture of the early Middle Ages, medical historians increasingly have given honorific medals to physicians of each generation after the late eleventh century for the developments at Salerno, the Islamic translations, and the so-called return to rational speculation.

To help correct this oversimplified view of medieval medical history, I wish to make some observations on the relationship between medical theory and practice during the entire period of the Middle Ages. My focus will be on drug therapy, because this was the way most medicine was practiced. The study consists of the following propositions: (1) Because both Roman and medieval

[5] Arturo Castigliono, *A History of Medicine*, trans. E. B. Krumbhaar, ed. 2 rev. (New York 1958); pages 13-30 cover prehistoric medicine whereas pages 288-299 cover early medieval medicine up to Salerno.

[6] A. Pazzini, *Storia della medicina*, 2 vols. (Milan 1947) 1.316-331; P. Winter, "Le moyen age," *Historie générale de la médecine, de la pharmacie, de l'art dentaire et de l'art veterinaire*, 3 vols. (Paris 1936-1949) 2.1-29; C. Daremberg, *Histoire des sciences medicales*, 2 vols. (Paris 1870) 1.254-269; George Sarton, *Introduction to the History of Science*, 3 vols. (Baltimore 1927-1947) 1.14-21. Interestingly, Sarton, who denounced the concept of the dark ages —"those ages were never so dark as our ignorance of them" (1.17)—also said, "The historian of science can not devote much attention to the study of superstition and magic, that is, of unreason, because this does not help him very much to understand human progress. Magic is essentially unprogressive and conservative; science is essentially progressive" (1.19). Recently, some historians of medicine believe that the study of "magic and superstition" is precisely where one must look for many changes in the historical process. For other historians who devote attention to challenging the "dark ages" in medicine, see, Loren C. MacKinney, "A Half Century of Medieval Medical Historiography in America," *Medievalia et humanistica* 7 (1952) 18-42, esp. 29-30.

[7] Bruno Gebhard, "Historical Relationship between Scientific and Lay Medicine for Present-Day Patient Education," BHM 32 (1958) 47.

medicine consisted of noninstitutionalized, informal practice, there was probably little change in the practice of medicine, at least in drug therapy, between the two eras. (2) Roman and early medieval medical education were substantially the same. (3) Although speculative medical theory was almost totally abandoned, fifth-century through tenth-century records show that medical progress was not solely dependent on written language.[8] Instead this evidence shows that a medical practice existed based upon a pharmacy that not only preserved the older practical knowledge but also recognized and used new drugs. (4) The movement, from the eleventh-century, to reestablish the preeminence of medical theory should not be given unqualified endorsement as a great leap forward because it embodied a retrogressive feature: it produced a gap between theory and practice which did little to aid the practicing physician because the new drug theory was unworkable. (5) As seen in a practical medical guide, the lapidary literature, and the *Pestschriften*, the general practitioner of the later Middle Ages reacted to the new learned infatuation with theoretical medicine by largely ignoring it. (6) In contrast to (5), as seen in some Italian rhetorical treatises and the *consilia*, theoretical medicine achieved a prestige that challenged the practical physicians and moved to exclude them from the profession. Although the results were mixed, the practical physicians made their contributions to modern medicine.

No notable division between late Roman and early medieval medicine exists. Part of the current misunderstanding of early medieval medicine stems from the assumption that institutionalized schools of medicine, with a determined curriculum and a licensing of practitioners, existed in Antiquity. If such there were, they were only isolated phenomena. Medical education was conducted by the physician father teaching his son or apprentice.[9] Thus, reports of the demise of ancient schools of medicine are, to say the least, exaggerated because we cannot be sure that they were ever born.[10]

In order to reveal a decayed age in medicine, some scholars have contrasted Varro's (first century B.C.) so-called nine disciplines with Martianus Capella's

[8] *Contra* Winter (n. 6 above) 9: "Les progrès de la médecine dependent donc de ceux de la linquistique."

[9] I. E. Drabkin, "On Medical Education in Greece and Rome," BHM 15 (1944) 333-351; Theodor Puschmann, *A History of Medical Education* (New York repr. 1966, first publ. 1891) 96, 121; Neuburger (n. 1 above) 1.279; John Scarborough, *Roman Medicine* (Ithaca 1969). H. I. Marrou, *A History of Education in Antiquity*, trans. George Lamb (New York ca. 1956) 265 passim, claims that the teaching of medicine was mostly clinical. The only exception, Marrou (341) says, is the official instruction of medicine given by the physicians (*archiatri*), who controlled the so-called public health service. The word *archiatri* is used in the sixth-century Ostrogothic State (Cassiodorus, *Variae* 6. 19). See Loren C. MacKinney, *Early Medieval Medicine with Special Reference to France and Chartres* (Baltimore 1937) 47-48.

[10] MacKinney (n. 9 above) 68-69, 71, 79; while William H. Stahl, in "Dominant Traditions in Early Medieval Latin Science," *Isis* 50 (1959), 92-124, holds the opinion that early medical science was lost in the medieval web of mysticism and superstition.

(ca. 5th century A.D.) seven "handmaidens," the trivium and quadrivium, and have noted that both medicine and architecture were curricular dropouts.[11] Varro's "disciplines" are misunderstood. He was not outlining a school curriculum but categories of *useful knowledge.*[12] By the "handmaidens" of philology, Capella meant pillars of wisdom. This reflects Seneca's Epistle 88, which contends that the purpose of *studia liberalia* or *artes liberales*, as contrasted with the *artes mechanicae*, is not to make money.[13] *Scientia* was "used to designate a discerning, penetrating, intellectual grasp of a situation or a given subject."[14] To Roman and early medieval people, medicine was an art, not a *scientia*; so Hippocrates had said[15] and so the early Middle Ages believed. It could no more be formally studied than woodcarving, plowing, or butchering. Medicine was neither a science nor chance but a skill, a trade. Isidore said medicine was not a "subject" because it deals in all areas, not singular themes.[16]

[11] As examples of the error of contrasting Varro with Capella: M. L. W. Laistner, *Thought and Letters in Western Europe, A.D. 500 to 900* (Ithaca 1931) 40; Stahl 98; L. C. MacKinney, *The Medieval World* (New York 1938) 51; and to a lesser degree, Neuburger (n. 1 above) 1.284. Varro's work, now mostly lost, is known by a very indirect, curious route (perhaps not correctly understood), especially via Jerome, *De vir. ill.* 54 (2.879.Vall.). Varro's work that names the "subjects" is *De imaginibus*, cf. H. J. Rose, *A Handbook of Latin Literature* (New York 1960) 226-227, and Martin Schanz, *Geschichte des römischen Literatur*, 4 vols. rev., ed. Carl Hosius (Munich 1927) 1.567-568.

[12] Marrou (n. 9 above) 341. Benedictus Crispus (d. ca. 732) wrote to Maurus, a student whom Crispus had instructed in the seven liberal arts: "You claimed that the knowledge of good medicine—which you thought of little value for anything—held no place or share in a liberal education. Now, however, since the irregularity of various illnesses more frequently overpowers you, you compel that very irregularity to broaden your knowledge of the arts, which formerly you did not blush to call wicked and vile. You require of me that I make you a rustic [i.e. a low-level medical man] and teach you the powers of medicinal herbs" Trans. Jerry Stannard, "Benedictus Crispus, an Eighth-Century Medical Poet," *Journal of the History of Medicine and Allied Sciences* (JHMAS) 21 (1966) 31. Stannard's translation is based on the Latin text as published in PL 197. 1125-1352. It is also published more recently by Franz Brunhölzl, "Benedetto de Milano ed il 'Carmen Medicinale' di Crispo," *Aevum* 33 (1960) 25-67, who expresses doubt about the author and the date of the poem.

[13] Ernst Robert Curtius, *European Literature and the Latin Middle Ages*, trans. Willard R. Trask (New York 1953) 36-39. Seneca (*Epistle* 88.1): "You wish to know my views concerning liberal studies. My answer is this: I respect no study, and deem no study good, which results in money-making."

[14] James A. Weisheipel, "Classification of the Sciences in Medieval Thought," *Mediaeval Studies* 27 (1965) 54. The medieval popularity of the Hippocratic statement, "Vita brevis, ars vero longa," represented an argument, or provided an excuse, not to learn theoretical medicine because the art was acquired by doing.

[15] Hippocrates *Περί τέχνης*; *Αφορίσμοι* I; cf. Ludwig Edelstein, "The Hippocratic Physician," *Ancient Medicine, Selected Papers of Ludwig Edelstein* (Baltimore 1967) 87-110.

[16] Isidore, *Etymologies* (*Ety.*) 4.13.1, Lindsay ed.: "De initio medicinae. Quaeritur a quibusdam quare inter ceteras liberales disciplinas Medicinae ars non contineatur. Propterea, qui illae singulares continent causas, ista vero omnium."

Early medieval medicine was practical. The distinction was dropped between medicine as a practice (art) and medicine as a theory (science), a distinction made by Aristotle and noted by Pliny who railed against illiterate practitioners knowing no theory.[17] Hellenistic theoretical medicine withered, its roots never deep in Roman soil, but there remained another level of growth, practical medicine.[18] Culturally this was due to a reaction in the early western Middle Ages against the "rational science" of Antiquity. As Christianity divided into eastern and western halves, the western monastic orders stressed the basic practical values as compared with the more ascetic and theoretical attitudes of eastern Christianity.[19] Only traces of Hellenistic and eastern theory are found in the Latin documents of the early Middle Ages.[20]

[17] Aristotle, *Politics* 1282a3: "There is the physician who is a craftsman (*δημιουργός*) and there is the scientific physician (*ἀρχιτεκτονικός*), and thirdly there is the educated man who had studied the art (*ὁ πεπαιδευμένος περὶ τὴν τέχνην*), cf. Drabkin (n. 9 above) 343. Pliny (*N.H.* 29.8, 17-18, trans. W. H. S. Jones) says "Medicine alone of the Greek arts we serious Romans have not yet practiced . . . [He continues to say that many medical men cannot either read or understand Greek medical works.] Accordingly, heaven knows, the medical profession is the only one in which anybody professing to be a physician is at once trusted. . . . . Physicians acquire their knowledge from our dangers, making experiments at the cost of our lives. Only a physician can commit homicide with complete impunity."

[18] Ludwig Edelstein, in "Recent Trends in the Interpretation of Ancient Science," *Journal of the History of Ideas* 13 (1952) 573-604, reprinted in *Ancient Medicine, Selected Papers of Ludwig Edelstein*, eds. Owsei and C. Lilien Temkin (Baltimore 1967) 401-439 (citations to book) believes that ancient science was in decay by A.D. 200 at the latest (416). He says, "Greek science advocated at all times assumptions about an invisible world of law and order; it was theoretical rather than practical" (421). "I can find no indication that knowledge of crafts and techniques was a decisive factor" (420). "I suggest that the failure of the empirical trend to establish itself securely was in great measure due to the lack of social integration of science" (434).

[19] Richard E. Sullivan, "Early Medieval Missionary Activity: A Comparative Study of Eastern and Western Methods," *Church History* 22 (1954) 17-35; Lynn White, jr., Review of Silvano Borsari, *Il monachesimo bizantino nella Sicilia . . . Speculum* 41 (1966) 116-7.

[20] Paul Diepgen, *Die Theologie und der ärztliche Stand* (Berlin 1922) 1ff., esp. 12 says that the church writers generally thought the purpose of the physician was to treat the body while the priest administered to the soul. The physician had a prestigious position in an orderly world conceived by God. Adolf Harnack, *Medizinisches aus der ältesten Kirchengeschichte* (Leipzig 1892) notes a Christian acceptance of medicine especially in view of Christ's parables and Luke being a physician. Loren MacKinney (n. 9 above, 61 and passim) believes that some of the writings by churchmen, which may seem antagonistic to medicine, represented an "official public attitude." Still this does not negate the numerous instances where church men were sympathetic towards physicians, relied upon them for aid, and studied their works. The Church never prohibited dissection, only cemetery breaking, see Mary N. Alston, "The Attitude of the Church towards Dissection before 1500," BHM 16 (1944) 221-238. The early Church Fathers respected the practice of medicine (n. 40 below). Augustine, as an example, makes frequent use of the *Christus medicus* concept with many medical similes; see Rudolph Arbesmann, "The Concept of 'Christus medicus' in St. Augustine," *Traditio* 10 (1954) 1-28. In *De doctrina christiana* 1.14.13 (H. J. Vogels, *Florileg. Patrist.* 24 [1930] 8ff.), Augustine wrote revealingly of pharmaceutical theory as follows: "A physician, in

What was left was the actual practice of medicine. Practice was the execution of health regimen, generally by drug and diet therapy. In pharmacy, practice was a constant tradition of unstructured testing of the relationships between drugs and ailments (a form of experimental controls), a mode of transmission of recipes, and a commitment to drug therapy. In contrast, theory was the conceptual scheme that supplied explanations for the physiological administration and action of drugs. The art of cooking is analogous to medicine as an art. Good cooks practice an art without an intellectual schema beyond a commitment to culinary tastes, a constant testing of results and a mode of transmission of recipes, written or unwritten. The good cooks of yesteryear frequently could not explain in coherent, quantifiable terms a particular recipe but were able to demonstrate by doing. Certainly early medieval physicians worked according to a conceptual framework—each person must have some rationale for what he is doing—but early medieval medical theory was so ignored that the practitioners themselves considered it well-nigh unimportant.

Even though medical theory was virtually lost in the West, the ancient legacy of pharmaceutical prescriptions was fairly efficiently transmitted. Dioscorides's *De materia medica* was translated into Latin before the sixth century[21] and this was by far the most complete authority for plants, animal products,

---

treating an injury to the body applies certain opposites, as cold to hot, dry to wet, or something else of this kind; in other cases he applies like remedies, as a round bandage to a circular wound, or an oblong bandage to an oblong wound, not using the same bandage for every limb but adapting like to like. Thus the wisdom of God, in healing mankind has employed Himself to cure it, being Himself Physician and Medicine both in one."

[21] The transmission of Dioscorides's *De materia medica*, which contains a description of around nine hundred pharmaceutical items through the Middle Ages is very complex. There was a translation into Latin before the sixth century on the evidence of Cassiodorus, *De institutio divinarum literarum* 31, who says: "Those monks who cannot read Greek can read many writers, such as Dioscorides, in Latin." The Latin translation, which is fairly faithful to the original Greek although the grammar is poor, is found in Munich MS (CLM) 337, eighth century, and Paris Bibliothèque Nationale lat. MS 9332, ninth century, fols. 243-321v. K. Hoffman and T. M. Auracher began editing CLM 337 (*Römanischen Forschungen* 1 [1882] 49-105) and the project was continued by H. Stadler (*Ibid.* 10 [1897] 181-247 369-446; 11 [1899] 1-121; 13 [1902] 161-243; 14 [1903] 601-636). Stadler had the advantage of the discovery of BN 9332 which he used for editing Books 2-5 but he did not reedit Book 1. BN 9332 lacks leaves now in Bern MS A 91.7.fols. lv-2v. Book 1, using BN 9332, is reedited by H. Miheuscu, *Dioscoride latine materia medica libro primo* (Iasi, Roumania 1938). Paris BN lat. 12, 995, ninth century, was not known to any editor, yet it has the most complete text of *De materia medica*. According to Charles Singer in "The Herbal in Antiquity and Its Transmission to Later Ages," *The Journal of Hellenic Studies* 47 (1927) 34-35, there is yet another Latin version of Dioscorides found in Vienna, Nationalbibliothek lat. MS 16, which he dated around A.D. 600. The Vienna MS 16, however, contains not the Latin Dioscorides but fragments of the Greek beneath a Latin hand from Bobbio. This manuscript is now at Naples, Biblioteca Nazionale, with the current shelf mark of MS lat. 2. Folios 61v-65v have the Greek.

and minerals in medicine. More popular than the full version, however, was a Latin abridged edition known as *Ex herbis femininis.*[22] The latter was a more practical guide to the average medical man. *Ex herbis femininis* listed only seventy-one herbs, but each was drawn for identification, in contrast to the more than eight hundred items in the Latin Dioscorides, which was largely not illustrated.[23] Further, *Ex herbis femininis* was associated in most manuscripts with the beautifully illuminated *Herbarius* of Pseudo-Apuleius.[24] One manuscript copyist in central Europe noted that some plants in Pseudo-Apuleius's text were not locally known; thus he omitted these and inserted in their place some local plants not in the regular text.[25] The author of *Ex herbis femininis,* who flourished around the sixth century, used the Greek text of Dioscorides for his basic text, but included only the herbs more commonly known to Europe. Moreover, he omitted some uses of herbs and added other medical benefits from no other apparent literary source. Further, he modified plant descriptions and nomenclature. The rubrics to some copies explain that the herbs described are those "most useful in medicine."[26] The texts of medieval pharmaceutical treatises generally are less descriptive of the herbs and minerals than classical texts, and thus require that the reader have some prior acquaintance with the subject before using the written works.

[22] I have located a total of twenty-seven manuscripts of *Ex herbis femininis*: five from the ninth century; two from the tenth century; three from the eleventh century; four, twelfth century; five, thirteenth century; three, fourteenth century; and four, fifteenth century. About as many MSS are extant from before the twelfth as afterwards. Given the statistical probability of greater loss of earlier MSS than later ones, this demonstrates the popularity of *Ex herbis femininis* during the early Middle Ages and its relative decline thereafter. The editor of *Ex herbis femininis,* probably someone living in Ostrogothic Italy, based his condensation on Dioscorides but he drew on his experience as well. The principal theme is the medicinal qualities of each herb with little or no description of the plant except as appears in the illustration. A text based on a limited number of manuscripts is published by Heinrich Kaestner, "Pseudo-Dioscorides de herbis femininis," *Hermes* 31 (1896) 578-636.

[23] The MSS of *Ex herbis* are generally of excellent quality with good illuminations of plants, which make it far easier to use than the complete *De materia medica* which is not illuminated in Latin MSS, except for a few sketches in Munich MS 337.

[24] Most MSS containing Pseudo-Apuleius's Herbal have immediately following it the text of *Ex herbis,* e.g., as in Florence, Laurent MS Plut. 73.41, eleventh century, Lombardic script, and Oxford, Bodl. MS 130, eleventh century. The text of Pseudo-Apuleius is published, *Antonii Musae de herba vettonica liber. Pseudoapulei herbarius. Anonymi de taxone liber. Sexti Placiti medicinae ex animalibus,* ed. E. Howald and H. E. Sigerist, "Corpus medicorum latinorum," vol. 4 (Leipzig 1927). Also see, Henry Sigerist, "Zum Herbarius Pseudo-Apulei," *Sudhoffs Archiv* 23 (1930) 197-204; Paul Diepgen, "Zur Tradition des Pseudo-Apuleius," *Janus* 29 (1925) 55-57, 140-160.

[25] Henry Sigerist, "The Medical Literature of the Early Middle Ages," BHM 2 (1934) 34; Erhard Landgraf, "Ein frühmittelalterlicher Botanicus," *Kyklos* 1 (1928) 3-36.

[26] Florence, Laurenziana, MS Plut. 73.16, thirteenth century, fol. 179: "In hoc libro Dioscoridis continetur herbas femina numero LXXI utilissimus pro usu medicinae"; also London, British Museum, MS Harley 1582, twelfth century, fol. 79.

Galen's and Hippocrates's prescriptions were generally transmitted either in individual treatises in Latin translation, in individual prescriptions with alteration, or as incorporated by later Roman writers whose works were more frequently used.[27] Galen's work on pharmaceutical theory was ignored and apparently not known either directly or indirectly until the eleventh century. The texts show that early medieval knowledge of drugs was, at least, about the same as that of the Romans.

The fact that the general run of the early medieval pharmacy texts are copies of classical works has led many historians to conclude incorrectly that the science of drugs was static.[28] Good medicine, however, aims at curing, not at novelty. Also for almost any ailment as diagnosed there were available numerous different recipes in the manuscript texts,[29] and in the very act of selecting which one recipe to employ a medical decision was made. Moreover, many new early medieval recipes are derived from folk medicine—Germanic, Celtic, Hispanic, and the like.[30] This in itself, plus the fact that new recipes

[27] The transmission of Hippocratic literature is treated by Pearl Kibre, "Hippocratic Writings in the Middle Ages," BHM 18 (1945) 371-412. Galen's transmission is both more complex and less well treated, see Augusto Baccaria, *I codici di medicina del periodo presalternitano (secoli IX, X e XI)* (Rome 1956) 445-448. Galen's treatise *De simplicibus medicinis,* which contains pharmaceutical theory, was not translated until the eleventh century at the earliest (n. 60 below), but Galen's recipes, like other classical authors', were included in the frequently consulted later Roman writers such as Cassius Felix (fl. 447), Marcellus Empiricus (fl. 410), Theodorus Priscian (fl. 367-383), and Sextus Placitus (fl. early fourth century). These writers both added new recipes and transmitted older ones. For evidence of the use of these recipes, see Thomas Oswald Cockayne, *Leechdoms, Wortcunning, and Starcraft of Early England,* 3 vols. (London 1864-1866, repr. 1961); Henry Sigerist, *Studien und Texte zur frühmittelalterlichen Rezeptliteratur* (Leipzig 1923) esp. 182-186; Julius Jörimann, *Frühmittelalterliche Rezeptarien* (Zürich 1925); and Wilfrid Bonser, *The Medical Background of Anglo-Saxon England* (London 1963).

[28] See MacKinney (n. 9 above) 35; *contra* Wilfrid Bonser, "General Medical Practice in Anglo-Saxon England," *Science Medicine and History* 2 vols. (Oxford 1953) 1.163. Sigerist, "The Latin Medical Literature of the Early Middle Ages," JHMAS 13 (1958) 146, says: "The greatest achievement of these anonymous compilers was that they kept the torch alight for almost eight hundred years."

[29] Many ailments diagnosed were simple ones, revealing the presence of the medical craft at a low level. Typical are remedies for coughing, prevention of conception, headaches, swollen eyes, lunacy, temptation of the devil, spider bite, too much traveling, dysentery, elvish tricks, stomach ache, pimples, and so on, in a form of potions, ointments, plasters, powders, pills and other such. Most recipes were for items we today could purchase at the patent medicine counter. See Sigerist (n. 27 above) 170; MacKinney (n. 9 above) 32. But, there are also relatively sophisticated remedies for strangury, abortions, consumption, erysipelas, mouth cancer, tumors (various types are differentiated), dysentery, scabies, and many others which reveal a presence of learned medical judgments.

[30] John H. Grattan and Charles Singer, *Anglo-Saxon Magic and Medicine* (Oxford 1952) 23, report the following distinguishable elements in the early English medical literature: Greek medicine filtered through Latin formularies of the late empire, Roman magic, "Pythagorean" devices, Latin liturgical elements, Byzantine theurgy, pagan Teutonic magic,

were compiled, show that the texts were actually used and not simply copied. After all, the great respected men of classical medicine, Galen, Hippocrates, Celsus, and the rest, had not themselves discovered the medicinal value of the herbs, minerals, and animal substances used. Thousands, nay hundreds of thousands, of experiments in folk practice had separated those substances with pharmacological action from the inert and harmful. The writers of medicine merely recognized the result of this trial-and-error science.[31] Frequently, they had not authenticated the action of each simple or compound drug they recommended. When one particular part of an herb, say a root, was found as being effective for some specific action, this information was orally transmitted whenever and wherever men communicated and one generation taught the other. This process takes place independently of literary transmission.[32] There was a continuous pratice of medicine which was independent of loss, attrition, or, eventually, the recovery of classical medical theory. Far from being a gray science in a gray, confused period, early medieval medicine was a partly empirical, partly traditional skill.

Finding convincing proof of an active medical profession in the early Middle Ages is difficult because of the nature of our written evidence. The assumption that one can know early medieval medicine simply in identifying the texts is faulty. Researches by Thomas Cockayne, J. H. Grattan, Charles Singer, C. H. Talbot, Jerry Stannard, Wilfrid Bonser, and others, but especially by the late Loren C. MacKinney, have noted an omnipresent practice by both literate and illiterate, lay and clerical medical men.[33] Recent studies of such

---

Christianized Teutonic ritual, Celtic magic and theurgy, "Hisperic" elements and South Italian classical survivals.

[31] For instance, Marcellus Empiricus, *De medicamentis liber* (Leipzig 1916), recorded prescriptions using (without editing) either the Greek or Latin word for a substance depending on sources. There is no indication that he knew that a substance with two names in his book was actually one item. He merely wrote remedies the way he learned them. His work combines Celtic medicine, superstition, and traditional knowledge; see Sarton (n. 6 above) 1.391.

[32] Obviously by the time we learn of a people's pharmacopea through the first extant records, the list of drugs is already extensive: thus, the writers are merely recording knowledge gained by folkways. Dioscorides (*De materia medica*, ed. Wellmann praef. 2-4) says he learned of drugs by traveling and talking to the people in various regions. Writers of his own times, he says (praef. 2) have "written about the powers of medicines and they, by their examination being conducted in a cursory manner, not by delineating a drug's effectiveness but by vain speculation, have elevated each medicine to a controversy by arguing point by point. They do not know one medicine from the other." Galen (*On simple medicines* 11.796-798, ed. Kühn) says the best method of learning about drugs is by going out in the field, not through books.

[33] For example, Cockayne (n. 27 above); Grattan and Singer (n. 30 above); Stannard (n. 12 above); Bonser (n. 27 above); MacKinney (n. 9 above); Puschmann (n. 9 above) 184-196; Talbot, *Medicine in Medieval England* (London 1967); Joseph Frank Payne, *English Medicine in the Anglo-Saxon Times* (Oxford 1904) 61-62 passim; Gerhard Baader, "Der Berliner Codes Phillipp. 1790, ein frühmittelalterliches medizinisches Kompendium," *Medizinhistorisches Journal* (MJ) 1 (1966) 150-155.

medical writers as Benedictus Crispus (d. ca. 732) and Walafrid Strabo (d. 849) show a very practical and very empirical knowledge of medicinal herbs.[34] A study of Jewish rabbis' responses note the prevalence of leeches, physicians, magicians, and sorcerers who practiced medicine.[35] The Visigothic and Ostrogothic law codes and tenth-century Welsh law give evidence of legal controls on practicing physicians.[36] Norse medicine shows absorption of classical and southern European medicine even before Christian conversion.[37] The phenomenal growth of the cult of Cosmas and Damian reflects the medieval belief in cure—exactly how is not determined.[38]

Some scholars have underrated the influence of the Church in medicine. One historian of medicine, Benjamin Lee Gordon, stated that the Church subverted medicine by campaigning instead for spiritual cures and that it pressed the few remaining nonclerical practitioners into compromising "rational medicine" with the admission to their practice of "prayers" and "charms." Contrary to Gordon's view that "no true progress can be made in such a stifling

[34] *Hortulus Walahfrid Strabo*, trans. Raet Payne (Pittsburgh 1966); Stannard (n. 12 above) 24-26. For Benedictus Crispus, see above, n. 12.

[35] H. J. Zimmels, *Magicians, Theologians and Doctors. Studies in Folkmedicine and Folklore as reflected in the Rabbinical Responsa (12th-19th Centuries)* (London 1952) 2.

[36] Darrel W. Amundsen, "Visigothic Medical Legislation," BHM 45 (1971) 553-569, observes that Visigothic laws, far from being static copies of Roman legislation, governed, on a changing basis, medical activity in order to protect patient and physician alike from abuses and to encourage responsible practice. He believes that the means were arbitrary by which legislators and judges distinguished who was a *medicus*; accepted *medici* were probably those known to the community. Visigothic laws are in MGH Legum Sectio 1. 1 (Hanover 1902); for Ostrogothic medicine, see Cassiodorus, MGH Auctores antiquiores 12.191 ff and MacKinney (n. 9) 4-5, 28; see also Pearl Kibre "The Faculty of Medicine at Paris, Charlatanism, and Unlicensed Practices in the Later Middle Ages" BHM 27 (1953) 3. A study by J. G. Penrhyn Jones, "Medicine in the Tenth Century. Facts from Welsh Medical Law," *Medicine Illustrated* 5 (1951) 84-86, shows that tenth-century Welsh physicians had a definite status. Physicians obtained a fixed salary but under some circumstances they could levy a personal charge. The physicians had a seat in the great hall of the palace at the Table of Honor. Evidence of surgical practice exists.

[37] Gredrik Grön, "Remarks on the Earliest Medical Conditions in Norway and Iceland with Special References to British Influence" *Science, Medicine, and History*, 2 vols. (London 1953) 1.142-153; Puschmann (n. 9 above) 186-197.

[38] The literature on Cosmas and Damian is vast. The best and most complete recent treatment is Anneliese Wittman, *Kosmas und Damian, Kultausbreitung und Volksdevotion* (Berlin) 1967. Wittman says the cult came from Byzantium to Sicily where it continues in modern times, and she has collected considerable documentation to prove that it was very present in Italy during the fifth and sixth centuries (54). By the ninth century it was in the Rhineland where it became widespread (76-118). A review of the literature is by Walter Artelt, "Kosmas und Damian—ein Literaturbericht," MJ 3 (1968) 151-155. For evidence of the cult in early medicine, see E. Wickersheimer, "Une vie des saints Côme et Damien dans un manuscrit médical du IXe siècle, suivie d'une recette de collyre attriubée à la mère des deux saints," *Centaurus* 1 (1950) 38-42.

atmosphere,"[39] most Church Fathers, including Saint Augustine, were sympathetic to medicine and even knew something of it; the Church was not antagonistic to man helping man to overcome pain.[40] In the early Middle Ages the Christian ethic advocated in the strongest way the care of the poor, miserable, downtrodden, and sick, an emphasis lacking in Graeco-Roman ethics.[41] Churchmen depended on knowledge that they said was supplied by God to help them help themselves. Monks were cured both by other monks, who learned medicine through reading, and by professional medical men, some of whom were in monastic residence.[42] To be certain, lay medicine not only existed during the early Middle Ages but the addition to it of the Christian ethic probably did much to stimulate medicine.

Early medieval medical practitioners were also willing to recognize innovations. A statistical analysis of a Latin ninth-century antidotary shows that it has 123 recipes, involving 361 different ingredients used a total of 944 times.[43] Of the most frequently cited drugs, a majority could have come only from the Orient; for example, aloes, myrrh, frankincense, pepper, and mastic. These prescriptions were not exclusively copied from classical texts nor were they merely handwriting exercises. Receptaries and antidotaries dating from the ninth through the eleventh centuries have ambergris, zedoary, and camphor,

[39] Gordon (n. 1 above) 43.

[40] See n. 20, above; Sister Mary E. Keenan, "St Gregory of Nazianus and Early Byzantine Medicine" BHM 9 (1941) 8-31, shows that many Fathers, such as St. Gregory and St. Basil—both of whom studied medicine—regarded it highly. Tertulian (*Ad nationes* 2.14; Arbesmann 19.3) once called Asclepius "a bastard" and "a beast so dangerous to the Word." Tertullian's other references to medicine reveal that he was not against medicine per se but against the concept of a pagan deity who was responsible for health. See also Mary E. Keenan, "St. Gregory of Nyssa and the Medical Profession," BHM 15 (1944) 150-161. Certainly later medieval writers, such as Rabanus Maurus, knew medicine and were sympathetic with the profession. For instance, Richer of Rheims studied classical medicine and his explanation of diseases was medical, not theological—Loren C. MacKinney, "Tenth Century Medicine as seen in the *Historia* of Richer of Rheims," BHM 2 (1934) 352-354.

[41] Vern L. Bullough and Bonnie Bullough, *The Emergence of Modern Nursing*, ed. 2 (London 1969) 32-35. The changed medieval ethic is to be contrasted with the Roman and Greek view of the poor and destitute which is very different, see A. R. Hands, *Charities and Social Aid in Greece and Rome* (Ithaca 1968). In contrast, Loren C. MacKinney, "Medical Ethics and Etiquette in the Early Middle Ages," BHM 26 (1952) 1-30 esp. 28, believed there is little difference between the ideals of classical Greek medicine and those of early medieval medicine.

[42] Grattan and Singer (n. 30 above) 12-13, 16-17; Loren C. MacKinney, "Early Medieval Medical Education," *Aiti del XIV congresso internazionale di storia della medicina* 2 (1954) 3-8 esp. 6. The studies reveal that there was some literacy among the professional or semi-professional lay practitioners.

[43] John M. Riddle, "The Introduction and Use of Eastern Drugs in the Early Middle Ages," *Sudhoffs Archiv* 49 (1965) 186-187, from St. Gall, Stiftsbibliothek MS 44 fols. 228-255, and published by Sigerist (n. 27 above). I have seen this MS. The Arabic names are in the same ninth century hand as the rest of the antidotary.

substances unknown in Graeco-Roman pharmacy.[44] One conclusion is justified: not only was there a continuous drug trade between the eastern and western Mediterranean worlds, but also information about new drugs was discovered in the West and used.[45] The names for herbs changed, thus illustrating continuous usage and not a static art.[46] The term apothecary (*apotheca*) evolved from ἀποθῆκαι, a Byzantine word for local depots in main harbors and road termini, and came into wide usage in thirteenth-century Italy, France, and Germany to mean "druggist." The fact that the term for an import-export house came to be associated entirely with the meaning "drug store" demonstrates emphatically the relation between trade and drugs during the early Middle Ages.[47]

[44] Riddle 189-198; cf. Brunhölzl (n. 12 above) 31 ff., and Stannard (n. 12 above) 41. The same observation was made for camphor appearing in an eleventh century MS by Piero Giacosa, "Un ricettario del secolo XI nel'Archivio Capitolare d'Ivrea," *Reale accademia delle scienze di Torino. Memorie* 2 (1886) 649. Evidence of use of eastern drugs and not merely those represented in formularies is found in a study by G. E. Trease, "The Spices and Apothecaries of the Royal Household in the Reigns of Henry III, Edward I, and Edward II" *Nottingham Medieval Studies* 3 (1959) 21-22, 38-52. I. H. Burkill, in *A Dictionary of the Economic Products of the Malay Peninsula*, 2 vols. (London 1935) 1.546, argues for the introduction of *dryobalanops* camphor or levo-camphor to the Romans "about the time of Christ, or soon after." J. Innes Miller in *The Spice Trade of the Roman Empire 29 B.C. to A.D. 641* (Oxford 1969) 41-42, accepts Burkill's statement but omits the qualification that this is not the substance known as camphor. Burkill says that *Cinnamonum* camphor, a dextro camphor, was manufactured by the Chinese and Japanese sometime "before the ninth century." *Cinnamonum* camphor is the camphor used in medicine whereas *dryobalanops* is mentioned by Dioscorides (n. 32 above) 4.187.

[45] Loren C. MacKinney, "Oleum savinium, An Early Medieval Synthesis of Medical Prescriptions," BHM 16 (1944) 276-288, esp. 286-287, based on evidence in Paris, BN lat. MS 6400 B, tenth century, fols. 86v-87.

[46] H. E. Sigerist, "Herbs Momordica," BHM 4 (1936) 511-513. Also *Ex herbis femininis* adds new names for drugs. At first the Anglo-Saxon leech had no precise way of quantifying his prescriptions but more accurate notations came from the continent and caused the leech to change; see Grattan and Singer (n. 30 above) 27-28.

[47] The Byzantine warehouses are discussed by Robert S. Lopez, "The Trade of Medieval Europe: The South," *The Cambridge Economic History of Europe*, 6 vols. (Cambridge 1952), 2.275, and their relation to drugs by Riddle (n. 43 above) 196. An edict of Frederick II refers to *apotheca* apparently in the sense of a storehouse for drugs: Wolfgang-Hagan Hein and Kurt Sappert, *Die Medizinalordnung Friedrichs II. Eine pharmaziehistorische Studie.* Veröffentl. d. Intern. Ges. F. Gesch. de. Pharmaz. N. F. 12 (Eutin 1957) 51. *Apotheca* or *Apothecarius*, in the sense of a "druggist," was used in Cologne as early as 1225 and certainly by the middle of the thirteenth century apothecary represented an official designation; Rudolf Schmitz, "Über deutsche Apotheken des 13. jahrhunderts. Ein Betrag zur Etymologie des apoteca-apotecarius Begriff," *Sudhoffs Archiv* 45 (1961) 289-302. In 1268 in Paris *apothécaire* is mentioned in *Le livre des metiers d'Etienne Boileau* 267 (2.16, 4.5), reprinted in *Les status et règlements des apothicaires*, 3 vols., ed. François Prevet (Paris 1950) 1.2. A University of Paris *chartularium* in 1271 (Prevet 1.3) speaks of an attempt to regulate an *apothecarius vel herbarius*. Finally the statutes of Marseille, dating between 1200-1263 (Prevet 3.2355) decree "De Medicis . . . et quod nullam societatem habebunt cum apothecariis et quod confectiones et syrpos quos conficient, vel conficere facient."

Pharmaceutical knowledge increased because western Europe as a whole was open to new ideas and techniques, and medicine was never isolated culturally. Modern research demonstrates that western Europe was in continuous contact with the East.[48] According to Peter the Deacon, Constantine the African (d. ca. 1085), who brought Arabic medical works to the West, had himself gone as far as India where presumably he studied medicine.[49] While we may doubt the details about Constantine's travel because Peter's account is untrustworthy, we may observe the direction from whence knowledge was expected to come. More and more emphasis is placed by modern historians on cultural and scientific change on an intercontinental basis, and medicine was but a part of early medieval society.

Although principally we have used pharmacy texts, the contributions of early medieval medical men were not restricted to pharmacy. For instance, C. H. Talbot observes that the Anglo-Saxon *Leechbook* of Bald (ca. 900-950) is derived frome earlier medical works but that the treatise modifies medical information. One example is the procedure for a liver operation in which the author, rather than merely copying an older text, made modifications by a "deliberate purpose pursued rationally."[50]

In summary, contrary to older opinions, early medieval medicine was a continuously developing art. There is no way to know whether or not cures effected by early medieval medical men were as good as those worked in the famed Doric-columned Aesculapian temple.[51] To be sure, there was a move-

[48] Lynn White, jr., *Medieval Technology and Social Change* (Oxford 1962) 14-38; *idem* "Medieval Borrowings from Further Asia," *Medieval and Renaissance Studies* 5 (1971) 3-26; *idem* "Tibet, India and Malaya as Sources of Western Medieval Technology," *American Historical Review* 65 (1960) 515-526; and *idem*, "Cultural Climates and Technological Advance in the Middle Ages," *Viator* 2 (1971) 171-201. S. D. Goitein, *A Mediterranean Society: The Jewish Communities of the Arab World as Portrayed in Documents of Cairo Geniza.* vol. 1: *Economic Foundations* (Berkeley 1967) 42-59 and passim; *idem*, "Letters and Documents on the India Trade in Medieval Times," *Studies in Islamic History and Institutions* (Leiden 1966), chap. 17. 329-350. The records indicate that both drugs and spices—spices were often drugs—account for the bulk of export items from India westwards. Michele Amari, *Storia dei Musulmani di Sicilia*, 3 vols. (Catania 1937-1939) 3.1. passim; Francesco Gabrieli, "La medicina araba e la Scuola di Salerno," *Salerno* 1 (1967) 12-23; Charles and Dorothea Singer (n. 2 above) 124 observe that, according to the chronicle of Achimaaz (850-1060), there were trade and family connections between southern Italy and Egypt.

[49] Charles Singer, "A Legend of Salerno. How Constantine the African brought the Art of Medicine to the Christians" *Johns Hopkins Hospital Bulletin* 28 (1917) 64-69, which has translation of Peter the Deacon's comments.

[50] Talbot (n. 33 above) 18-19.

[51] Astrology was connected with medical practice, to be sure, but the early medieval medical texts do not have the emphasis on astrology that later ones do. See Henry Sigerist, "*The Sphere of Life and Death* in the Early Mediaeval Manuscripts," BHM 11 (1942) 293-303. The *Sphere* is a medical device used to determine whether or not the patient will recover by figuring with the stars. Isidore (*Ety.* 4.13.4) says that a medical man needs to know astrology: "Postremo et Astronomiam notam habetit, per quam contempletur rationem

ment away from the rational theory of the Hellenes, which was, after all, only a veneer on Roman medicine, towards a medicine in the early Middle Ages which emphasized the empirical cures. The relationship was closer to "magic and experimental science," as Lynn Thorndike expressed it, than to theory.

If such were the contributions of the early Middle Ages, what then was the thrust of the later Middle Ages in medicine? It was towards making medicine a science, not just an art or practice.

Two developments are chiefly responsible for reversing medicine's focus. First, Carolingian education made medicine a part of a liberal arts training, and, in so doing, made it broader and shallower.[52] Noteworthy is one of the first references to Salerno, in the late tenth century, which, while discussing the supposed superiority of a Carolingian-trained liberal arts physician over a Salernitan, emphasized the essentially clinical character of early Salernitan medicine in contrast to a liberal arts training:

> The Salernitan, though untrained in letters, had by reason of his natural intelligence acquired wide practical experience. . . . One day they were considering the different aspects of *dynamidia*, and were discussing the effectiveness of pharmacy, surgery, and botany. The Salernitan being unfamiliar with the strange names, blushingly avoided any explanation.[53]

Second, with the impact of Islamic science and the new Greek-to-Latin writings, Salernitan writers of the second half of the twelfth century begin returning theory to medicine.[54]

Constantine's *De gradibus* brought back Galen's pharmaceutical theory but the full impact of a return to speculative thought had to await the thirteenth

---

astrorum et mutationem temporum." Roger Bacon (*On the errors of physicians*, 144-145, ed. and trans. E. T. Withington, *Essays on the History of Medicine Presented to Karl Sudhoff* [Oxford 1924]) wrote: "A fourth defect [of physicians] is that they do not study the heavenly bodies upon which all alternation of bodies in the lower world depends, while purgations, venesections and other evacuations and constrictions, and the whole of medical practice are based on the study of atmospheric changes due to the influence of the spheres and stars. Wherefore a physician who knows not how to take into account the positions and aspects of the planets can effect nothing in the healing arts except by chance and good fortune."

[52] MacKinney (n. 9 above) 94-95.

[53] Richer of Rheims, *Historia* 2.59, quoted by MacKinney (n. 42 above) 4-5.

[54] Paul O. Kristeller, "The School of Salerno," BHM 17 (1945) 156-157. Francis Bacon, *Nov. organon* 1.85, ed. F. H. Anderson, says the great technical and practical discoveries are "older than philosophy and the intellectual arts. So that, if the truth must be spoken, when the rational and dogmatical sciences began, the discovery of useful works came to an end." Recently a noteworthy study was conducted by Brian Lawn in *The Salernitan Questions* (Oxford 1963), who relates the development of lists of questions as teaching aids in medicine.

century.[55] The twelfth-century Salernitan works, including Nicholas's *Antidotarum* and Mattheus Platearius's *Circa instans*,[56] are—or were in early editions—practical guides to drugs with little theory: practical enough in fact so that apothecary guild rules of the fourteenth and fifteenth centuries required a copy of Nicholas's *Antidotarum* or something similar to be in every druggist's shop.[57] So likewise the non-Salernitan Western works on medicine by Macer Floridus, Marbode, and Hildegard, were very practical, nonspeculative works to serve the needs of a growing economy moving toward urbanization.[58] Responding to newly fashionable scholastic method, the authors of the late twelfth-century and thirteenth-century medicine reflect a steady trend toward theory.[59]

Late Salernitan writings (ca. 1100 to ca. 1300) brought philosophical speculation back to Europe, but the actual practice of medicine may not have been appreciably advanced after the first wave of assimilation. With the translation

[55] Talbot (n. 33 above) 38-55.

[56] In the case of Nicholas's *Antidotarum*, there were many versions from what originally was a simple treatise containing 50 to 60 prescriptions to a lengthy treatise with complex, polypharmacy prescriptions as editors in each generation added their contributions to the nucleus. H. Sigerist (n. 27 above) 187-195 says that Nicholas never existed; other authorities are prepared to accept a man by this name. Constantine himself is even proposed as the original author—Giuseppe Ongaro, "Gli antidotari Salernitani," *Salerno* 2 (1968) 35-43. The *Circa instans* apparently has an equally obscure beginning—Sarton (n. 6 above) 2.241-242), and Hans Wölfel, *Das Arzneidrogenbuch Circa instans* (Berlin 1939).

[57] Prevet (n. 47 above) 1.21 "Ordinatoines facultatis medicinae Paris de apothecariis [Circa an. 1322, Parissiis] La faculté de médecine pour le pourfit commun: Premièrement que tout li apothicaire et espicier de Paris soient appelé cascus an pardevant nous une fois et jurechent qu'ils feront loiablement à leur pouvoir le mestier de l'apothèque et de l'espicerie et ke il aront l'Antidotaire Nicolas corrigiet et semblant autel l'un comme l'autre." Similarly in 1422 the Faculty of Medicine of Paris added a regulation: "Primo juraverunt quod habebunt Cinonima correcta [Synonima Serapionis] et Circa instans Plateari." (Prevet 1.35) See Loren C. MacKinney, "Medieval Medical Dictionaires and Glossaries," *Medieval and Historiographical Essays in Honor of James Westfall Thompson* (Chicago 1938) 264-265.

[58] Macer's *Herbal* (late eleventh century) is most recently studied by Bruce P. Flood, Jr., "Macer Floridus: A Medieval Herbalist" (Ph. D. dissertation, University of Colorado, Boulder, 1968) and Göstal Frisk, ed., *A Middle English Translation of Macer Floridus de viribus herbarum* (Uppsala 1949); I have recently completed a study of Marbode of Rennes's (1035-1123) medical works, which will soon be published by *Sudhoffs Archiv*, and I found them to be close to the prevailing empirical, popular medical practice. G. M. Engbring, "Saint Hildegard, Twelfth-Century Physician," BHM 8 (1940) 777-778, observes, "A much more important source of her medical knowledge was the tradition of her monastery, the knowledge of herbs and treatment of various ailments handed down, either by word of mouth, or in jottings and recipes."

[59] Talbot (n. 33 above) 42. Michel R. McVaugh, in "Quantified Medical Theory and Practice at Fourteenth-Century Montpellier," BHM 43 (1969) 400, believes that, despite the theory, "thirteenth-century medicine remained strictly empirical in its use of specific simples and formulary compound drugs for specific ailments."

of Galen's *De simplicibus medicinis*,[60] together with the even more complex theories of Avicenna's *Canon*, Haly Abbas's *Pantegni*, *Liber Theorice*,[61] and others, medieval medical theory becomes so complex as to be unworkable. During the height of scholastic medicine, physicians confronted by a patient had to make a series of judgments that no human could execute in practice.[62] The factors to be determined in the administration of drugs were roughly as follows:[63] Each simple was active in one of four degrees according to heat, coldness, dryness, or wetness. Accordingly a drug is administered by opposites; that is, a feverish patient needs a drug that is cooling. But the intensity of a drug was measured by degrees; thus for a very high fever on a four-degree scale, a drug that is cool in the third degree may be prescribed. But a drug has not one but two characteristics, according to its composition; for example, it may be cold in the second degree and dry in the first. Thus a disease that had an excess of heat and dryness must not have a simple drug administered

[60] Karl Sudhoff, in "Die kurze 'Vita' und das Verzeichnis des Arbeiten Gerhards von Cremona," *Sudhoffs Archiv* 8 (1914) 78, and Moritz Steinschneider, in *Die europäische Übersetzungen aus dem Arabischen bis Mitte des 17. Jahrhunderts* (Graz 1956) 18, name the translator as Gerard of Cremona; but Rudolf Creutz, in "Der Arzt Constantinus Africanus von Monte-Cassino," *Studien und Mitteilungen zur Geschichte des Benediktiner Ordens* (SMGBO) 47 (1929) 19, and Heinrich Schipperges, in *Die Assimilation der arabischen Medizin durch das lateinische Mittelalter* (Wiesbaden 1964) 26-27, 32, name Constantine as the translator of a treatise with a similar title. Perhaps these are two separate works.

[61] Avicenna was translated by Gerard of Cremona (Steinschneider 21), and Haly Abbas or "Ali ibn Abbas," *Pantegni liber theorice* was translated by Constantine (Schipperges 35).

[62] Some thirteenth- and fourteenth-century writers were aware of the dangers of using theory when unchecked by experience, e.g., as following: "Medicina simplex . . . perferenda est composite . . . quia effectus expertarum medicinarum non expertis componendis vią rationis et experimenti, et cum intellectus operantis concludere nequeat silogizando effectus omnes elementales et celestes complexionatorum ex quibus conficitur medicamen. Experimenta enim innotuit deus largifluus servis suis effectus aloquos compositi"; Arnold of Villanova, *Antidotarium* (Lyon 1509) fol. 243vb.

[63] In making this all too brief summary, I have taken the theory from the following sources and simplified it: (1) Constantine, *De gradibus*, from Munich MS lat. 267, fourteenth century fol. 118rv, and printed edition in *Opera* (Basel 1536) 342-344; (2) Galen, *De simplicibus medicinis* in *Galeni . . . opera* (Venice [?] 1490) fols. 238v-310v; (3) Haly Abbas (trans, Constantine), *Pantegni, liber theorice* in *Issac Israeli omnia opera* (Lyon 1515) 1. fols. 1-9. 10, fols. 51v-61v; (4) Avicenna, *Liber canonis* (Venice 1507, fasc., repr. Hildesheim 1964) 2. 1-2. fols. 81-88., (5) *Apud antiquos* in Michael McVaugh, "Apud Antiquos and Mediaeval Pharmacology," MJ 1 (1966) 18-23; (6) Maurus of Salerno *De flebotomia*, ed. R. Buerschaper (Borna-Leipzig 1919) esp. for diurnal considerations; cf. Morris H. Saffron, *Maurus of Salerno*, trans. American Philosophical Society (Philadelphia 1972) 14-15. These theories are to be contrasted with the all too simple pharmaceutical theory pronounced by Isidore (*Ety.* 4.5.1): "Sanitas est integritas corporis et temperantia naturae ex calido et humido, quod est sanguis; unde et sanitas dicta est, quasi sanguinis status"; and (*Ety.* 4.9.3,7): "Pharmacia est medicamentorum curatio. . . . Contraria enim contrariis medicinae ratione cúrantur." See Michael Rogers McVaugh, "The Mediaeval Theory of Compound Medicine" (Ph. D. dissertation, Princeton University 1965).

which is both cold and dry but one that is cold and wet, unless a counterdrug is given, such as one that is wet in the first degree.[64]

Writers of theoretical medicine argued whether a drug had an absolute scale or whether its qualities were relative to the individual patient; thus a high fever in an old patient needs a less severe cold medicine than in a more naturally sanguine younger patient. But also an individual patient's constitution (*complexio*) has remarkable variations such as age, zodiac sign according to birth and appearance of the malady, personality, individual membranes, sex, and race. For each drug, there are diurnal variations that must be considered. In addition, the question arose that if simples had all the possible combinations, then what was the advantage and action of a compound?[65] Did a combination of simples, that is to say a compound, merely act as the accumulated merits of the simples therein or did the compound itself assume different characteristics because of the union? Moreover, a disease was seldom treated as a unit; instead the symptoms were individually treated. Pneumonia, for instance, would theoretically have various drugs administered to treat each of its symptoms separately, such as high temperature, an intermittent chill, pain in the chest, rusty sputum, cyanosis, and bloody urine. Not only were there four degrees for each drug but each degree has three *numeri* or subdivisions, and as many as twelve total.[66] One drug may have as many as twenty virtues.[67] Naturally a good physician had also read the horoscope.[68]

[64] The complexity in prescribing drugs was probably what led to the search for "wonder drugs" or occult medicines, the knowledge of which was thought to be unknown or concealed by the ancients. These universal drugs, e.g., ambergris and lignum aloes, were also sometimes known as cordials by virtue of the allegation that they strengthened the heart. Their qualities were so mysterious and transcending that the normal, complex process of drug administration could be suspended. Roger Bacon, *De retardatione accidentium senectutis*, ed. A. G. Little and E. Withington; cf. "Introduction," xxxviii-xlii.

[65] *Circa instans* (n. 56 above) 1: "Quidam non ociosa proponitur cur medicine fuerint invente composite cum omnis virtus, que compositis inest, in simplicibus reperiatur." Roger Bacon, *Antidotarius* ed. A. G. Little and E. Withington (Oxford 1928) 105, observed that complex medicines have complex operations: "Et nec est admirandum si in medicina composita est operatio duplicata, que in simplicibus non habetur, quia a duobus suam trahit proprietatem, scilicet a prima compositione que ab elementis fit, et a secunda que ab arte, quod simplex non facit." And he added that a compound may have greater or lesser powers than the sum of its components (113).

[66] McVaugh, "Apud antiquos" (n. 63 above) 20, lines 76ff.

[67] Bartholomeus, *Practica*, in Salvatore de Renzi, *Collectio Salernitana*, 5 vols. (Naples 1856 4.325: "Unde Ypocras: Vita brevis, ars vero longa, vita brevis ad artis comprehensionem, ars vero longo propter multitudinem et rerum difficultatem huic arti subiacentium. Multitudo manet; de difficultate autem patet. Difficile est quidem medicinarum virtutes invenire, cum unius herbe virtutes sint (?) la co (?) anplius (?), cum nondum invente sint ex eius nisi XX aut plus minus et sic de ceteris."

[68] Cf. n. 51 above; see also C. Talbot, "A Mediaeval Physician's *Vade Mecum*," JHMAS 16 (1961) 213-233, and Vern Bullough, "Medieval Bologna and the Development of Medical Education," BHM 32 (1958) 212.

All these determinations must be made by the humble physician. It is no small surprise that we begin finding recipes with more than a hundred ingredients—the physician, burdened with all those factors, was trying to touch on all contingencies.[69] The immediate value of Islamic pharmacology was certainly not its theory.[70]

Considering the combination and variation of each drug, all this would be complex enough, but there was little certainty as to the drugs themselves. First, there are discrepancies between various authorities as to the degrees of each drug. Second, Islamic medicine added hundreds of new drugs;[71] and third, the translator had often transliterated Arabic names for drugs into the Roman alphabet without seeking to determine the Greek, Roman, or vernacular equivalent. For example, during the thirteenth century there were five words in circulation which meant "amber": *karabe* (Arabic), *succinum* (Latin), *lugerion* (latinized Greek), *electrum* (latinized Greek), and *Bernstein* (German).[72] In some learned and elaborate pharmaceutical prescriptions of the thirteenth to fifteenth centuries, which list about one hundred drugs, there appear two

[69] For examples of elaborate polypharmacy, see Mesue, *Iannis Mesuae medici charissimi opera* (Venice 1581); Nicholas Myrepsos (d. ca. 1280), *Nicolai Alexandrini* (Inglostadt 1543); Peter of Abano (d. 1316), *De aegritudinibus cordis in universiali* as published in Mesue, *Opera* (Venice 1581); and later versions of Nicholas, *Antidotarium.* For the complexity of using the pulse for diagnosis, see Boyd Hill, Jr., "A Medieval German Pulse Tract," *Medical History* (MH) 9 (1965) 72-76. The problem of identifying the drugs would seem to be met by the large number of medical dictionaries and glossaries which were a product of this confused period. (See MacKinney, n. 57 above). My own experience in working with these works, however, is that far from solving nomenclature problems of the writers own times, the authors were pedantically infatuated with earlier authorities. I refer to the following: Simon of Genoa (fl. late thirteenth century), *Synonima Simonis Genuensis* (Milan 1473); Giacomo de Dondi of Padua (d. ca. 1359), *Aggregator de medicinis simplicibus* (Venice 1543), Matteo Silvatico (ca. 1342) *Opus pandecta medicine Matthei Silvatici* (1521); Platearius, "*Der Traktat Liberiste* (die sogennanten Glossae Platearii) aus dem Breslauer Codex Salernitanus," ed. Erwin Müller (dissertation, Würzburg 1942).

[70] Max Meyerhof, in "Arabian Pharmacology in North Africa, Sicily and the Iberian Peninsula," *Ciba symposia* 6 (1944) 1872, comments: "In looking back at the various epochs of Arabian medicine one may conclude that despite the tremendous number of books that they wrote, the Arabs did not advance essentially beyond the Greeks in the theory of pharmacology. They faithfully adopted Galen's theory of the three [sic] degrees of pharmacological action, and in their systematic manner added only further subdivisions. . . . The true service rendered by the Arabs, however, is that they enriched materia medica." One possible later benefit of Islamic pharmacological theory is cogently argued by Michael McVaugh, in "Arnald of Villanova and Bradwardine's Law," *Isis* 58 (1967) 56-64, who believes that the mathematical skills developed by the pharmacological theorists influenced the Merton College's or Bradwardine's Law on Motion.

[71] Alexander Tschirch, ed., *Handbuch der Pharmakognosis*, 3 vols., ed. 2 (Leipzig 1910) 1.2.594-615.

[72] J. M. Riddle, "Pomum ambrae and Ambergris in Plague Remedies," *Sudhoffs Archiv* 48 (1964) 111-122; *idem*, "Amber and Ambergris in materia medica during Antiquity and the Middle Ages" (Ph. D. Dissertation, University of North Carolina, Chapel Hill 1963).

or more words in the same recipe for the same herb or mineral.[73] The conclusion is simple: no one compounded such prescriptions. Would an apothecary or physician have two or more jars on his shelf with the same ingredients in each jar and differentiated only by the outside labels? Not likely. What we have is a learned man who is copying from various sources all the drugs he can find for a specific ailment. In other words many of these documents were not used in medical practice because they could not be used. Medical theory in pharmacy was becoming less related to practice.[74] An Arabic handbook written about 1150 has about three thousand medical plants but the Geniza documents of about the same period mention only about one hundred and twenty medical items in various everyday prescriptions, business, and other letters.[75] The working pharmacopoeia must have been much smaller than the learned knowledge of pharmacy. This would explain the manuscripts, known as quid pro quo, which are guides for substituting drugs, the earliest of which appears in the thirteenth century.[76] Under the burden of an unworkable theory, despite language problems, the general practitioner shows evidence of attempting to relate experiences, probably chiefly by ignoring what he did not understand.

According to Heinrich Schipperges,[77] Islamic medicine was largely clinical until the mid-tenth-century, when it began turning towards theory. Following the same pattern as Islamic medicine, late twelfth-century Europe moved from clinical medicine toward "learned medicine."[78] The Arabic writings were

[73] See n. 69 above; Riddle, "Amber and Ambergris in materia medica" (n. 72 above); and Magister Salerno, *Compendium*, in De Renzi (n. 67 above) 3.52-68.

[74] Roger Bacon (n. 51 above) 141-148 says of his day: "Another defect is due to ignorance of simple drugs, so that the physicians do not know what they use. . . . The generality of physicians cannot recognize their simple drugs but trust ignorant apothecaries who, as the physicians themselves know, aim only at deceiving them. . . . A second reason for the ignorance of natural philosophy is the perversity of translation. . . . One is ignorant of languages from which medicine is taken. For the authentic books are full of Arabic, Greek, Chaldean (Persian?) and Hebrew, so that one cannot know what the authorities mean, as is clear in numberless places. And because they do not know Greek, Arabic and Hebrew from which innumerable terms are extracted in the books of the Latins, owing to their ignorance of these, also they can neither understand nor practice medicine."

[75] S. D. Goiten, "The Medical Profession in the Light of the Cairo Geniza Documents," *Hebrew Union College Annual* 34 (1963) 189.

[76] London BM MS Harley 2378, pages 208-213; Prague, Univ. Knihovna MS XII F 11 (2349), thirteenth-fourteenth century, fol. 189v; Vatican MS 5373, thirteenth-fourteenth century, fols. 36v-41; Vienna, Nationalbibliothek MS Pal. 5371, fifteenth century, fols. 121v-3; Brno, Univ. Knihovna, MS Mk 107, fifteenth century, fols. 173-4v; Copenhagen, Kongelige Bibl. MS 1653 (760), thirteenth century, fol. 148.

[77] Heinrich Schipperges, "Die arabische Medizin als Praxis und als Theorie," *Sudhoffs Archiv* 43 (1959) 317-328. This same opinion is held by Talbot (n. 33 above) 35-37.

[78] Paul O. Kristeller in "Beitrag der Schule von Salerno zur Entwicklung der Scholastischen Wissenschaft im 12. Jahrhundert," *Artes Liberales von der antiken Bildung zur Wissenschaft des Mittelalters*, ed. Josef Koch (Leiden 1959) 84-90, believes that by the mid-twelfth century the school at Salerno was turning towards theory, philosophical speculation, and systema-

well received but only partially understood. Hunain ibn Ishaq's *Isagoge in artem parvam*, translated by Constantine, opens with: "Medicina dividitur in duas partes, id est in theoricam et practicam."[79] And Avicenna, translated by Gerard of Cremona, began his *Canon* with this repeated statement that medicine is divided between theory and practice. Avicenna's translator continues by explaining that a division exists between *scire* and *operari*.[80] The Islamic writers warned that experience was necessary, but, because of the division of medicine in two parts, emphasis and dignity were given to theoretical medicine. In discussing why theoretical consideration ought to be dominant in determining and defining a medicine's usefulness, the Latin translation of Haly Abbas went so far as to say that one could neither know nor understand a drug's medicinal action by experimenting.[81] Ricardus Anglicus said practical medicine was "greatly inferior and more undignified."[82] Roger Bacon wrote:

> A third defect is that the generality of physicians give themselves up to disputes about numberless problems and useless arguments, and

tization in medicine. This process was progressive to the extent that medicine could be placed beside theology and law as a higher faculty. In his earlier article ("The School at Salerno," BHM 17 [1945] 138-194, esp. 155), Professor Kristeller says medical historians have emphasized the practical side of early Salernitan medicine rather than the "speculative element," which he regards as progressive. Professor Kristeller argues convincingly for the contribution of speculative medicine to philosophy but it is less clear that people suffering from disease benefitted. Talbot (n. 33 above, 44) comments: "If the medical writers of the school of Salerno can be credited with an important role in the diffusion of Aristotelian doctrines in the West, it can only be viewed from the medical point of view as the introduction of a wooden horse."

[79] As quoted from Basil MS D I 6, thirteenth century, fol. 1 by H. Schipperges (n. 60 above) 33.

[80] *Liber canonis* 1.1.1, fol. 1 "Potest autem aliquis dicere quod medicina dividitur in theoricam et practicam sed tu totam ipsam posuisti theoricam: cum dixisti quod est scientie . . . Cum ergo de medicina dixerimus, quod eius est theorica et ex ea est practica, non est existimamdum quod velimus dicere quod una divisionum medicinae est scire et altera operari." There was certainly recognition that practice and theory go hand-in-hand, as is shown by Haly Abbas, 1.3., fol. lv: "Omnis ergo medicine aut theorica est: aut practica theorica est perfecta noticia rerum solo intellectu capiendarum: subiecta memorie rerum operandarum. Practica est suiectam theoricam demonstrare in propatulo sensum et operatione manuum secundum praeuntia theorice intellectum."

[81] *Liber pantegni-practice* (10.1.fol. 127b) asserts that theoretical considerations are more important than practical experiences in determining a medicine's usefulness because life is too short to experience all. He concludes: "Experientes vero non potuerint hoc cognoscere vel comprehendere cum semper fere uno et eodem medicamine multo et longo experto tempore et infirmorum multiplicitate." And Roger Bacon (n. 65 above 103-104) said of judging compound medicines: "Sed iudicium quod habet ex simplicibus non potest sciri nisi per ratio cinationem." But he added a balance: "Sed quod habetur ex tota forma sua non potest sciri nisi per experimentum." And he emphasized one point of Haly Abbas: "Et de medicina composita intelligendum est illud quod Haly supra Tegni dicit, quod quelibet medicina duobus, modis ab artifice debet experiri, scilicet per experimentum ratiocinationis et per experimentum certitudinis."

[82] Quoted by Talbot (n. 33 above) 62.

> give no time to experience as they ought. Thirty years ago they used to give all their time to experience, but now by the art of "Topics" and "Elenchi" they multiply infinite casual questions, and still more infinite dialectic and sophistic arguments in which they get absorbed, so that they are ever seeking and never discovering the truth. For discovery is by the path of sense, memory and experience especially in the applied sciences of which medicine is one.[83]

The new Latin translators were more prejudiced toward theory than the Islamic writers. In the main, the Latin translators of the medical works, such as Constantine and Gerard, were not themselves practicing physicians. Constantine had been a merchant who saw a need in the West for medical works, and so he put some into Latin.[84] Consequently, the translators in the selection of their material chose the more theoretical, philosophical works and omitted the more clinical.[85] In a letter to the Abbot Desiderius of Monte Cassino, Constantine reveals his concern that so few considered medicine a science.[86] Constantine, for instance, selected only the theoretical books of Haly Abbas to translate and left to later translators the practical books. One can only speculate what might have happened had the more clinical Arabic writers, who were more influenced by East Asian science, been the Latin West's first contact with the mass of Arabic medical authorities.[87] What cultural

[83] Bacon (n. 51 above) 144.

[84] Ferrarius, quoted by R. Creutz, "Die Ehrenrettung Konstantins von Afrika," SMGBO 18 (1931) 40-41, from Erfurt MS Ampol. Oct. 62[a], thirteenth century, fol. 49v-50: "Constantinus autem sarracenus exstitit. Mercator tamen, qui mercationis causa huc venit et multas mercationes secum attulit qui cum per plateam pergeret. Ad curiam sancti Petri ascendit in qua erat peroptimus medicus, frater principis, qui abbas de curia nuncupabatur. Constantinus ergo ipsum urinas iudicantem intuens et nostram linguam penitus ignorans, servis sarracenis pretium tribuit, ut ei iudicaret interpretarentur. . . . Constantius ergo rediens in Africam tribus continuis annis physicae diligentem adhibuit operam, et demum, multos accipiens libros, huc rediit."

[85] I am grateful to Professor Lynn White, jr., for this observation.

[86] PL 150.1563-1526: "Multi reverendissime Pater, dubitant, medicina scientiane sit necne, dumque ipsam ad artibus et scientiis excludunt, excluduntur ipsi a praestantissima artium medicina; dum enim tempus inutilibus quaestionibus sophisticis terunt inutiliter, fit ut unquam ad veram untilemque speculationem artis perveniant. Acuti homines disputant, illam non esse scientiam, quae magis quam ulla alia de naturae operibus tractat; cohaerent autem omnia opera naturae certissimo ordine, et erorum principia sunt certiora aliis, nec facile inveniunt artem quae ita ordine procedat, et ita aliud ex alio intelligatur. Absolutum nemo profiteatur se philosophum nisi teneat haec, alia enim omnia huic, ut omnis philosophiae sacram excipimus philosophiam fini, deserviunt."

[87] Joseph Needham, *Clerks and Craftsmen in China and the West* (Cambridge 1970) 15: "Here we come upon a very interesting fact. It is not that there was no contact between Arabic civilization and East Asian science; quite the contrary. But for some reason or other, when the translations were being made from Arabic into Latin, it was always the famous authors of Mediterranean antiquity who were chosen and not the books of Islamic scholars concerning the science of India and China."

impact would Rhazes have produced if he had been introduced into the West before Avicenna?[88] As it was, when Rhazes was translated, he was placed in a conceptual framework molded by Avicenna and his like.[89] Roger Bacon noted this when he wrote:

> Avicenna was a philosopher rather than a physician, as the translator of his book says, and at the end of his translation he regrets that he took the trouble, especially as he found the works of Rhazes and others complete both in practice and theory. So the Arabs do not use Avicenna's works chiefly, but others, and the Latins who practice according to his book often go wrong, as the experienced know.[90]

The problems for the Western practitioners were even greater than those of their Islamic counterparts. Even though Islamic writers advocated clinical medicine, Western translators and writers were more interested in theory which, when understood, was too elaborate for the general practitioner. As the general practitioners became aware, albeit very slowly, of "how behind" they were in modern medicine, some doubtlessly felt obliged to try to understand the new theories and to change accordingly. By trying, some may have compromised old but valid ways. Generally speaking, early medieval pharmacy was the simple knowledge that this-or-that drug is good for such-and-such ailment. The new learned medicine was a bittersweet pill and was not taken as directed.

Despite these problems practical medicine continued. At any time there are probably more physicians than all other men of science put together, and the body of medical literature is proportionally large.[91] By far the greater part of the late medieval literature, contrary to that of the earlier period, is theoretically oriented, and this makes it difficult for modern scholars to learn of the rank-and-file physician. The happy find of a late fourteenth-century physician's *vade mecum* gives us a rare opportunity to view the practice of an ordinary physician and to expand our knowledge beyond what C. H. Talbot

[88] Mirko Draxen Grmek, in "Influsso di Avicenna sulla medicina occidentale del medio evo," *Salerno* 1 (1967) 6-21, recognizes that the impact of Avicenna on Europe may be construed as being retrogressive. "Averroes is Avicenna gone mad," writes Talbot (n. 33 above, 35) about the contributions of a later philosopher whose works were translated and taken as a medical authority. R. Creutz (n. 60 above, 7) gives as a reason for rejecting Peter the Deacon's account of Constantine's travels that Constantine would have been in Bagdad a hundred years after the death of Rhazes. If he had known Rhazes's works—and surely he would have, had he been to Bagdad—might Constantine not likely have selected Rhazes for translation? See also, Owsei Temkin, "A Medieval Translation of Rhazes's *Clinical Observations*," BHM 12 (1942) 102-117.

[89] Grmek (n. 88 above, 16) quotes Arnold of Villanova as saying of Avicenna: "Qui in medicina majorem partem medicorum latinorum infatuat."

[90] Bacon (n. 51 above) 150.

[91] Sarton (n. 6 above) 2.64.

calls the "highly successful and celebrated doctors."[92] It is a brief digest, designed to hang from a physician's belt as he made house calls. Written at Oxford, the manuscript contains information needed for a diagnosis; it has a calendar, canons of the eclipses of the sun and moon, a table of the planets, rules for phlebotomy, and descriptions of urine. From this manuscript we learn that, hundreds of years after the discoveries at Salerno, the ordinary physician who owned it was not discernably affected by theoretical medicine of his modern period.[93]

Another means of gaining a glimpse of practical medicine is to study the lapidary literature, most of which were guides to the use of minerals in medicine.[94] The lapidaries were less subject than the herbals to scholastic discourse. Perhaps the reason is their closer adherence to magic; consequently they have been less studied than the herbals as an antecedent to modern science. Then again, of all medieval literature, the *Pestschriften* are relatively more clinical than other late medieval medical writing; they contain generally empirical judgments by medical men faced with the trauma of the Black Death when none of the old theories seemed to work.[95] Psychologically we can picture a man, who had made hundreds of house calls to no avail only to see death, and who wants to record his thoughts before he too was stricken.[96] One would think, if some evidence were not to the contrary, that those physicians who lived through such an experience would throw away old books and begin anew. But there was a return by them to the old ways,[97] and the reputation of doctors who had apparently done next to nothing seems to have increased following the Death.

Most of the late medieval documents have a heavy theoretical basis. A study of early fifteenth-century *consilia*, that is, medical opinions, written by a very learned Italian physician, reveals that the prestigious physician frequently

[92] Talbot (n. 68 above) 213.

[93] *Ibid.* 213-233, esp. 217.

[94] John Riddle, "Lithotherapy in the Middle Ages. . . . Lapidaries Considered as Medical Texts," *Pharmacy in History* 12 (1970) 39-50.

[95] Karl Sudhoff (*Sudhoffs Archiv* 4-17 [1910-1925] with index in 17) lists some 281 *Pestschriften* and discusses 141 with the texts of many published. British plague-tracts are listed by Dorothea W. Singer and Annie Anderson, *Catalogue of Latin and Vernacular Plague-Texts in Great Britain and Eire* (London 1950). The best study so far—much needs yet be done—is A. M. Campbell, *The Black Death and Men of Learning* (New York 1931). See also John Riddle, "Pomum ambrae" (n. 72 above).

[96] Perhaps the reason for this outburst of writing was the same as the one that caused a seventeenth century rabbi to explain why he was writing his medical book: "In a town in which there is no doctor available, but a scholar or wise man is found, he will be able by the help of this book to understand, to study and to search for a remedy for the sick"—quoted by Zimmels (n. 35 above) 15.

[97] Morris H. Saffron, review of Vern Bullough, *The Development of Medicine as a Profession*, *Speculum* 44 (1969) 450.

did not even see the patient.[98] The advice was written in response to a referral from another physician or a wealthy patient. The nature of the advice was a learned discourse on this or that point with frequent citations of the chief Islamic and classical authorities. These consilia seem more like a lawyer's brief with authorities quoted as if they were some former decisions of precedent, rather than a major concern for the health of the patient. A triumph is scored if there is some resolution of an apparent contradiction between, say, Avicenna and Galen. Sold to the patient for a high sum, possibly the entire treatise describes only a symptom and omits a diagnosis, much less a prognosis.[99] A great paradox exists here. Probably at no other period in history have physicians enjoyed such respected and prestigious places in society,[100] and the physicians, if we judge literally and quantitatively, were practicing some medicine suspect by modern clinical standards.[101] By the fifteenth century, medical texts were largely philological, not clinical. The medicine of most of our documents is more concerned with scholastic discourse than with the patient. Surely, if medicine were implemented as written, the short-run loss was with the patient. Probably, medicine was not so practiced, however.

Measuring the interaction between theory and practice is extremely difficult. On one hand the theoreticians seemed to have the upper hand. There existed side by side with them a larger number of practitioners—now called charlatans and quacks—who carried the burden of responsibility for caring for the sick and injured. They, however, were under ever-increasing attack.[102] The prestige

[98] Dean Putnam Lockwood, *Ugo Benzi, Medieval Philosopher and Physician* (*1376-1439*) (Chicago 1951) 47.

[99] These judgments were formed by Lockwood (47-54) but Lynn Thorndike, in "Consilia and More Works in Manuscript by Gentile da Foligno," MH 3 (1959) 8, submits a contrary opinion: "Unlike the commentaries upon Avicenna and other past authorities, the *consilia* faced existing conditions, dealt with present problems, and show us what actual practice was like." Many of the *Pestschriften* are in the form of *consilia* and exemplify Thorndike's judgment. Nonetheless, my reading of the general evidence supports Lockwood's thesis. See also Henry Sigerist, "Karl Sudhoff the Mediaevalist," BHM 2 (1934) 24.

[100] Lynn Thorndike, "When Medicine Was in Flower," BHM 33 (1959) 110.

[101] As examples of medical men who were not concerned with practice but in recovering past theories, see Pearl Kibre's studies, "Cristoforo Barzizza, Professor of Medicine at Padua," BHM 11 (1942) 389-398; *idem*, "Giovanni Garzoni of Bologna (1419-1505), Professor of Medicine and Defender of Astrology," *Isis* 58 (1967) 504-514.

[102] For example, E. A. Hammond, "Physicians in Medieval English Religious Houses," BHM 32 (1958) 105-120; *idem*, "Incomes of Mediaeval English Doctors," JHMAS 15 (1960) 167-169; *idem*, "The Westminster Abbey Infirmarer's Rolls as a Source of Medical History," BHM 39 (1965) 261-276; Claudius F. Mayer, "A Medieval English Leech Book and Its 14th-Century Poem of Bloodletting," BHM 7 (1939) 381-391; Ida B. Jones, "Popular Medical Knowledge in Fourteenth-Century English Litterature," BHM 5 (1937) 405-451, 538-588; Charles F. Mullett, "John Lydgate: A Mirror of Medieval Medicine," BHM 22 (1948) 403-415. One obvious group of non-university-trained practitioners were the numerous Jewish medical men who were in the main excluded from the university. Nonetheless, their reputation as physicians was high; cf. Cecil Roth, "The Qualification of Jewish Physicians in the

of university medicine produced an ever-growing attempt to regulate all practitioners and bring them up to "standards." Although we are used to associating this with progress, the professionalization campaign may have had harmful side effects and, in any case, served only to accentuate the split begun at Salerno.[103] The elaborate medical works of late Salerno and Montpellier, the polypharmacy treatises and the consilia, represent attempts to intellectualize medicine while the *vade mecum*, the lapidaries, and the *Pestschriften* show little success in obtaining goals. Rhazes once wrote a letter entitled: "The Reason Why the Ignorant Physicians, the Common People, and the Women in the Cities are More Successful than Men of Science in Treating Certain Diseases, and the Physicians' Excuse for This."[104] The conflict between theoretical and practical medicine could not have been a happy one. On one hand, the practical medical man had his bases for working challenged while the university-centered doctor did not succeed in making medicine a pure science and in expelling the nonformally trained from the ranks. There were always some, like Nicholas of Montpellier (late thirteenth century or early fourteenth century) who assailed Galen for saying, "Physician, how can you cure, if you are ignorant of the cause?" Nicholas, as others must have, advocated abandoning the "new learning" in medicine and relying instead on the old, tried, traditional remedies.[105]

In the late fourteenth century and the early fifteenth century an Italian debate reveals the failure of the complete professional aspirations of theoretical medicine. The debate concerned whether law or medicine was the higher learning. Both law and medicine were likened unto one another because lawyers and physicians do similar things, namely, examine the specifics of a case and apply the proper legal or medical authorities. These scholastic debators concluded that medicine had not succeeded in detaching itself from the magic and the mechanical arts and thus had not become sufficiently

---

Middle Ages," *Speculum* 28 (1953) 834-843. Antonin, Archbishop of Florence (1389-1459), says that the qualities of a good physician should be *honestas*, *maturitas*, and *practicalis* (Diepgen, n. 20 above, 10).

[103] Vern Bullough, "The Development of Medical Guilds at Paris," *Medievalia et humanistica* 12 (1958) 34. A University of Paris regulation of 1271 forbids the illegal practice of medicine: "Statutem facultatis medicinae contra illicite practicantes, scilicet ne qui Judaeus in aliquam personam fidei christianae chirurgice seu medicinaliter operari praesumat et ne quis chirurgus, apothecarius vel herbarius metas artificii sui excedat," Prevet (n. 47 above) 1.3. But it was not until the fifteenth century that a licentiate in arts was required before a licentiate in medicine at Paris, see Bullough, "The Medieval Medical University at Paris," BHM 31 (1953) 201.

[104] Ibn al-Nadim, *Fihrist*. ed. and trans. Bayard Dodge, 2 vols. (New York 1970) 2.708.

[105] As cited by Lynn Thorndike, *A History of Magic and Experimental Science*, 8 vols. (New York 1923-1958) 2.768-769.

intellectualized. Since law was not subject to such degradation, law was considered "higher" than medicine.[106]

One branch of medicine, surgery, seems to have advanced steadily through this same period when pharmacy was slipping.[107] Such noted surgeons as Guy de Chauliac (d. ca. 1368) even modified Hippocratic and Galenic humoral theory.[108] Why? Because surgery was considered always a craft or an art, it was consequently little subjected to a theory unrelated to practice.[109] For this

[106] Coluccio Salutati, *De nobilitate legum et medicinae*, ed. Eugenio Garin (Florence 1947) chapters 2, 4, 8, 11: "Verum doces: nonne nobilior est progressu legibus medicina? . . . Verum in isto crescendi cursu nobilior legum progressus fuit, qui numquam a ratione discesserit, quam medicine, que cepit at incantationibus magicis et in experimenta procedens tandem ad rationem pervenerit, quam multotiens vanam ostendit vel experimentorum evidentia, vel rerum exitus, qui numquam fiunt, ratione deprehensus. Ergo quintadecimem conclusionem adiciam: quod magnitudo legalis scientie, ad quam leges ad initio modice pervenerunt, conflictatione solum et examine rationis sine dubitatione processit," chap. 2. Allessandro Braccesi (Paul O. Kristeller, "An Unknown Correspondence of Alessandro Braccesi," *Classical Mediaeval and Renaissance Studies in Honor of Berthold Louis Ullman*, 2 vols. [Rome 1964] 2. fol. 138v of Bodl. MS Auct. F. 2.17), writing to a friend to persuade him not to go into medicine, says: "Cognitantem me diutus non in medicine artis facultatem, quippe que ipsa per se nobilis est atque insignis, sed in eius professores ignaros quidem as ineruditos aliquid scribere, ad id facile presentia inpulisset consilium tuum mi frater, quod de medicorum disciplina consequenda te iam cepisse mihi nuper aperuisti si modo per ocium licuisset, Nam etisi antea sponte ad hanc rem satis animatus esse videbar, tamen post cognitam huiusmodi voluntatem tuam magis eram ad scribendum incensus." See also Francesco Petrarca, *Investive contra medicum*, ed. Pier G. Ricci (Rome 1950); and, for analysis, R. de Rosa "Die Stellung der Medizin in der Frührenaissance. Das Problem der Beziehung zwischen Theorie und Praxis im Streit der Wissenschaften " *Aktuelle Probleme aus der Geschichte der Medizin*, "Proceedings of the 19th International Congress for the History of Medicine" (Basel 1966) 259-266.

[107] Talbot (n. 33 above) 88. The existence of surgery during pre-Salernitan times is well attested—MacKinney (n. 9 above) 38 and passim; MacKinney, "The Beginnings of Western Scientific Anatomy: New Evidence and a Revision in Interpretation of Mondeville's Rome " MH 6 (1962) 233-239; Payne (n. 33 above) 62; and Grattan and Singer (n. 30 above) 12. A. Pazzini ("Significato della storia della medicina e genesi delle nuove idee e scoperte," *Congresso Italiano di storia della medicina* 15 [1957] 7-15) says that medieval surgery did not originate in Salerno but descended from Tuscan-Aemilian centers—cited by Bartolomeo Olivieri, "Questioni intorno all' spongia soporifera,'" *Salerno* 2 (1968) 44-45; cf. Henry Sigerist, "A Salernitan Student's Surgical Notebook," BHM 14 (1943) 505-516 and Corner 15. By far the most thorough study of surgery is Karl Sudhoff, *Beiträge zur Geschichte der Chirurgie im Mittelalter*, 2 vols. (Leipzig 1914-1918). Sudhoff (2.93-1021) gives a list of surgical writings in Latin during the early Middle Ages.

[108] Margaret S. Ogden, "Guy de Chauliac's Theory of the Humors," JHMAS 24 (1969) 272-291, esp. 272.

[109] In *Antidotarius* 1.14, Henry of Mondeville, a late thirteenth-century to early fourteenth-century surgeon, wrote: "Ex dictis actoribus [Averrohoes, Avicenna, Haly Abbas] patet quod cyrurgia est multum practica et valde parum theorica et quod operando addiscitur. Ex quibus sequitur quod curyrgicus, ut sit, non teneatur qualitates singularum medicinarum simplicium aut compositarum cognoscere exquisite nec etiam graduare praecise " ed. Julius Leopold Pagel, *Die Chirurgie des Heinrich von Mondeville* (Berlin 1892) 515.

reason theoretical medicine considered surgery outside medicine. The acceptance of surgeons (barbers) into medicine's professional image of itself was long in coming, except possibly in Italy.[110]

To be certain, theoretical medicine was not without its merit, although it has been oversold. In the long run, theoretical medicine benefited the patient because it created a body of learning that required formal training,[111] a perceived requisite to modern medicine. Scholastic or theoretical medicine was so voluminous, so rigorous to learn, so intricate to implement that it required the best minds, not the neighborhood midwife, the old woodsman who could repair a broken bone of dog or man alike, or the leech who knew the herbs. According to a new definition of *scientia*, medicine became partially a "science" as Constantine had wanted it to be, and it was studied by some of the best students in most of the universities,[112] but it lost some of its older characteristics as an art. One reason the Church began to forbid its clergy from practicing medicine is simply that medicine demanded too much time to learn, much less to practice.[113]

Let me conclude. Relative to the early Middle Ages (ca. 500-1000) and the early Salernitan period (ca. 900-1100), retrogression in competence of medical practice is suggested by a literal interpretation of most theoretical works, but we must try to understand who was doing the writing and for what purposes. Some modern scholars, as observed above, suggest that early pharmacy lit-

[110] Vern L. Bullough, in "The Development of Medical Guilds" (n. 103 above, 33-40, esp. 37) says that the royal ordinance dealing with surgery was issued by Philip IV in 1311 and the year 1356 saw the recognition of surgeons as a faculty. See also Vern Bullough, *The Development of Medicine as a Profession* (New York 1966) 59ff., where he cites a 1239 regulation at Montpellier specifically excluding surgeons from the university. (Cf. Bullough, "The Teaching of Surgery at the University of Montpellier in the Thirteenth Century," JHMAS 15 [1960] 202-204; and Kibre [n. 36 above, 1-20, esp. 6ff.].)

[111] Bullough, *The Development* (n. 110 above) 4-5.

[112] Armand Maurer, "Ockham's Conception of the Unity of Science," *Mediaeval Studies* 20 (1958) 98-112, esp. 108. As examples of the word *scientia* applied to medicine, see Prevet (n. 47 above) 1.25; Bullough, *The Development* (n. 110 above) 4ff.; and Karl Sudhofff, "Eine Verteidigung der Heilkunde aus der Zeiten der 'Mönchsmedizin,'" *Sudhoffs Archiv* 7 (1913) 225. Dean P. Lockwood (n. 98 above, 7) says that even in Ugo Benzi's time of the early fifteenth century, the distinctly medical portion of the body of knowledge required for a physician to know was hardly enough "to occupy one intelligent person's time." When one observes the complexity of the theory, the difficulty of acquiring texts, and the amount of material to be absorbed, I believe that a medical student of the late Middle Ages had more material assigned to master than does his modern-day counterpart. But Lockwood observes (6) that there were physicians contemporary with Ugo, but younger than he, who professed only medicine and it had little philosophical content.

[113] This explanation is advanced by E. A. Hammond, in "Physicians" (n. 102 above, 119-120) who says, however, "no single explanation is adequate." Hammond's thesis is accepted by Bullough, "A Note on Medical Care in Medieval English Hospitals," BHM 35 (1961) 74. Pearl Kibre (n. 36 above, 4) says that by mid-fourteenth century the prohibition of clerics to practice medicine was being liberalized.

erature was little more than handwriting exercises. Yet many of these same scholars marvel at the return in the late twelfth century to speculative medicine and, thereby, assume that the documents of the period reflect a "progressive" medicine. My observations are different. Many of the elaborate, polypharmacy treatises of the thirteenth and fourteenth centuries could only have been mental exercise, while, as postulated above, the early medieval pharmacy literature reveals actual use by practitioners. By the late thirteenth-century medical theory challenged the simpler practices of the general medical men. To determine, however, actual progress or decline in medicine may be impossible. Nevertheless, late medieval pharmacological theory could not have initially improved pharmaceutical practice. Most of the ordinary physicians recoiled from the prolix arguments and the theoretical orientation of procedure. In the West, when the gap between theory and practice was increasing, the general medical man did not loose his strong empirical prejudices and, with them, his self-confidence to practice medicine, despite the move to professionalize medicine.

In the West, what we call modern medicine owes much more to the practical physician than has been acknowledged. The precursors of Paré and Paracelsus are as much the unnamed, unsung general practitioners as the illustrious men like Avicenna and Peter of Abano. What rescued Western medicine from undue subservience to theoretical medicine was the anti-intellectualism that characterized the early Middle Ages and was reinforced by the *devotio moderna* and mysticism of the late Middle Ages. The anti-intellectual movement, represented by Saint Francis of Assisi, blocked extreme emphasis on theory of knowledge.

Around A.D. 830 Al-Hahiz observed, "The curious thing is that the Greeks are interested in theory but do not bother with practice, whereas the Chinese are very interested in practice and do not bother with theory."[114] Carolingian education, Salerno, and the translators brought Hellenic theory back into vogue. In the West, however, while not remaining impervious to it, the general medical practitioner remained a bit "Chinese": he assimilated little of the frequently unworkable theory. He was a doer, little of a reader, and seldom a writer. He was as much a contributor to modern medicine as was his highly acclaimed intellectual rival who speculated as to causes.

[114] Needham (n. 87 above) 39.

ADDENDA

VI p. 160, n. 11. Added words in italics: Varros' seven liberal arts were in his work *Disciplinae. Vid. Cambridge History of Classical Literature. II Latin Literature*. E.J. Kenney and W.V. Clausen, eds. (Cambridge: Cambridge University Press, 1982), p. 286.

VI p. 175, line 13. Added words in italics: "This would explain the manuscripts, known as quid pro quo, which are guides for substituting drugs, the earliest *one* of *which that is attributed to Dioscorides* appears in the thirteenth century."

VII

Book Reviews, Lectures, and Marginal Notes

Three Previously Unknown Sixteenth Century Contributors to Pharmacy, Medicine and Botany—

Ioannes Manardus, Franciscus Frigimelica, and Melchior Guilandinus*

IN accepting with thanks the Edward Kremers Award, I would like to share with you some aspects of my research having to do with historical developments in the profession of pharmacy. In working on a long project on Dioscorides, the Greek author of *De materia medica*, I discovered three written documents by early sixteenth century authors which were not intended for publication. One is a letter which serves as a book review, another is lecture notes, and the third is notes penned in the margins of a published book. I believe that I can see in these unexplored writings indications of changes occurring in the fields of pharmacy, medicine and botany before such changes are measured in more celebrated works deliberately written for publication.

*The 1979 Edward Kremers Award Address, Anaheim, California.

Part I: Ioannes Manardus; Book Reviewer

Letters to authors or about the authors served as the principal method of reviewing books during the Renaissance. Sentiments range from wholesome praise, abject flattery, bitter, biting criticisms and even on occasion judicious evaluations. Sixteenth century "book reviews" in personal letters by the gentle humanists were often more vituperative than they are in many of today's learned journals, excepting a few like PHARMACY IN HISTORY. Such an example of the sixteenth century epistolatory reviews is found in the letters of Ioannes Manardus.[1] The first letter was written to Marcellus Virgilus Adrianus. By October 15, 1518, Marcellus, a Florentine and benefactor to Machiavelli, completed and published locally a Latin translation of Dioscorides' work,[2] thereby fulfilling his childhood ambition.[3] In the same year Antonius Varchionsis praised Marcellus' work in his preface to Euripedes published in Florence.[4] In Ferrara, Ioannes Manardus' reaction was different. Errors, mistranslations, misreadings, misjudgments, stupidities: Manardus listed them all in reviewing Marcellus' first book of the Dioscorides. Manardus enumerated them in a letter written in 1519 to Marcellus. Familiarly he began the letter with an excuse for not having written earlier. "... a little after your Dioscorides came to me, a troublesome foot illness rendered me unable for many days to stand up from the bed."[5] Manardus did not say whether he was reading Marcellus' translation in manuscript or a printed copy. But implicitly, one assumes that Manardus had only a manuscript copy. We do not know how tardy Manardus was with his reply. If his letter were to prevent error prior to publication, we could value Manardus' willingness to help; otherwise, he is vindictive. Manardus said he went through the first book "without catching my breathe" because it had timely remedies.[6] Since his letter to Marcellus concerned only the first book of Dioscorides, it is more than charitable, in fact, reasonable, to suppose that Manardus was reading a manuscript copy of Marcellus' translation. He probably did not know that it had been published in Florence late in the previous year. To some extent Manardus tried to be polite and diplomatic. He said that he was uplifted by the difficulties of the translation which required exacting diligence and serious judgment. But—and how often does the conjunction "but" separate the ritual praise from the serious criticisms in book reviews—in a spirit of frankness he knew Marcellus would wish to know about his errors. Manardus knew, he said, that Marcellus' purpose in translating Dioscorides was for the good of all Europe and not personal ambition. Marcellus, he added, your work can profit from my observations and our friendship will continue.[7]

Ioannes Manardus (Giovanni Manardo) had impressive credentials to respond to Marcellus. He was born in Ferrara on July 24, 1462. His father was a notary and a great uncle, Antonius Manardus, an apothecary. The home town boy stayed close to Ferrara most of his life. He received a doctorate in arts and medicine on October 17, 1482, and became a lecturer. His advancement was said to have been blocked because of his attacks on astrological and theoretical medicine. Between 1513 and 1518 Manardus went to Hungary as a royal physician to the Magyar crown but returned to Ferrara in 1518 where he became a professor of medicine in 1524. A seemingly unflawed career was marred when at the age of seventy-three his marriage to a young girl produced public censors.[8]

We know of Manardus' letter to Marcellus because it was published. Almost certainly Manardus had no intention to publish it when he wrote it. Manardus' *Epistolae medicinales* were published in Ferrara in 1521 and reissued again, Paris, 1528; Strasbourg, 1529; and Bologna, 1531; but the edition did not include this letter to Marcellus. In Lyon in 1532, four years before Manardus' death, eleven years after Marcellus' death, Francois Rabelais edited Manardus' letters and included Manardus' letter to Marcellus as well as two later letters on Dioscorides. Had Manardus intended publishing the letter he would likely have included them in his own editions and, more to the point, his text would have been more helpful to the general reader. Indeed one wonders how useful Manardus' letter would be to a general reader. In order to make sense out of the letter, one also has to have before him a copy of a good Greek text of Dioscorides and Marcellus' translation. Otherwise, it will not make sense. Manardus' first correction was Marcellus' translation of Dioscorides' "Preface." In harvesting plants for medicines, Dioscorides explained that sap and resin are best taken from stems when they are ripe. Marcellus translated Dioscorides' word ἀκμή which in this context means "ripe," "full strength," "zenith," or "culmination," into the Latin "integra aetate": thus, "Succus ex herbis colligendum in nova caulium producrione eodemque modo ex foliis liquores lachrymasque sectis integra aetate caulibus excipiendos."[9] *Integra* can mean "whole," "entire," "complete," "unmutilated," "fresh," or "new." Manardus explained that ἀκμή when used by Hippocrates in the *Aphorisms* meant, "at the height." Similarly Galen used the word in relation to disease at the crisis period.[10] Manardus seems to think that Marcellus' meaning might cause sap or resin to be collected too early, say in the spring.

Manardus observed that this was the only error in Marcellus' translation of the "Preface." Now the assault begins. Under the first entry on the herb *Iris* (I, 1), Manardus discussed the various kinds of iris and in a context that suggests that he might have been reacting to Marcellus' commentary and not his translation alone. He corrected Marcellus' translation of ὤχρα for a color of the plant; ὤχρα means "pale" possibly ranging to "yellow," so says Liddell-Scott. Marcellus translated it as *virides* or "green" whereas Manardus says it should be *pallidos* or "pale," "... as it is known to be by physicians (*medici*)."[11] Parenthetically the word ὤχρα was only in a few texts of Dioscorides and probably there as an interpolation. In a similar vein, Manardus employed Ruellius' earlier (Paris 1516 ed.) Latin translation of Dioscorides as well as other authorities, such as Hippocrates, Plato, Celsus, Galen, and Hermolaus Barbarus' *Commentary on Pliny*. He used them in order to get better shades of meanings from words, as an example as when he translated Dioscorides' entry on *iris*.[12]

Under *acorus*, or *sweetflag*, chapter two, Marcellus translated: καὶ εἰς ἐγκαθίσμα ὡς ἶρις πρὸς τα γυναικεῖα ("and [it is taken] in a sitz-bath, as with iris for female disorders"), as "utiliterque Iridis modo insidentibus Acoro muliebria id est menses foventur."[13] Manardus said Marcellus should not have translated γυναικεῖα ("female disorders") as "muliebria (= female disorders) that is fomenting the menses." *Muliebria* means not only menses, Manardus said, but as it is commonly (*universale*) known the term applies to a variety of female problems ("sed diversa mulierum malla"). The lexography of Galen, Hippocrates and Herophilus was cited as proof. Better for medicine that the full range of meanings be made clear.[14]

Marcellus translated Dioscorides' entry on *asarum* to read: "Coronaria et odorata herba Asaron est (Asarum is suitable for cornets and is aromatic)."[15] *Asarum* is probably *Asarum europaeum L.*, a member of the birthwort family. Manardus said that he could not find that Dioscorides had said that it was suitable for cornet or garlands. Further Manardus observed that not all of these plants can be described as being aromatic.[16] Two Greek manuscripts of Dioscorides, however, yield a reading which supports Marcellus' translation. The famous 6th century Juliana Anicia palempsest, and the 7th century Neapolitan manuscript have: *βοτάνη εὐωδηςστεφανωματική*...[17] Marcellus could not have seen the Juliana Anicia manuscript since it was not yet in Europe,[18] therefore he must have employed, directly or indirectly, the Neapolitan text. Manardus was quite correct in pointing out that he could not find such a reading but he was likely using one of the Greek printed editions of Dioscorides, probably the Aldine 1499 edition or 1518 edition.

Manardus enumerated a considerable and impressive listing of corrections. The letter was lengthy, some 60 pages in the *editio princeps*. Manardus was more than a humanist; he was a humanistic physician who sought medical knowledge in a careful, scholarly study of the medical classics. Presumably from his career his knowledge was tested clinically. His purposes were not confined to philology and certainly not restricted to a dogmatic defense of the ancients. Instead, he sought pharmaco-medical benefits for his and future generations through scholarship. And it was in scholarship that he found his Florentine "friend" lacking. Manardus ended his letter to Marcellus with the sentiments that he hoped that he would accept his remarks (*censorem et arbitrum*) on Dioscorides' first book. "I question the first book then," Manardus concluded, "so that you might consider the advantages and good [my criticisms afford] and you might know me to be among those who mistrust you, and even that you might consider withdrawing from this endeavor. Farewell. From Ferrara. 1519."[19]

Fortune has preserved Marcellus' letter in defense of his translation. One blow followed another. While probably still under the initial glow of a new author, Marcellus received the blow of Manardus' criticisms and a blow from a horse which left him incapacitated. He does not reply until March 8, 1520, citing the horse kick as the reason he had not written earlier. Marcellus felt his critic wrong for complaining about the book he did not write. "I translated Dioscorides, not Galen and others," Marcellus explained. Although he specifically answered some of Manardus' criticisms, he excused himself partly on the ground that he was not a physician nor a follower of the art. It was merely his intention to make known the uses of the simples in Dioscorides.[20]

Authors' reactions to critical reviews are universally human. From his grave Marcellus might have felt some vindication when his translation received five more editions including an edition by Ioannis Soteris in Cologne, 1529, with a parallel Greek text from the 1518 Aldine printing.[21] Also it received fairly general respect among Dioscoridean authorities throughout the sixteenth century, a century in which there were many such authorities.

Manardus was not to allow Marcellus to have the last word. Rabelais'

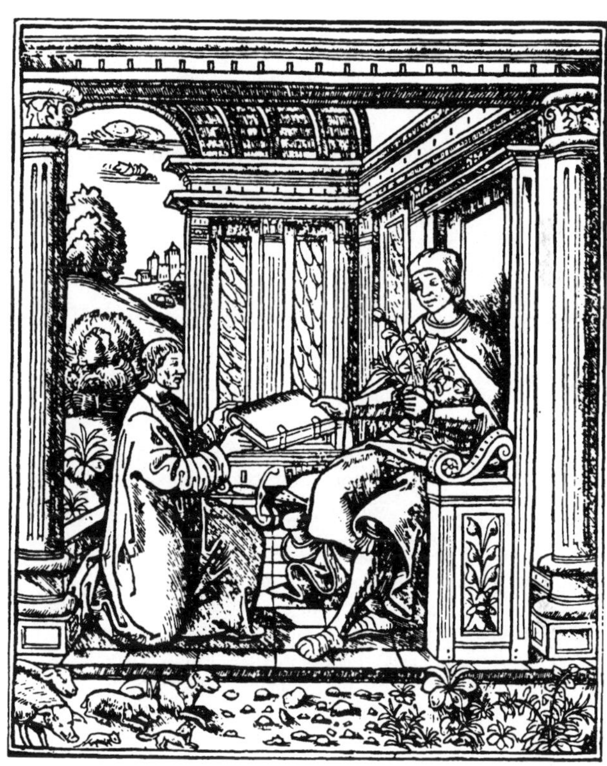

Frontispiece of a 1528 Lyon edition of Dioscorides.

edition of Manardus' letters contains two more letters correcting more errors, justifying former corrections in Book One and, since now he had read the entire translation, expanding the corrections to all five books, plus a falsely attributed work. The second letter is relatively short, some twenty-two pages, but it is undated.[22] Manardus' third letter, the largest with one hundred and twenty-one pages, is addressed to Bartholomaeus Tingus Pastoriensis and dated January 15, 1523, at Ferrara. In this letter Manardus is aware that Marcellus had died (Dec. 1, 1521).[23] Manardus' second letter is undated and is addressed to an unnamed friend who at Manardus' request had defended Marcellus,[24] thereby bracketing its date not earlier than 1521 and before 1523. Manardus explained that when he received his friend's letter he was discouraged and distraught, more in the mood to surrender than to fight. Although he wrote the reply it remained unsent for more than two years.[25] It is not our purpose here to review these later letters, since they, or at least the third one, was written for the purpose of publication. What niceties and restraints as were present in Manardus' review written directly to Marcellus are gone now that he is dead. Manardus' attack was devastating. Still Marcellus' work survived and continued to be read. In one way this is reassuring but, if Manardus is correct in many or most of his corrections, our reassurance as an author might be different if we had been a patient of a physician or apothecary using Marcellus' translation of Dioscorides.

Part II: Franciscus Frigimelica, Lecturer

Note taking, perhaps for lectures, perhaps for a book someday, perhaps as a private aid to organize one's ideas, is one way in which pharmacy has been practiced throughout the ages. Virtually unnoticed are the notes of Franciscus Frigimelica. He obviously worked hard on pharmacy but his effort has escaped modern notice, and we know even less about him than we do of his work. There are two manuscripts of a commentary he wrote to the first four books of *De materia medica*. The earlier and most complete is dated April 7, 1530,[26] while the other is dated October 17, 1553, at Padua and Bologna.[27] The latter version, now at Erlangen, arrived there from a purchase of the medical faculty's library at Padua. However, this manuscript contains a shorter, abridged version of the longer version, which is currently found in a manuscript at Oxford. It was in the library of Matteo Luigi Canonici (1727–1805) whose manuscripts were purchased by the Bodleian Library in 1817. The Oxford manuscript may very well be the autograph notes Frigimelica made for his lectures. But where did he lecture? Even though the Erlangen manuscript says he lectured at Bologna, Umberto Dallari does not list him on the faculty there.[28] J. Facciolati's *Fasti Gymnastii Patavini*[29] clearly gives us his *curriculum vitae*. Born in Padua on January 15, 1491, Franciscus Frigimelica received a doctorate in arts and medicine from Padua on April 1, 1518, and between 1518 and 1525 he taught sophistic and moral philosophy and lectured during these years on Aristotle, Galen and Dioscorides. He is listed as lecturing simply on medicines from 1525 to 1532 and on theoretical and practical medicine thereafter. Padua indulged its master; Frigimelica rose through the ranks without publication. His only work published during his lifetime was a tract in Italian on the 1535 plague in Padua. Four of his works, all medical, were published posthumously. The commentary on Dioscorides, a work on headaches and a commentary on Aristotle's *De sensu et sensato* have remained in unnoticed and unstudied manuscripts.[30] Even a bibliophilic mania of the botanist and Dioscoridean expert Conrad Gesner failed to learn of Frigimelica's work when Gesner wrote an essay published in 1559 on contemporary, European Dioscoridean scholarship.[31] In his comments Gesner charitably included mention of those who said they intended to work on Dioscorides, a deed even a fearless bibliographer would not dare do today.

Earlier Renaissance attention to Dioscorides began as part of the humanistic interest in the restudy of classical works. The approach mostly was philological. What did Dioscorides actually say to us concerning plants and things? What did this or that term mean? And, more often than not, what is the plant or plants of today which correspond to Dioscorides' Greek words? Hermolaus Barbarus, Ioannes Baptista Egnatius and Marcellus Virgilius Adrianus studied Dioscorides from this perspective. Frigimelica's approach was different. He used Dioscorides as the means of contributing his pharmaceutical knowledge because Dioscorides is the best, he explained, and he teaches us most about medicines. His commentary is filled with prescriptions, each carefully conveying the measurements and preparation instructions.[32] Dioscorides' own work was unfortunately wanting in this area. Using Dioscorides' unfathomable arrangement, Frigimelica follows the first four books of *De materia medica*, thereby omitting the fifth book with information about the medicinal usages of minerals. Why minerals should be omitted is without Frigimelica's explanation. Possibly, like many of us, he just never finished his lectures to include the material. His purpose was certainly more pharmaceutical than botanical because he seldom discussed the plants except occasionally to aid in identification. In the Oxford manuscript Frigimelica discusses some 377 plants and 33 animal products in some seventy-five folios. Whereas some entries are relatively short, many are elaborate pharmaceutical discourses on the drug use of the products. For example, in Dioscorides' Book Two, Frigimelica's comments on milk and eggs are lengthy, running to several folios. Since animal products were an integral part of Frigimelica's pharmacopoeia, his omission of minerals in Dioscorides' Book Five is a failure of time, not of doctrine.

The entry on *acorus*, our *acorus calamus L.* or *sweet flag*, will illustrate Frigimelica's method. He began by stating *acorus* is presently called *calamus aromaticus*.[33] During the middle ages the term *calamus aromaticus* came to be applied to the drug from the root of the *acorus* plant and possibly from the root of the *iris pseudacorus L.* as well.[34] Seemingly when the plant as a whole is mentioned by Frigimelica the plant *acorus* is meant; when the drug derived from the root is meant, then Frigimelica used the term *calamus aromaticus*. Frigimelica did not explain this. He had two prescriptions, one calling for a dramma of *calamus aromaticus*, another for two drammae of *acorus*. If this manuscript were a text for a lecture, then we can be reasonably sure that either Professor Frigimelica would have given his students some further explanation or else they would have been confused. At least from our perspective of the sixteenth century pharmacy, the distinctions between *acorus* and *calamus aromaticus* are not clear in the sources. Pity the poor student who must be expected to know this!

With the short statement that *acorus* is called *calamus aromaticus*, Frigimelica begins the pharmacy. The drug is good, he said, for all internal illness where a fever is not present. The recipe[35] is:

℞ pul. calami aromatici ________________ ʒ.i.
Zucc.(ari) rosati ________________ ʒ.5.

Calamus oil, a distillate of acorus, is currently used in bitters for alcoholic drinks[36] so Frigimelica's prescription of five parts more of rose-colored sugar to one part acorus root is understandable. A spoonful of sugar helps the medicine go down.

Next Frigimelica related the use of *acorus* as a diuretic when pulverized and given with good wine and as a provoker of menstruation "quod habeas pro secreto apud mir frequentissimo reperto," he explains. Frigimelica's next recipe is for debilitated membranes and preserving youth.[37]

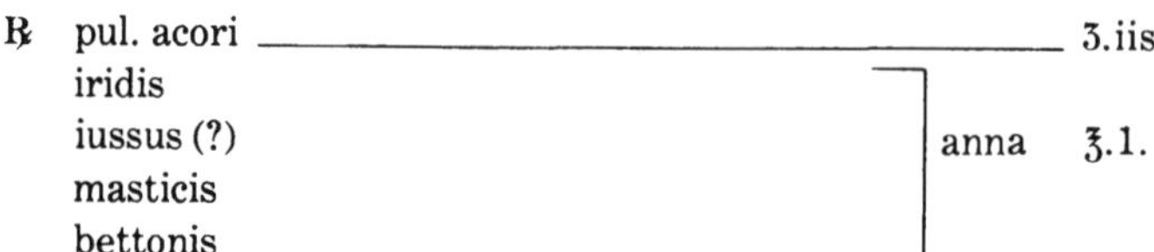

℞ pul. acori ——— ʒ.iis
iridis
iussus (?)
masticis
bettonis] anna ʒ.1.

This is prepared, mixed with a double portion of wine and taken in the mouth. Thus ended Frigimelica's discussion of acorus. It is important to observe what he did not say. He has no discussion about the plant's identity, nomenclature, description or plant habitat. Frigimelica did not report the usages of the plant given by Dioscorides, Galen, Avicenna or, as far as I have learned, any other authority. Frigimelica has no acknowledgement of Galenic degrees. Galen, whom Frigimelica occasionally quoted, said of *acorus* that its action was because of its warming and drying action[38] and Avicenna refined the activity to the first degree of warming on the familiar four degree scale.[39] In fact Frigimelica's method seems consistent throughout because he rejects the medieval scholastic refinement of the Galenic theory in favor of a simpler, less cumbersome empirical approach to pharmacy. Frigimelica seems to have been in the vanguard of the Renaissance rejection of Galenic pharmaceutical theory.

Although an assessment of Frigimelica's originality deserves a deeper study, I can report that his pharmaceutical commentary appears innovative. Sometimes his commentary appears conventional in respect to his contemporaries' concerns with Dioscorides' text. Under *ancusa* or our *true alkanet* he says only that it is similar to *bugolossus*, or our *burrage*.[40] By similar we presume similar in medicinal usages. Under *bugolossus*, he observed that this herb is "most frequently used by us," and related, without any prescriptions or descriptions of preparation, that it warms the heart and its roots are good for melancholy.[41] On the other hand under *theraebinthus*, or our *terebinth pistache*, he explained that the tree is the source of *theraebinthinina*, a resin which we call *turpenthin*. He gave two recipes for compounding it including one for *dolores articulorum*, presumably arthritis, which he called for two ounces of turpentine, one of juniper oil and one dramma of salt.[42] Then he said "common women and common medical people" make a salve using turpentine for scabies.[43] From my reading of sixteenth century university medical professors' works, I would argue that is most unusual for one of them to employ folk practices. Few of Frigimelica's colleagues at other universities would approve such research as being professional. For whatever reasons or combination of accidental circumstances, Frigimelica's work on Dioscorides appears unnoticed in the records of his time. A judgment of his work needs further study. Until then he is merely another teacher on a faculty roster whose influence, if any, came through his anonymous students.

Part III: Mechoir Guilandinus, Note Taker

Anonymity does not describe our third and final sixteenth century scholar, Mechior Guilandinus, but a mix of obscurity and intrigue does. On the shelves of the Biblioteca Nazionale Marciana[44] is a copy of Petrus Haultin's 1549 Paris edition of Dioscorides, which contains in its covers a Greek text and Ruellius' Latin translation, but so do other cities have a surviving copy, cities such as London and Washington. San Marco's copy is distinct. Throughout its margins, tops, bottoms, left and right sides, and interlinearly are glosses made by Mechior Guilandinus. I have a colleague whose love for books leads him to consider as a scholarly crime the act of writing and underlining in books. My discomfort, when he sees my heavily annotated library, is alleviated somewhat when I think of the insight into the mind and thought of past scholars afforded by their desecration of the sacrosanctity of a book. I must find comfort, if only because I also write in books.

Guilandinus' origins are obscure.[45] He was born around the same year that Manardus dealt the blow to Marcellus; that is he was born about 1520, somewhere in Prussia, perhaps Königsberg. Linguistically his family name was likely Wieland, later Latinized as Guilandinus, Italianized as Guilandini. Where he learned his Latin or Italian or even whether he had any formal education is unknown. The first known event in his life places him in southern Italy where, in his own words, he was so poor that he lived on roots which he sold along with medicinal herbs carried on a donkey from town to town. It's a long way from Prussia to Calabria and there is no reason to blame or credit the Hapsburgs for this transfer. His itinerant medicine show eventually took him to Rome where he attracted the attention of the Venetian ambassador, who took him to Venice as his client. Guilandinus found a new patron in Senator Marin Caballo, who sponsored him to undertake a trip in 1558–1560 to Greece, Syria and Egypt to procure rare plants. He planned to go to America to find new flora but in the port of Cagliari he was captured and held by Algerian Corsairs in North Africa. His friend, P. Gabriel Falloppio, Professor of Anatomy and Surgery at Padua, ransomed him. In 1561 Falloppio secured for Guilandinus the directorship of the Botanical Gardens in Padua, and he remained there the rest of his life. In 1557 Guilandinus published his treatise on plants.[46] Between 1558 and 1562 he was engaged in a bitter controversy arising out of his criticisms of Petrus Matthiolus' famed translation of Dioscorides. The attack led to Matthiolus' counterattack and a third party's defense of Guilandinus made by Paulus Hessus.[47] The fight did not prevent him from receiving the Chair of Botany at the University in 1562. He died on December 25, 1589.

Exactly when Guilandinus wrote his unpublished glosses on Dioscorides is not known. Obviously it had to have been after the release of the 1549 Paris edition. The most recent published writers who are mentioned in the notes are Dodoens and Cornarius. Presumably, Dodoens is Rembert Dodens (1516–1585) whose first botanical work on cereals, vegetables and fodders was published in 1552, followed by an extensive herbarium in 1554.[48] There is one note on Cornarius. Janus Cornarius translated and commented on Dioscorides in a work written in 1555 and not published until 1557. It was in 1554 that Petrus Andreas Matthiolus published his famous extensive commentary in Latin on Dioscorides. The fact that Guilandinus did not cite it, although once he mentioned Matthiolus by name,[50] leads me to conclude tentatively that most of Guilandinus' notes were made between 1550 and 1554. Matthiolus during this period was the town physician at nearby Görz. His earlier work in Italian on Dioscorides was known and his preparation on the more extensive Latin commentary must have taken him on trips to Venice and the Paduan Botanical Gardens. The Director of the Gardens from 1546 to 1561 was Aloysius Anguillara (Luigi Anguillara), who is also mentioned in several places in Guilandinus' notes.[51] Since Guilandinus' normal practice was to cite both author, work and pagination in his cross-references and since for neither Matthiolus nor Anguillaria is a title given, it seems probable that their names are as a result of personal conversations about plants and their usages. For instance beside the plant Λιμωνιον or *Limonium* Guilandinus wrote: "Anguil (laria) thinks it commonly called aquatic plantain."[52] Had he been citing Anguillara from a written work he likely would not have used "putatur." The extensiveness of the notes makes it likely that they are the result of years of note taking in explicating Dioscorides' text. It is reasonable to suppose that from 1550 to 1554 Guilandinus made marginal notes to Dioscorides as he built the knowledge and expertise to write his own monograph. The note to Cornarius may have been a late addition. The fact that there is only one mention each of Cornarius and Matthiolus is my reason for supposing the bulk of the notes were written earlier.[53] The extensive contributions these writers made would seemingly have caused Guilandinus to have considered their ideas in greater detail had they been known at the time of his writing.

In this light, his interests, the method of his mind, and the revelation as to work habits make a study of Guilandinus' notes interesting. Beside Dioscorides' first entry on *iris* (I, 1) where the Greek word Ἶρις is transliterated by Ruellius as *Iris*, Guilandinus added in Greek "Ἶρις ἀγρία, Χγρις."[54] He observed that in Book IV, p. 202 (entry 22, Wellmann ed.) Dioscorides described a plant ξυρίς which is very similar in spelling and description. Guilandinus indicated that Dioscorides first entry on *iris* is the *wild iris* which is similar to or the same as his later entry on *xyris*. Most earlier authorities on Dioscorides had identified Dioscorides' first entry as the *Illyrian iris*;[55] on the other hand, Matthiolus (Venice ed. 1554) says Dioscorides had two varieties in the first entry, *wood iris* and *domestic iris*.[56] Modern authorities believe that Dioscorides first entry is either *iris germanica L.* (common iris) or *iris florentina L.* (fleur-de-lis) or both and the second entry, the one in Book IV, is *iris foetidissima L.* (stinking iris or gladdon).[57] Such is the maddening difficulty in interpreting Dioscorides in any age but, as Manardus said, he is the best there is—prior to the sixteenth century that is. That Dioscorides' *iris* is *wild iris* which is the same as *xyris* is proven by Galen in his *Book on Simples*, Guilandinus wrote, giving the book and paragraph citation.[58] Thus, the first word of Dioscorides' text, the first correction by Guilandinus. No blind worshipper of authority for this misplaced Prussian.

In the cramped margin Guilandinus next quarreled with both Dioscorides' Greek text and Ruellius' translation: in describing the stemmation of flowers from the stalk Dioscorides' Greek used παράλληλα ("side by side") whence Guilandinus corrected the Greek by supplying "ἐπαλλαγή [fitting into one another] id est promiscuus [that is distinct]." Ruellius' translation was: "Flores in caule equalibus inter se spatiis distant [The flowers on the stem are separated equally from one another]."[59] It was not what Dioscorides said, but what he should have said, Guilandinus inferred. Certainly Ruellius' translation was not entirely accurate. Guilandinus' correction, however, was not made on the basis of textual criticism but inaccuracy in a real life description. This sort of observation is a departure from the method of early writers such as Manardus.

Although the bulk of Guilandinus' notes have more to do with the botany than the pharmacy of plants, Guilandinus did not confine himself to botany.

For instance under *iris*,[60] where Ruellius translated as "somnum conciliatur (inclines one to sleep)," Guilandinus has a lengthy note at the bottom of the folio calling attention to Apollonius' prescription for iris. Apollonius says iris cures a headache arising from a hangover (*πρὸς κεφαλαλγίαν τηὶν δὶα μὲθην καὶ ακπατοποσίαν*).[61] Guilandinus added to Dioscorides and Apollonius the casual connection that by inducing sleep the headache is made well.

The majority of the notes are simply cross references to other authorities, normally with work and pagination given as well. Specifically he cited Hippocrates, Aristotle, Theophrastus, Nicander, Philander, Cato, Columella, Scribonius Largus, Pliny, Archigenes, Galen, Oribasios, Marcellus (Empiricus?), Scholiast of Theocritus, (pseudo-) Apuleius, Rhasis, Serapion, Avicenna, Hermolaus Barbarus (*Castigationes Plinii*), Leonardus Fuschsius, Valerius Cordus (*Commentary on Dioscorides*), Agricola, Anguillara, Matthiolus, Dodoens, and Cornarius. The prodigious reading Guilandinus made in preparing these notes on Dioscorides reveals that the mind at work is that of a first class scholar. The glosses are thorough, erudite and empirical. Although they are relatively scant on the animal and mineral sections of Dioscorides, nonetheless his interest was not confined to plants. His readings were wide enough to have read Georgius Argicola whose *De re metallica* was published in 1530.

Guilandinus did not hesitate to challenge even Dioscorides as when he incorrectly described plants. Dioscorides used the word *καυλὸυς* in describing the stemmation of the mountain nard instead of the better word *κλάδους*.[62] Where Dioscorides said that *balsumum* is grown only in a valley in Judaea and in Egypt, Guilandinus noted that this is not true.[63] Where Dioscorides said that the *Σρατιώτης* (*stratiotes aloides* or *water soldier*), an aquatic plant, lives without roots, Guilandinus wrote *falsum*, it is untrue.[64] Sometimes he corrected Ruellius' translation as when Ruellius used *rubra* (red) for *πορφυρὰ* (purple) for the color of a lily flower.[65] Guilandinus' hundreds of corrections, though each may seem relatively modest, reveals the work of this medicine man and botanist, how carefully and thoroughly he searched the authorities, and, more importantly, how ready he was to challenge when his observations of nature differed from their pronouncements.

From Manardus' epistolatory book review, to Frigimelica's lecture notes, to Guilandinus' marginal notes we have examined their little known works. Directly their contributions in these works were minimal because we do not know if anyone was influenced by them. Only in the case of Manardus do we know that his work was read. They did not change pharmacy or botany or medicine or natural science. Each of these works has its own level of obscurity; they demonstrate the change in the fields which is taking place generally during the early sixteenth century, perhaps before it is seen in the more celebrated published works. From Manardus' precision in translating Dioscorides' text to Frigimelica's almost exclusive concern with the pharmacy in Dioscorides to Guilandinus' heavy emphasis on the pure botany, we can see how Dioscorides' work in the period 1519 to 1555 has provided the springboard by which a humanistic interest in a text led to a refinement of pharmacy and the foundation of botany.

(See References — next page)

References

1. The three letters discussed here are in Io Manardus, *Epistolorum medicinalium tomus secundus, nunquam antea in Gallia excusus*. Franciscus Rabelaesus, ed. Lugduni, apud Seb. Gryphium, 1532, Letter 1, pp. 112-172; Letter 2, pp. 172–194; Letter 3, pp. 194–315. Details of their publications in nine subsequent editions, as well as a description of the letters, are found in my forthcoming article, "Dioscorides," *Catalogus Translationum et Commentariorum*. P.O. Kristeller, ed. (Washington: Catholic University Press), vol. IV, pp. 50–54. (Riddle, "Dios.")
2. *De medica materia libri sex....* (Florentine, per haeredes Philippi Juntae, 1518).
3. W. Ruediger, *Marcellus Virgilius Adrianus aus Florenz; ein Beitrag zur Kenntnis seines Lebens und seines Wirkens* (Halle 1898), p. 1.
4. Preface to *Hecuba et Iphigenia Euripidis Erasmo interprete* (Florence 1518), reported by A. M. Bandini, *De Florentina Juntarum typographia*. 2 vols. in 1 (Lucca 1791), I, 38–454, 126.
5. *Epistolarum medicinalium*. vol. II, Book VIII, p. 112. (*Ep. med.*)
6. *Ibid.* II, Book VIII, pp. 112–113.
7. *Ibid.* II, Book VIII, pp. 113.
8. For short biographies and a listing of his works, see Riddle, "Dios.," pp. 53–54; and J. H. Cotton, in: *Dictionary of Scientific Biography*, vol. IX, 74–75. Also see analyses of some of his various contributions in: *Atti del Convegno Internazionali per le celebrazione della nascita di Giovanni Manardo, (1462–1536)* (Ferrara 1963).
9. Marcellus (1518 ed.), fol. 1v.
10. *Ep. med.*, II, Book VIII, pp. 113–14.
11. *Ep. med.*, II, Book VIII, p. 115; cf. Marcellus (1518 ed.), fol. 3.
12. *Ep. med.*, II, Book VIII, p. 114.
13. Marcellus (1518 ed.), fol. 5; Manardus' Greek text is the same as that modern edition by Max Wellmann, *Pedanii Dioscuridis Anazarbei De materia medica libri quinque*, 3 vols. (Berlin 1958 repr.), I, 2, p. 8.
14. *Ep. med.*, II, Book VIII, pp. 117–118.
15. Marcellus (1518 ed.) I, 9, fol. biii (book and entry numbering of Marcellus ed.).
16. *Ep. med.*, II, Book VIII, p. 123.
17. Alternate reading in Wellmann, I, 10. The Juliana Anicia Ms is now Vienna Ms Greek. 1 and the Neopolitan Ms is Vienna Ms suppl. Greek 28.
18. See Riddle, "Dios.," pp.4–5, 92.
19. *Ep. med.*, II, Book VIII, p. 172.
20. Marcellus' letter is in Milan, Ambrosiana, Ms S81 Sup., fols. 192–197v, and is available on microfilm in the USA from the Ambrosiana Collection, University of Notre Dame. See a discussion of the letter in Riddle, "Dios." pp. 35, 50, and Ruediger, *Marcellus*, p. 18.
21. Following the *editio princeps*, 1518, Florence, there was 1523, Florence; 1528, Florence; 1529, Cologne; 1532, Basel; and 1538, Venice.
22. *Ep. med.*, II, Book VIII, pp. 192–194.
23. *Ep. med.*, II, Book VIII, pp. 194–315.
24. *Ep. med.*, II, Book VIII, p. 172: "Cuidam viro doctissimi pariter et amiciss. qui Marcelli defensionem rogatus accoeperat."
25. *Ibid.*

26. Oxford, Bodleian Ms Canon, lat. misc. 31, anno 1530, fols. 1-75v, and described by Riddle, "Dios.," pp. 54-55.
27. Erlangen, Universitätsbibliothek, Ms 909, anno 1553, fol. 48-76, and described by Riddle, "Dios.," p. 55.
28. Dell' anzianato nell' antico comune di Bologna (Bologna 1887).
29. 3 pts. in 1 (Patavii 1757) pt. 2, 291, 311, 313, 337, 342 and 363.
30. For a biography and further references, see Riddle "Dios.," p. 55.
31. Preface, fols. iii-ix, anno 1559, in: *Valerii Cordi Simesusii Annotationes in Pedacii Dioscoridis...De materia medica*, Tigurini, 1561.
32. Oxford, Bodl. Ms Canon, 1st misc. 31, fol. 1; the preface in the Erlangen Ms is wanting.
33. Fol. 1v.
34. Wolfgang Schneider, *Lexikon zur Arzeneimittelgeschichte*, 7 vols. in 9. Vol. 5 in 3 pts.: *Pflanzliche Drogen* (Frankfurt a. M. 1974), V, pt. 1, pp. 42-44; K. Rüegg, *Beitrag zur Geschichte der officinellen Drogen Crocus, Acorus Calamus und Colchicum* (Disser., Basel 1936).
35. Oxford, Bodl. Ms Canon, lat. misc. 31, fols. 1v-2.
36. George Usher, *A Dictionary of Plants Used by Man* (London 1974), p. 19.
37. Oxford, Bodl. Ms Canon, lat. misc. 31, fol. 2.
38. Galen, *On simple medicines*, vol. XI, p. 820, Kühn ed.
39. *Canon*. Liber II, tract. II, cap. 46 (fol. 91v, Venice 1509 ed.).
40. Oxford, Bodl. Ms Canon, lat. misc. 31, fol. 66.
41. *Ibid.*, fol. 71 v. Dioscorides distinguished αγχόυδα (IV, 23 Wellmann) probably *Anchusa tinctorii L.* or *true alkanet*, from βούγλωσσου or *Borago officinalis L.* or *burrage*. Galen (XI, 852 Kühn ed.) said burrage is warming, incites myrth, and is good for coughs. Schneider (*Lexikon* V, pt. 1, pp. 92-93) lists alkanet's uses together with those of burrage, but he noted that Bock. around 1550, identified alkanet with Dioscorides' *echium*.
42. Oxford Bodl. Ms Canon. lat. misc. 31, fol. 14v.
43. *Ibid.*, fol. 15: "... mulieres vulgares et vulgares medici."
44. Ms Gr. V, 3 (1280). I should note that I have examined this only on microfilm.
45. For biography and references, see Riddle, "Dios.," pp. 86-87.
46. *De stirpium aliquot nominibus vetustis ac novis*, (Basel 1557).
47. Paulus Hessus, *Defensio XX. problematum Melchioris Guilandini adversus quae Petr. Andreas Mattheolus ex centum scripsit... Adjecta est Petr. Andreae Matthaeoli adversus XX. problemata Melchioris Guilandini disputatio...* (Patavini 1562).
48. Dodoens is mentioned on fols. 193v, 201v, 231v, and 233v (Marciana Ms Gr. v. 3 [1280]. The last note gave a title, *Libellus de frumentariis* which presumably, is *De frugum historis, liber unus* (Antwerp 1552). For a biography, a list of words with references, see Marcel Florkin, "Dodoens," *Dictionary of Scientific Biography*, IV, 138-140.
49. Cornarius is noted on fol. 233v (Marciano Ms Gr. V. 3 [1280]). A description of his work is in Riddle, "Dios.," pp. 39-40.
50. Fol. 229 (Marciana Ms Gr. V 3 [1280]).
51. Fols. 154v, 197 r & v, 201, 232v (*ibid.*).
52. Fol. 201 (*ibid.*).
53. The notes to Dodoens, Cornarius, Matthiolus, and Anguillara all appear between the 154v-233v, with one note to Dodoens and the only one to Cornarius both together on the same folio. This suggests to me that they might be later than the bulk of the other notes. A close personal examination of the notes might reveal what the microfilm would not about the ink and handwriting.
54. Fol. 4 (Marciana Ms Gr. V. 3 [1280]).
55. Among them, the late eleventh or early twelfth century Latin Alphabetical Redaction (unnumbered folio, Colle 1478), Hemolaus Barbarus' translation (fol. 1, Venice 1516), and Ioannes Ruellius' translation (I, 1, Paris 1516).
56. Fol. 17.
57. Schneider, *Lexikon*, V, pt. 2, pp. 201-207; P. Font Quer, *Plantas medicinales el Dioscorides renovado* (Barcelona, 1962), pp. 916-920.
58. Fol. 4 (Marciana Ms Gr. V. 3 1280).
60. *Ibid.*
61. Galen, *Composition of medicines*, XII, p. 514, Kühn ed., in quoting Apollonius.
62. Fol. 2v (Marciana Ms Gr. V. 3 [1280]): Dioscorides I, 9, Wellmann, ed.
63. Fol. 13 (Marciana Ms Gr. V. 3 [1280]): Dioscorides I, 19, Wellmann, ed.
64. Fol. 227 (Marciana Ms Gr. V. 3 [1280]): Dioscorides IV, 101, Wellmann, ed.
65. Fol. 178 (Marciana Ms Gr. V. 3 [1280]): Dioscorides III, 102, Wellmann, ed.
66. Peter Dilg, "Die Botanische Kommentarliteratur Italiens um 1500 und ihr Einfluss auf Deutschland," in: August Buck and Otto Herdings, eds., *Der Kommentar in der Renaissance, Kommission für Humanismusforschung*, no. 1 (Bonn, 1976), 225-252; Karen Meier Reeds, "Renaissance Humanism and Botany," *Annals of Science*, XXIII (1976), 519-542; and Reeds' "Botany in Medieval and Renaissance Universities" (Cambridge, Mass., unpubl. Harvard Dissert., 1975); and Charles G. Navert, Jr. "Humanists, Scientists and Pliny: Changing Approaches to a Classical Author," *American Historical Review*, LXXXIV (1979), 72-85.

VIII

Albert on Stones and Minerals

In common with a host of nature's observers before him, Albert knew that all things are either animal, vegetable, or mineral. Few before Albert, however, devoted study to minerals. Those that did were either lapidarists, astrologists, magicians, encyclopedists, or medical men interested in their therapeutic effects. No previous writer observed and recorded information on the entire compass of minerals, enough so that one could say to a modern scientist's satisfaction, "this is a pioneer work in mineralogy." To some extent Albert was aware that he was venturing in a new branch of *scientia*, one without a previous tradition, because he could cite no authorities who combined the theory of mineral formations and their properties together with the practical knowledge of the lapidarists, alchemists, pharmacists, miners and other practitioners in stone and metals lore. Aristotle had written on minerals but Albert could find only excerpts, and Avicenna's work, it seemed to Albert, treated the subject too briefly and insufficiently.[1] Albert wrote the *Book of Minerals* in five books. He wrote neither merely to record and synthesize all prior authorities, nor merely to add his own observations. The task was too great, the subject too vast. What he intended, in his own words, was that "on the basis of what has been said [in his work], anything else [relating to minerals] that has not been mentioned here

[1] Albert, *De mineralibus* I, tr.1, c.1 (ed. Borgnet 5: 1b; trans. Dorothy Wyckoff [Oxford, 1967], p. 9).

Reprinted from James A. Weisheipl, ed. *Albertus Magnus and the Sciences. Commemorative Essays, 1980*, pp. 203–234, by permission of the publisher. © 1980 by the Pontifical Institute of Mediaeval Studies, Toronto.

can also be readily understood."[2] This is what a branch of science is all about. Albert provided a theoretical structure for the organization and explanation of data in a category of physical nature and to that extent founded a "scientia de mineralibus."[3]

In 1967, Dorothy Wyckoff published a detailed English translation and commentary to Albert's *Minerals*.[4] Her work is so thorough, so scholarly, and so clear that we can do little more than supplement her contributions. Wyckoff, a mineralogist by profession, a classicist by avocation, saw in Albert's study an important step in the field's foundation, for few before her saw Albert's work as anything but a curious blend of scholasticism, lapidarist folklore, and alchemy.[5]

Albert's *Minerals* has a logic in the design of presentation, as we shall see more fully below. In the first book Albert outlined his procedure. In keeping with the logic of Aristotle and the conventional, Empedoclean explanations of the compositions of minerals, he explained that minerals are not alive and have no souls, but are compositions of earth or of water. Stones are the subject of his first discourse. Even the driest stones formed of earth have water which binds the stone together. Some stones are congelations primarily of water, and this provides an explanation of glass and quartz. He rejected the explanation of alchemists who said that stones "born" in water were necessarily stones formed of water, because they might be solidifications of the earth material in water.[6] The power of the elements is the *material cause*. The *efficient cause* is the production of stones through a *mineralizing* power which is, he observed, a mysterious natural process produced by heavenly powers and difficult to explain except through analogy. Albert rejected previous theories of stone production including those of the alchemists who said that

---

[2] *De min.* v, tr.1, c.9 (ed. Borgnet 5: 102b; trans. Wyckoff, p. 251). Unless otherwise noted all quotations in English from Albert's *De mineralibus* are of Wyckoff's translation.

[3] *De min.* III, tr.1, c.1 (ed. Borgnet 5: 60a): ". . . et complebimus in eius totam istius scientiae de mineralibus intentionem" (Wyckoff, p. 155).

[4] *Albertus Magnus Book of Minerals*, trans. by Dorothy Wyckoff (Oxford, 1967).

[5] As late as 1955 a commentary on a translation of Agricola dismissed Albert as well as all other medieval writers of lapidaries with the observation: "There was no important work on mineralogy from the time of Pliny until Agricola published his *De natura fossilium* in 1546 and the shorter introductory work *Bermannus* in 1530. During the intervening fourteen centuries that spanned the rise and fall of the Roman Empire and the Dark and Middle Ages, writers on mineralogical subjects merely elaborated on the information and misinformation contained in Pliny's *Natural History*." Mark C. Bandy and Jean A. Bandy, trans., *George Agricola De Natura Fossilium*, Geological Society of America Special Paper 63 (Menasha, 1955), p. v.

[6] *De min.* I, tr.1, c.3 (ed. Borgnet 5: 4a-b; Wyckoff, p. 20).

stones were purely an accidental production by dry heat, for example a brick produced from clay by baking. Were this so, Albert said, stones would not differ one from another, and there were obvious differences in properties, appearance and powers. Only a discerning mineralizing power can effect the variety of stones. Further, if all stones were merely dry heat, they could be dissolved by moist cold, and "we do not see this happen" (quod non vidimus contingere).[7]

Albert's preference for Aristotelian theories of stone formation was occasionally an *impedimentum* to his insight into minerals. Favoring Aristotle's explanation over vague hints to the contrary in Avicenna, Albert believed that rocks originated where they were formed, that is, *in situ*.[8] Were he to have expanded on Avicenna he might have observed the corrosive effects of water wearing smooth river pebbles or erosion on sedimentary rock layers or the action of glaciers. River pebbles are formed, Albert said, by the action of the heat of the earth on river bottoms which bakes the mixture of earth permeated by water in the pores so that vapor cannot escape, thereby cooking, as it were, a river stone.[9] More acceptable to modern theory is the following statement:

> From all this it seems impossible to report anything certain about the [kind of] place that produces stones. For [stones occur] not in one element only, but in several, and not in one clime only, but in all. . . .For all things produced must have a certain place of production, and away from this they are destroyed and dispersed.[10] (Wyckoff trans.)

A description of the destruction and dispersion (*corrumpuntur et destruuntur*) of stones would have opened new vistas but, from this, it is unclear whether Albert thought the destruction and dispersion was a natural process or accidental.

Similarly Albert came close to developing a classification scheme for stones. Given the ancient, especially Aristotelian, propensity for systemization and classification, one would have expected earlier attempts at classification. Albert seemed to have had thoughts in this direction, but he aborted them. As an example he said there was a

---

[7] *De min.* I, tr.1, c.4 (ed. Borgnet 5: 7a; Wyckoff, p. 21). On the Aristotelian background for Albert's ideas here, see James A. Weisheipl, *Development of Physical Theory in the Middle Ages* (Ann Arbor, 1971), pp. 37-38.

[8] *De min.* I, tr.1, c.7 (ed. Borgnet 5: 9b-10b). See also Wyckoff's discussion on the problem together with references to Aristotle and Avicenna, pp. 16, 26-27, 36-38.

[9] *De min.* I, tr.1, c.8 (ed. Borgnet 5: 11a-b; Wyckoff, p. 31).

[10] *De min.* I, tr.1, c.7 (ed. Borgnet 5: 10b; Wyckoff, p. 29).

group (*genus*) of marbles which included porphyry, alabaster and so on, and that there were other groups.[11] In discussing the cause of colors in nontransparent, nonprecious stones, he said there were four groups, namely flint, tufa, freestone and marble.[12] And yet, he did not develop a systematic classification scheme, bowing instead to the convenience and custom of relating information about specific stones in alphabetical order. "This method," Albert said elsewhere about alphabetization, "is not suitable in philosophy."[13]

Following Aristotle's method Albert dealt with the *formal* cause, namely whether *forma* and *species* can be applied to stones. In modern times, the same question reformulated is whether stones have individual chemical composition, and how categories of similar physical qualities relate to one another, for example, whether all transparent stones are crystalline. "We find," Albert said, "in stones powers which are not those of any element at all," but powers based on "the particular mixture of their elements."[14] Albert followed the Avicennian pharmaceutical theory, although probably not directly from Avicenna's works. Avicenna held that a compound has as its characteristics not only the sum of its constituent elements but, as a result of a "fermentation," unique, specific qualities as well. Thus one cannot predict the qualities of an object, such as a stone, by ana lyzing its chemical makeup. Its *forma specifica* can be known through experience in its use.[15] Albert's doctrine is important because, as will be seen later in his discussion of the qualities of individual stones, each has unique powers which are empirically tested.

Albert implicitly rejected a major pharmaceutical theory over which controversy was raging, probably in the 1240s in Paris where Albert lived before writing the *Minerals*.[16] In the *Minerals*, Albert did not seem to accept the Galenic theory on degrees of intensity for the active and passive qualities of simples and compounds. In a few

---

[11] *De min.* I, tr.1, c.6 (ed. Borgnet 5: 9a; Wyckoff, p. 26).

[12] *De min.* I, tr.2, c.3 (ed. Borgnet 5: 17a; Wyckoff, p. 44).

[13] Cited as *Animals* XXII, tr.2, a.1 by Wyckoff, p. 68; Albert explained that the alphabetical order for stones was most convenient inasmuch as medical men followed this custom in describing simples (*De min.* II, tr.2).

[14] *De min.* I, tr.1, c.6 (ed. Borgnet 5: 8b; Wyckoff, p. 24).

[15] Ibid. "Experience" as the means of knowing the specific qualities can be seen in *De min.* II, tr.1, c.1 (ed. Borgnet 5: 24a, 30a; Wyckoff, pp. 56, 68-69). For more precise statement and corroboration, see Avicenna, *Canon.* V, tr. spec., fol. 507v (Venice 1507); *Canon.* I, fen.2, summa 1, cap.15, fol. 33v; Michael R. McVaugh, *Arnaldi de Villanova, Opera Medica Omnia*, vol. 2: *Aphorismi de gradibus* (Granada-Barcelona, 1975), pp. 18-19.

[16] McVaugh, *Arnaldi*, 2: 31-32.

instances throughout the whole of *Minerals* Albert does allude to the active qualities of warmness and coldness and the passive qualities of dryness and wetness. One of each is possessed by everything, be it animal, vegetable or mineral.[17] Although Albert doubtless knew of Roger Bacon's pronouncements on the subject and may have known of Peter of Spain's attempt to place the physical actions of substances on a high theoretical plane,[18] he made little attempt to incorporate the current controversy in the *Minerals*, and only later in *Plants* did he accept the basic rudiments of Galenic theory.[19] On the surface it seems strange that Albert, given his Aristotelian penchant for systematization, was not attracted to Galen's theory which provided an explanation and perhaps predictive indicator for the physiological action of minerals. In fact, Albert must have consciously rejected this theory. He extensively employed Constantine's (d. ca. 1085) *On degrees* as a source for individual stones in Book Two of the *Minerals*, but Albert omitted Constantine's ascription of intensity of action for the minerals even when quoting directly.[20] We can only conclude that Albert was not satisfied by the theory and, while not speaking against it, was unwilling to employ its rationale for the explanation of various minerals' behavior. Probably he did so because the theory did not satisfy his strong empirical bias[21] or his assumptions.

---

[17] *De min.* IV, tr.1, c.1; IV, tr.1, c.2 (ed. Borgnet 5: 84a, 85b; Wyckoff, pp. 204, 207) Albert gave the degrees of intensity of qualities (and elsewhere) when relating qualities, but simply as cold and dry, and without "degrees"; see *De min.* II, tr.1, c.3; V, tr.1, cc.4, 5, 7, and 8 (5: 27a, 100a, 102a, 102b; trans. Wyckoff pp. 62, 245, 249, 250). It is curious that all citations to Albert's intensity of qualities come in the last two books, thereby raising a question whether, if the work were composed over an extended period and Books IV and V were written last, Albert had not by then come to accept to some small extent Galen's drug theory.

[18] McVaugh, *Arnaldi*, 2: 32; Lynn Thorndike, *A History of Magic and Experimental Science* (New York, 1923), 2: 488-510. We know of no definitive dating of Peter's *Summule logicales*, which contains his pharmaceutical theory, but Heinrich Schipperges (*Die Assimilation der arabischen Medizin durch das Lateinische Mittelater*, in *Sudhoffs Archiv*, Beiheft 3 [Wiesbaden, 1964], p. 180) places it as the earliest of his works. L. M. De Rijk places the date of Peter's *Summule* in the early 1230s (Peter of Spain, *Tractatus, or Summule logicales* [Assen, 1972], pp. lvii-lxi).

[19] For example, Albert, *De veg.* III, tr.1, c.6; VI, tr.1, c.2.

[20] For example, Albert, *De min.* II, tr.2, c.7, *granatus* (ed. Borgnet 5: 38a; Wyckoff, p. 96) quoting directly and by name Constantine's citation of Aristotle; whereas in Constantine's work *De gradibus* (*Opera* [Basel, 1536], p. 352), the degrees are given in sections on drugs intensive to the first degree; "Quos omnes Aristoteles cal[ida] et sic[ca] dixit esse." Compare also *De min.* II, tr.2, c.6, *falcones* (ed. Borgnet 5: 37a; Wyckoff, p. 92) with Constantine *De gradibus* [Basel, 1536], p. 383.

[21] *De min.* II, tr.1, c.1 (ed. Borgnet 5: 24a; Wyckoff, p. 56).

Albert looked to Hermes who, "of all the ancients," gave "the most probable reason for the powers of stones."[22] One by one Albert related the various authorities' explanations before summarizing those of Hermes. The heavenly power operated through stars and constellations to impress powers into every specific form of stone.[23] "Nevertheless this statement," Albert cautioned, "is not enough for natural science (*physicis*), although perhaps it may be sufficient for astrology and magic. For natural science discusses the cause that acts upon matter."[24] The implanted powers in stones (and metals) are both indirect and accidental. It is indirect because the power goes through the intermediary of the elements and the fermentation. The power is accidental in so far as not all objects in their various locations receive the same distribution. Thus stones have accidental properties, such as color, transparency, hardness, fissility, porosity and size, according to their mixture.[25] What Albert calls mixture is today called chemical composition. Thus each type of stone is unique. Even individual stones of the same class may differ from one another as, for instance, a *saphirus* which is said to lose its power to cure abscesses once it has cured one. But even here there are variations from the norm because Albert claimed that he had personally seen a *saphirus* cure two abscesses in a four-year interval.[26]

Tractate Two of Book Two is the most familiar section of the *Minerals* because it is the traditional lapidary. Often in many manuscripts this section of the *Minerals* was separated and stood as an independent treatise.[27] The names of some ninety-nine "precious stones" as well as their descriptions and powers are related by Albert as they are known "either by experience or from the writings of authorities."[28]

In this section Albert gave advice on how to conduct successful business deals, win battles, test for virginity, prevent storms, protect

---

[22] *De min.* II, tr.1, c.3 (ed. Borgnet 5: 27b; Wyckoff, p. 63). But Albert often disagreed with Hermes on other matters of detail, e.g., *De min.* III, tr.1, c.3 and 8; IV, tr.1, c.4 (ed. Borgnet 5: 63a, 69b, 87a; Wyckoff, pp. 162, 171-172, 213).

[23] *De min.* II, tr.1, c.2-3 (ed. Borgnet 5: 24a-28a; Wyckoff, pp. 58-64).

[24] *De min.* II, tr.1, c.3 (ed. Borgnet 5: 27a; Wyckoff, p. 63).

[25] *De min.* I, tr.2, c.1-8 (ed. Borgnet 5: 14a-21b; Wyckoff, pp. 36-53).

[26] *De min.* II, tr.2, c.17 (ed. Borgnet 5: 44b; Wyckoff, p. 115).

[27] Inc.: "Supponamus autem nomina praecipuorum lapidum et virtutes secundum . . ." — Cambridge, Univ. Lib. MS Dd III 16, fol. 7v-15v (with Book II, tractate 3, on sigils); London, British Libr. MS Sloane 1009, fol. 68v-72v; Toledo, Bibl. del Cabildo MS 157, fol. 78 ff.; Vienna, Nationalbibliothek MS Pal. 2303 (s. xiv), fol. 62-64v; MS Pal. 12,901 (s. xiii-xiv), fol. 94-125v.

[28] *De min.* II, tr.2, c.1 (ed. Borgnet 5: 30a; Wyckoff, p. 68).

against robbery, reduce or eliminate fever, stop breathing, confer happiness, and cure scabs, dropsy, heart attacks, kidney stones, bladder stones, hemorrhoids, belching, stomach ache, jaundice and diarrhea. In short, stones can control almost any aspect of the environment as well as most physical ailments as diagnosed. But for someone unfamiliar with medieval tradition it comes as a surprise to read of the saint advising the use of stones to thieves for successful robbery,[29] to women to prevent conception or to produce a miscarriage,[30] to men to betray secrets,[31] and to all people to arouse sexual desire.[32] The initial shock is mitigated perhaps when one reads that there are stones which counteract these powers, such as stones which drive away phantoms,[33] keep travellers safe from robbery,[34] help childbirth,[35] restrain sedition,[36] moderate licentiousness[37] and check hot passions and desires.[38] Generally most stones are recommended for qualities of making people happy and alleviating pain and illness. In this section more than any other Albert was relying on previous authorities, including Marbode (1035-1122), bishop of Rennes, and possibly as well the Venerable Bede.[39]

Albert, true to his prefatory remarks, has throughout related his personal experience in attesting to the stones' powers. Albert often differentiated what his authorities say and what he learned through experience. When he said chalcedony is good for fanciful illusions for those afflicted with melancholy and causes and preserves the powers of the body, he added, "The last is a matter of experience" (*hoc ultimum est expertum*).[40] For him it worked. He said about

---

[29] *De min.* II, tr.2, c.13, *ophthalmus* (ed. Borgnet 5: 42b; Wyckoff, p. 110).

[30] *De min.* II, tr.2, c.8, *jaspis*; c.13, *oristes* (ed. Borgnet 5: 39b, 43a; Wyckoff, pp. 100, 110).

[31] *De min.* II, tr.2, c.15, *quiritia* (ed. Borgnet 5: 44a; Wyckoff, p. 114).

[32] *De min.* II, tr.2, c.1, *alectorius* (ed. Borgnet 5: 31b; Wyckoff, p. 73).

[33] *De min.* II, tr.2, c.3, *chrysolitus* (ed. Borgnet 5: 34b; Wyckoff, p. 83).

[34] *De min.* II, tr.2, c.8, *hyacinthus* (ed. Borgnet 5: 38b; Wyckoff, p. 98).

[35] *De min.* II, tr.2, c.6, *galaricides* (ed. Borgnet 5: 38a; Wyckoff, p. 95).

[36] *De min.* II, tr.2, c.5, *epistrites* (ed. Borgnet 5: 36a; Wyckoff, p. 90).

[37] *De min.* II, tr.2, c.7, *gelosia* (ed. Borgnet 5: 37b; Wyckoff, p. 94).

[38] *De min.* II, tr.2, c.17, *sardonyx* (ed. Borgnet 5: 45a; Wyckoff, p. 117). In the case of onyx, a stone which has bad effects (*De min.* II, tr.2, c.13, *onyx, onycha* [ed. Borgnet 5: 42a-b; Wyckoff, pp. 108-110], the stone is specifically counteracted by *sardinus* (II, tr.2, c.17 [ed. Borgnet 5: 45a; Wyckoff, p. 117]).

[39] Wyckoff, *Albertus*, pp. 266-268. Venerable Bede's lapidary is an example of a group of lapidaries, the so-called "Christian Symbolic Lapidary," a discussion always of twelve stones, which may differ. There is less uniqueness in this type of lapidary, thus making it unclear whether Albert ever used Bede on stones.

[40] *De min.* II, tr.2, c.3, *chalcedonius* (ed. Borgnet 5: 33a; Wyckoff, p. 78).

carnelian that "it has been found by experience that it reduces bleeding, especially from menstruation or hemorrhoids."[41] In powder form chrysolite helps one with asthma but in relating information, Albert failed to embrace with his own testimony his source's assertion that it expels stupidity and confers wisdom.[42] We might assume that he omitted his personal verification not because he doubted that chrysolite had these powers but either because he simply had not experimented with it or because of an economy of space. He challenges the credulity of his modern reader by telling of his experience with the stone *ramai*. He said experience gives certain proof that through its powers (". . .virtus pro certo experta est. . .") it overcomes looseness of the bowels and especially the bleeding of dysentery and menstruation.[43] He related first hand experience with powers of the stones rock crystal (*crystallus*, II. 2, 3), dragonstone (*draconites*, 4), jet (*gagates*, 7), amber (*ligurius*, 10), onyx (*onycha*, 13), sapphire (? *saphirus*, 17), emerald, (? *smaragdus*, 17), topaz (*topasion*, 18), and *virites* (?, 19). In no other lapidary does the author attempt to relate personal experience to the testimony of others on stones' powers. In addition, Albert attempted to straighten out descriptions of stones and testify to their locations, for example, dragonstone, perhaps a fossil ammonite (*draconites*, 4), eaglestone (*echite*, 5), pearl (*margarita*, 11), emerald (? *smaragdus*, 17), and *specularis* (?, 17). It is clear from his section on stones, and is even clearer in the section on metals discussed below, that Albert has not simply compiled previous sources but has added observations and judgments of his own which constitute a distinct contribution to the subject.

A modern mineralogist, more concerned with minerals themselves than with methodological problems, would observe that opal has two to four different names in Albert's work, differentiated by coloring patterns, *ophthalmus* (13), *pantherus* (14) and maybe *hiena* (8) and *agates* (1). Each one has different powers. Similarly there are four names, descriptions and powers for amber: *chryselectrum* (4), *succinus* (17), *ligurius* (10), and *kacabre* (9, maybe jet as well). Under *chryselectrum* he said that the story of its being a "solidification of an ignoble substance. . .is not true," but under *ligurius* (10), meaning in Greek "lynx-urine," he accepted the tale that the lynx, jealous of its urine, buries it and it subsequently hardens into amber. A modern expert, reading Wyckoff's translation, would wonder whether Albert

---

[41] *De min.* II, tr.2, c.3, *cornelius* (ed. Borgnet 5: 33b; Wyckoff, pp. 81-82).

[42] *De min.* II, tr.2, c.3, *chrysolitus* (ed. Borgnet 5: 34a; Wyckoff, p. 82).

[43] *De min.* II, tr.2, c.16, *ramai* (ed. Borgnet 5: 44a; Wyckoff, p. 44).

might not have known that *exacolitus* (5), *filacterium* (6), and *gecolitus* (7) were scribal errors in his authorities' texts for stones otherwise already discussed?[44] Why does Albert, he would think, attribute sexes to two stones, *balagius* (2) and *peranites* (14), when there is no hint of stone sexuality in Books One and Two where the theory of stones and minerals are discussed? Again, why would Albert advise and believe that stones have such wondrous powers — preternatural powers, in the modern view?

From a logical and rational point of view, many of Albert's theoretical explanations could be considered scientific even in the twentieth century. The acceptance of the assertion of stones' powers will be better understood by a physican and psychologist than by a mineralogist or even a gemologist. Albert accepted the claims of Costa ben Luca (Qustā ibn Lūqā, fl. late 9th c.)[45] who argued in a treatise called *On physical ligatures, incantations and suspensions around the neck* that, contrary to a fundamental aversion among the Greeks to magic and the occult, many of the body's afflictions are not because of bodily disorders, but are attributable to mental disorders. To some extent the mind controls the body, as Indian medical people have claimed and even some Greeks allowed. A belief in a cure is frequently itself a cure for the body's ill. It is superfluous to argue a stone's power because experience demonstrates the power, the mind believes it, and, therefore, it has the power.[46] It works. Costa ben Luca's work was known to Albert, but Albert seems to have had trouble in citing it because sometimes he calls it by title[47] and only

---

[44] Trans. Wyckoff, pp. 91-92, 95.

[45] See Fuat Sezgin, *Geschichte des arabischen Schrifttums*, 3 vols. (Leiden, 1970), 3: 270-274; Albert Dietrich, *Medicinalia Arabica* (Gottingen, 1966), p. 198; Carl Brockelman, *Geschichte der arabischen Literatur*, 2 vols. (Leiden, 1943) 2: 222-224.

[46] *De physicis ligaturis*, Brit. Libr. MS Add. 22,719 (s. xii), fol. 200v (-202v). The Latin translation is printed in *Opera Constantini* (Basel, 1536), pp. 317-320, and in *Opera Arnaldi de Villa Nova* (Venice, 1505), pp. 344-345. Both Constantine and Arnald are credited in various manuscripts as being Costa ben Luca's translator for *De physicis ligaturis*. The British Library's twelfth-century manuscript of the text, and the use of Costa by Constantine for *De gradibus* and by Marbode for *De lapidibus* makes it certain that the translation, if not by Constantine, was prepared by the eleventh century and certainly available to Albert.

[47] With the information coming from Costa ben Luca's *De physicis ligaturis*, Albert cites the work as "in physicis ligaturis" in *De min.* II, tr.2, c.3, *chrysolitus*. But in three other citations Albert seemingly cites the same work as "in incantationibus autem et physicis ligaturis", but the information does not come from Costa ben Luca's work; cf. *De min.* II, tr.2, c.5, *epistrites*; c.7, *galarcides* ("in libro de ligaturis physicis"); c.13, *oristes*, (ed. Borgnet 5: 36b, 38a, 43a; Wyckoff, pp. 90, 94, 110). Possibly Albert had yet another text (or texts) for *On physical ligatures*, and he merely compressed them into the one title, which was confused with Costa ben Luca's work.

once by name, *Constabulence*, where the quotation makes certain the text is related to Costa ben Luca's.[48] Further, at least two other of Albert's authorities accepted Costa ben Luca's assertions, namely Constantine the African and Marbode.[49] If one reads the lapidary section of Albert's *Minerals*, the tractate on images and sigils (II, tr.3) and to some extent the books on metals (III, IV), with Costa ben Luca's ideas in mind, then the powers inherent in stones, sigils, and metals make sense as psychotherapy. Much will make sense, not all. Thus when one reads that the dragonstone bestows victory[50] (II. 2, 4 *draconites*), then possibly the power of suggestion was operative.[51] Self-confidence derived from the stone's power. What about the second quality of dragonstone that it dispels poisons? Would a twentieth-century psychiatrist be willing to state unequivocally all *toxicity* or a *belief* in toxicity could not be willed away by faith in a cure or prophylactic?[52] So, when Albert says of carnelian (II. 2, 3, *cornelius*), "It has been found by experience that it reduces bleeding, especially from menstruation or hemorrhoids. It is even said to calm anger," one might readily agree to a possible psychotherapeutic effect of the latter and be cautious in challenging the efficacy of the former.[53]

The lines between the physiological and psychological (spiritual to Albert) are not clear, nor is it clear always whether the various stones are pharmaceutically active or inert as a placebo. Hematite, Albert advises, is "a powerful styptic, and therefore experience shows that if crushed, mixed with water, and drunk it is a remedy for a flux of the bladder or bowels, or menstruation; and it also heals a flux of bloody saliva."[54] Hematite is a red oxide of iron containing ferric chloride

---

[48] *De min.* II, tr.3, c.6 (ed. Borgnet 5: 55b-56a; Wyckoff, pp. 146-147).

[49] John M. Riddle, *Marbode of Rennes' (1035-1123) De lapidibus*, in *Sudhoffs Archiv*, Beiheft 20 (Wiesbaden, 1977), pp. 9, 16-20.

[50] *De min.* II, tr.2, c.4, *draconites* (ed. Borgnet 5: 35a; Wyckoff, p. 87).

[51] For an exploration of this phenomenon in a modern context, see Jerome D. Frank, *Persuasion and Healing: A Comparative Study of Psychotherapy* (Baltimore, 1961).

[52] For a recent reappraisal of medieval psychiatry and a revision upward in appreciation of medieval approaches to mental disorders, see Jerome Kroll, "A Reappraisal of Psychiatry in the Middle Ages," *Arch. Gen. Psychiatry*, 29 (1973), 276-283.

[53] *De min.* II, tr.2, c.3, *carneleus* (ed. Borgnet 5: 33b; Wyckoff, pp. 81-82). Arthur K. Shapiro, a physician, ("The Placebo Effect in the History of Medical Treatment: Implications for Psychiatry," *Amer. Jour. of Psychiatry*, 116 (1959), 298-304, esp. 299) defines the placebo effect "as the psychological, physiological or psychophysiological effect of any medication or procedure given with therapeutic intent, which is independent of or minimally related to the pharmacologic effects of the medication or to the specific effects of the procedure, and which operates through a psychological mechanism."

[54] *De min.* II, tr.2, c.5, *ematites* (ed. Borgnet 5: 36a-b; Wyckoff, p. 90).

which acts as an astringent.[55] But in comparing Albert's stones with modern pharmaceutical compounds there is always an element of uncertainty especially when we cannot even know what Albert's stone was, as for instance with *ramai*. Albert said that *ramai* was certain to overcome looseness of the bowels and especially the bleeding of dysentery and menstruation.[56] If we do not know what *ramai* was, we are unable to confirm or reject, however timidly, the alleged physiological actions. In most instances the actions may be those of a placebo but, as is recognized by modern medicine, placebo's have positive results in short-term psychotherapy.[57]

An interesting and largely typical example of Albert's recommendations is coral about which he said:

> And it has been found by experience that it is good against any sort of bleeding. It is even said that, worn around the neck, it is good against epilepsy and the action of menstruation, and against storms, lightning, and hail. And if it is powdered and sprinkled with water on herbs and trees, it is reported to multiply their fruits. They also say that it speeds the beginning and end of any business.[58] (Wyckoff trans.)

Coral is almost entirely calcium carbonate. Modern experts affirm, as any gardener knows, that calcium carbonate helps plants. Probably it would aid in coagulation either as a topical application or, possibly, internally.[59] For epilepsy, on the other hand, it is more difficult to determine how the disease would respond to calcium carbonate. An epileptic has an acidosis condition, which is an abnormally high production of acids or an abnormal decrease of alkalinity. Modern therapy would include a ketogenic diet in treatment because it produces acetone or ketone bodies which are helpful to an epileptic. An alkaline such as coral would be beneficial, but Albert advises its use as a necklace! The examples show that the ancients did know some

---

[55] Ferric oxide has no currently recognized astringent qualities but ferric chloride does. Pliny (*Nat. Hist.* xxxiv. 45. 152-153, ed. H. Rackham [Cambridge, 1952], 9: 238) recommends iron rust to unite, dry, and staunch wounds.

[56] *De min.* ii, tr.2, c.16 (ed. Borgnet 5: 44a; Wyckoff, pp. 114).

[57] In five separate studies when patients with various emotional states were given placebos, fifty-five percent showed significant symptomatic improvements: Lester H. Gliedman, Earl H. Nash Jr., Stanley D. Imber, Anthony R. Stone, and Jerome D. Frank, "Reduction of Symptoms by Pharmacologically Inert Substances and by Short-term Psychotherapy," *A.M.A. Archives of Neurology and Psychiatry*, 79 (1958), 345-351.

[58] *De min.* ii, tr.2, c.3 (ed. Borgnet 5: 33b; Wyckoff, p. 81).

[59] We are grateful to Prof. Samuel Tove, a biochemist at N. C. State University, in assisting in this judgment.

specific effects of the substances they dealt with and that their experiments tended to further this knowledge although in other respects they were credulous and accepted claims that could not be verified.

In trying to understand his attitude to stones, it is important for the history of science to realize the hermetic origins of much of Albert's thought. For in speaking of the occult (our term) powers of the *liparea* stone, he said, "If this is true, it is very marvellous, and undoubtedly is to be ascribed to the power of the heavens: for, as Hermes says, there are marvellous powers in stones and likewise in plants, by means of which natural magic could accomplish whatever it does, if their powers were well understood."[60] Albert knew of Evax, king of the Arabians, whose letter to Emperor Tiberius (14-37 AD) claimed that God had placed in each variety of stone certain powers beneficial to man.[61] These powers were made known to the Egyptians and almost lost in a fire which burned the library, presumably the Alexandrian library. The secrets were rescued and held in a trust by the Arabians. These secrets are there for man's discovery. Marbode said that for man each herb has certain powers, but even greater than those in herbs are the powers in stones.

Is not this line of thought, stemming from the hermetic tradition accepted by Albert, just as important in the history of modern science as the thinking of the more highly acclaimed natural philosophy which sought logical explanations for natural things, but whose theories were more separated from observation and empiricism? For Albert, God was not in each rock, but he had put certain powers into them through secondary causes, including the celestial bodies. Those powers, whatever they are, can be discovered only by observation of their effects.

Albert saw a division between natural science and the science of magic; the latter he saw as a legitimate field of inquiry but inferior to natural science.[62] When explaining why images of things are formed

---

[60] *De min.* II, tr.2, c.10 (ed. Borgnet 5: 402; Wyckoff, pp. 102-103).

[61] For text of the Evax letters, see Riddle, *Marbode*, pp. 28-31.

[62] When explaining that he was to omit a discussion of a method for the discovery of metal ores, an omission we regret, Albert said that the science dealing with this "depends not upon [scientific] demonstration, but upon experience in the occult and the astrological." He called that science, "the science of magic called treasure findings" (*De min.* III, tr.1, c.1 [ed. Borgnet 5: 60a; Wyckoff, p. 154]. After relating Hermes' reason for powers of stones, Albert stated: "Nevertheless this statement is not enough for natural science, although perhaps it may be sufficient for astrology and magic" (*De min.* II, tr.1, c.3 [ed. Borgnet 5: 27b; Wyckoff, p. 63]). But throughout this work Albert gathers information from magicians, astrologers, and incantators, e.g., *De min.* II, tr.2, c.8, *iaspis*; c.11, *magnes*; II, tr.3, c.5 (ed. Borgnet 5: 39b, 40b, 53b; Wyckoff, pp. 100, 104, 141).

in the patterns of gem stones and not in other things, for example in mineral ores, bones, etc., he theorizes that gemstones are more amenable to heavenly impression during their formation. He said, "These things are not pure science, but because they are good doctrine they are included here."[63]

Why should an image of a king's head appear in a marble slab which Albert saw when he was a young man in Venice? Albert had satisfied the curious spectators to the scene who wondered why the king's forehead was disproportionately large. Young Albert explained that, while the mineralizing power was forming the marble, the vapor at the forehead rose disproportionately higher, like a cloud.[64] He accepted the mysteries of the mineralizing power and the general power of nature. He was only a spectator, an observer, who called witness to the holy mysteries to his fellows. They all need only learn and know the powers God had given them in the secrets of things.

Another significant feature of the *Minerals* is the extended attention which Albert devoted to a consideration of metals and to materials which he classified as "intermediates," possessing the characteristics of both metals and stones. Three of the five books and nearly half of the space in his treatise were assigned to these topics, and in the discussion of metals Albert made many noteworthy observations. More than in the books on stones, he was forced to draw on his own experience since the sources available to him had even less to say about metals than about stones. Albert explained the problem facing him, and his method of solution, at the beginning of Book III.

> In [writing] this as well as the preceding books, I have not seen the treatise of Aristotle, save for some excerpts for which I have inquired assiduously in different parts of the world. Therefore I shall state, in a manner which can be supported by reasoning, either what has been handed down by philosophers or what I have found out by my own observations. For at one time I became a wanderer, making long journeys to mining districts, so that I could learn by observation the nature of metals. And for the same reason I have inquired into the transmutation of metals in alchemy, so as to learn from this, too, something of their nature and accidental properties. For this is the best and surest method of investigation, because then each thing is understood with reference to its own particular cause, and there is very little doubt about its accidental properties.[65] (Wyckoff trans.)

---

[63] *De min.* II, tr.3, c.2 (ed. Borgnet 5: 51a; Wyckoff, p. 134).

[64] *De min.* II, tr.3, c.1 (ed. Borgnet 5: 49a-b; Wyckoff, pp. 128-129).

[65] *De min.* III, tr.1, c.1 (ed. Borgnet 5: 59a-b; Wyckoff, p. 153).

To discuss metals, then, Albert sought to avail himself of the best sources of information he could obtain. From Peripatetic and Arabic philosophers Albert took elements with which to create a comprehensive theory explaining the formation of metals and their distinctive properties. The writings of the philosophers were not sufficient, however. From miners Albert learned much about where metallic ores and intermediates were found and the characteristics of ore bodies in relation to surrounding geological formations. That information, supplemented by personal observation, was cited to support various features of his theory. When miners could tell him little about the properties of metals, Albert turned to the alchemists, who knew of metals through their efforts to effect transmutations. By drawing upon the experience of two contemporary groups whose interest in and constant association with metals made them most knowledgeable on the subject, the miners and alchemists, Albert was able to effect a unique synthesis. Books III through V of the *Minerals* contain information on mineralogy and on metals which helps to bridge the gap in our knowledge of these subjects between the writings of Pliny in the first century and the sixteenth-century works of Biringuccio and Agricola. By focusing attention on metals it also represents a milestone in the literature, one which establishes the content, and to some extent the format, of later studies.[66]

Considering first the topic of mining and mineralogy, it is surprising that today we know as little as we do about the expansion of mining and the use of metals in the twelfth and thirteenth centuries. As John Nef, in his analysis of medieval mining, has noted,

> The increasing curiosity about the material world and the increasing agricultural, commercial, industrial and artistic needs for gold, silver, iron, lead, copper, tin and alloys of these metals made men eager to explore beneath the soil, to examine and to exploit the substances they

---

[66] Following Albert, the first major work devoted to metals was the *Pirotechnia* of Vannoccio Biringuccio (1540). Biringuccio began with a preface describing the location of ores, a book devoted to the ores of metals, and a book discussing "semi-minerals," a number of which, like marchasite, alum, and arsenic, are Albert's "intermediates," before proceeding to the discussion of assaying and smelting (Vannoccio Biringuccio, *Pirotechnia*, trans. by Cyril Stanley Smith and Martha Teach Gnudi [New York: American Institute of Mining and Mineralogical Engineering, 1941]). Agricola's primary work on mineralogy was *De natura fossilium* (1546). While devising a more "modern" classification system for minerals based on natural properties, Agricola's format followed Albert in treating metals in a separate section subsequent to the general discussion on "stones." See Georgius Agricola, *De natura fossilium*, trans. M. C. Bandy and J. A. Bandy, Geological Society of America Special Paper 63 (Menasha, 1955).

> found. Not until the eve of the Reformation, when fresh waves of settlers pushed into the same regions, was there another comparable movement of exploration and discovery.[67]

The discovery of gold in the river sands of the Rhine and the Elbe, the opening of silver-bearing ore bodies in the Carpathians and Erzgebirge, in Devon and Alsace, elicited the attention of commercial interests and civil authority, but drew scant notice from the schoolmen. Albert is practically the only major medieval figure to discuss the state of mineralogy before the sixteenth century. Although he had little to say about the technology of mining, which had little bearing on his main thesis, he did wrestle with the difficult problem of ore formation, thereby providing excellent descriptions of many primary ores. His own field observations, made on visits to such famous mining sites as Goslar and Freiberg, constitute an important contribution to our understanding of medieval mineralogy.

A full consideration of Albert's discussion of ores and of mining lore has been made by Dorothy Wyckoff in her article, "Albertus Magnus on Ore Deposits."[68] It suffices here to repeat the major points established by Wyckoff. Of primary concern for Albert was the need to establish, in the scholastic tradition, the causes for the occurrence and properties of metals "in a manner which can be supported by reason."[69]

The basis for the organization of Albert's *Minerals* was a synthesis of Peripatetic concepts of matter, central to which was the doctrine of the four elements, earth, water, air and fire, and Arabic alchemical ideas, which emphasized the importance of quicksilver and sulfur. The order of discussion was dictated by the degree of complexity involved. "First, then, we shall investigate stones, and afterward metals, and finally substances intermediate between these; for in fact the production of stones is simpler and more obvious than that of metals."[70] The material substance of stones, which are infusible, is some form of earth or some form of water. Metals, on the other hand, exhibit properties not possessed by stone, in that they are fusi-

---

[67] John U. Nef, "Mining and Metallurgy in Medieval Civilization" in *The Cambridge Economic History of Europe* (Cambridge, 1952) 2: 437. See also the important paper by Nadine F. George, "Albertus Magnus and Chemical Technology in a Time of Transition," in this volume, 235-261.

[68] Dorothy Wyckoff, "Albertus Magnus on Ore Deposits," *Isis* 49 (1958), 109-122.

[69] *De min.* III, tr.1, c.1 (ed. Borgnet 5: 59a; Wyckoff, p. 153).

[70] *De min.* I, tr.1, c.1 (ed. Borgnet 5: 1a; Wyckoff, p. 9).

ble and malleable, and these properties arise from the admixture of quicksilver and sulfur which, in turn, are combinations of the simple elements. The efficient cause for the production of metals was, according to Albert, heat which digests the unsuitable materials and allows for the combustion of the opposed passive properties of moisture, associated with quicksilver, and dryness, associated with sulfur, which give metals their unique characteristics.[71] A key concept in the genesis of metallic ores was that the nature of the formations in which the ores were "generated" influenced the proportions and the degree of purity with which the simple elements were mixed, thus determining the particular metal to be found:

> In order to know the cause of all the things that are produced, we must understand that real metal is not formed except by the natural sublimation of moisture and earth, such as has been described above. For in such a place, where earthy and watery materials are first mixed together, much that is impure is mixed with the pure, but the impure is of no use in the formation of metal. And from the hollow places containing such a mixture the force of the rising fume opens out pores large or small, many or few, according to the nature of the [surrounding] stone or earth; and in these [pores] the rising fume or vapour spreads out for a long time and is concentrated and reflected; since it contains the more subtle part of the mixed material it hardens in those channels and is mixed together as vapour in the pores, and is converted into metal of the same kind as the vapour.[72] (Wyckoff trans.)

Thus it is that gold and copper, both partaking of the redness imparted by sulfur, differed in their first properties because of the relative purity and admixture of the constituents. Gold had both pure quicksilver and sulfur mixed in the ideal proportions, and, for Albert, the nature of the place was a determining factor in the final product.

> But gold which is formed in sands as a kind of grains, large or small, is formed from a hot and very subtle vapour, concentrated and digested in the midst of the sandy material, and afterwards hardened into gold. For a sandy place is very hot and dry; but water getting in closes the pores so that [the vapour] cannot escape; and thus is concentrated upon itself and converted into gold. And therefore this kind of gold is better. And there are two reasons for this: one is that the best way of purifying sulfur is by repeated washing, and the sulfur in watery

---

[71] *De min.* III, tr.1, c.5 (ed. Borgnet 5: 65b-66a; Wyckoff, p. 167).

[72] *De min.* III, tr.1, c.10 (ed. Borgnet 5: 72b-73a; Wyckoff, pp. 182-183).

> places is repeatedly washed and purified; and for the same reason the earthy quicksilver is often washed and purified and rendered more subtle. Another reason is the closing of the pores underneath the water along the banks; and thus the dispersed vapour is well-composed and condensed, and is digested nobly into the substance of gold, and hardens into gold.[73] (Wyckoff trans.)

For copper, however, its occurrence in intrusive veins meant that the vapor could not be concentrated so that heat could digest the unsuitable materials. The resulting effect was a degraded mixture which was similar to gold in appearance, but inferior in form and properties.

> Let us assume, then, that the quicksilver is good, not full of dross and dirt, but still not completely cleansed of extraneous moisture; and that the substance of the sulfur is full of dross, burning hot and partly burnt, and in this condition it is mixed with the quicksilver, both in substance and in quality. Then undoubtedly it changes the quicksilver to a red color; and because neither is sufficiently subtle, they cannot be mixed well. And this will make copper, which is not at all well mixed, and much dross is separated from it, and it evaporates greatly in the fire.[74] (Wyckoff trans.)

The reference to an excess of dross and the occurrence of impure sulfur most likely stems from firsthand experience with the copper ores of the Rammelsberg at Goslar. There the sulfide ore of copper, chalcopyrite, appears in places in graded beds containing other heavy metal sulfides, and in a portion of the old bed, intercalated with slate in a network of ores including pyrite, galena and sphalerite.[75] The separation of copper from such an ore body would have involved repeated roastings, with material loss, and the copious release of sul-

---

[73] *De min.* III, tr.1, c.9 (ed. Borgnet 5: 73b; Wyckoff, p. 184). Albert believed that metals were formed where found, and so missed the true significance of alluvial gold deposits. However, nearly three hundred years later Biringuccio repeated many of Albert's observations on stream deposits while only suggesting the possibility of water transport to account for them. It was left to Agricola to suggest the true explanation of the formation of alluvial deposits.

[74] *De min.* IV, tr.1, c.6 (ed. Borgnet 5: 90a; Wyckoff, p. 223).

[75] Pyrite, galena, and sphalerite are the sulfides of iron, lead, and zinc respectively. A full discussion of the constitution of the Rammelsberg ore beds can be found in F. H. Bayschlag, J. H. L. Vogt, and P. Krusch, *The Deposits of Useful Minerals and Rocks: Ore Deposits*, trans. S. J. Truscott (London, 1914-16), 2: 1145-1148.

furous fumes.[76] Albert's theory, then, has been carefully constructed to conform with observed phenomena, graphically demonstrating that he was engaged in a scientific investigation into the nature of minerals, rather than elaborating on the knowledge of metals in the encyclopedist tradition.

The discussion of ores in the *Minerals* was not intended to include their identifying characteristics and properties. For one thing, Albert, like all writers on the subject before the sixteenth century, did not make a clear distinction between metals and their ores as having separate chemical identities. The occurrence of ores was used to illustrate the general theory for the constitution of metals. Yet, the descriptions are sufficiently precise for us to be able to identify those ores of which Albert had firsthand knowledge, and to determine where his information had been derived from other sources. In particular, his descriptions of mercury and tin clearly indicate a lack of familiarity with the ores of those metals. His treatment of tin ore nevertheless is of interest because of the possible light it throws on the date of composition of the *Minerals*.

Albert's discussion on tin ore is very brief: "Two [kinds of] tin are found, namely a harder and drier kind which comes from England or Britain, and a somewhat softer kind which is found more abundantly in parts of Germany."[77] In both regions the tin-rich lodes are associated with granitic intrusions. In England the Cornwall-Devon complex had been mined since pre-Roman times, and by the thirteenth century extensive underground mining of the granitic matrix already was being undertaken. The German mines occur in a broad, north-south zone intersecting the Erzgebirge (Ore Mountains) along the Saxony-Bohemia border not far from Freiberg.[78] Mining for tin had begun near Graupen, in Bohemia, by the end of the twelfth century,

---

[76] Agricola gives a detailed description of the complex process used to reduce copper pyrites to the metal. As a preliminary step, "The cokes of melted pyrites are usually roasted twice over. . . first. . . in a slow fire and afterward in a fierce one." The preliminary roasting drove off some of the sulfur, but additional roasting and refining was necessary to convert the black, brittle matte from the initial treatment to relatively pure blister copper. From Albert's descriptions it is clear that he had witnessed the process. Georgius Agricola, *De re metallica*, trans. by Herbert Clark Hoover and Lou Henry Hoover (London, 1912), p. 349; see also Hoover's footnote on the refining process, p. 407.

[77] *De min.* IV, tr.1, c.4 (ed. Borgnet 5: 88b; Wyckoff, p. 217).

[78] The geomorphology of the Cornwall-Devon complex is described in Charles F. Park, Jr., and Ray A. MacDiarmen, *Ore Deposits*, 3rd ed. (San Francisco: W. H. Freeman & Co., 1975), pp. 163-173; that of the Erzgebirge, in Beyschlag, Vogt and Krusch, *Useful Minerals*, 1: 425-429.

and, according to Albert's contemporary, Matthew Paris, tin ores had been discovered in Germany in 1241.[79] Certainly, this would refer to deposits on the northern slope of the Erzgebirge. From Albert's description, however, it appears that early tin mining in Saxony-Bohemia was confined to the exploitation of alluvial concentrations of the major tin ore, cassiterite. This was still largely true four hundred years later when Agricola described a number of "ancient" methods for working alluvial tin deposits.[80] By comparison to the Cornish hard rock mines the Saxon deposits of ore then would be "soft," as Albert described them.

From Albert's failure to describe cassiterite, the principal tin ore in the deposits of Saxony, one can only conclude that he never saw active tin mining.[81] This omission indirectly tends to support the completion date of 1250 for the *Minerals*. If Albert had visited the silver mines at Freiberg during his youth, as seems probable, there would have been little reason to make a side trip over the mountains into Bohemia to visit the then relatively minor tin works. However, if, as Dorothy Wyckoff has suggested, Albert continued to seek information for the book on his travels as prior provincial in 1254-1256 a visit to the cloister of Andelhausen near Freiberg or to the chapter house of St. Michael at Litomerice in Bohemia, just south of the Erzgebirge, almost certainly would have included examination of nearby tin mines.[82] The absence of a firsthand account of tin ores in the *Minerals* would seem to imply, then, that Albert had completed his work before 1254.[83]

---

[79] *Matthew Paris's English History From the Year 1235 to 1273*, trans. J. A. Giles (London, 1852), 1: 373.

[80] Agricola, *De re metallica*, trans. Hoover, pp. 336-341. Agricola noted that of eight common methods for mining tin, only two were of recent origin. The passage contains an illustration showing a miner digging into the side of a stream bank to tap an alluvial deposit with a mattock, indicative of the softness of the deposits.

[81] At one point Albert claimed to have seen tin incorporated with stone, but no details are given. This, however, was probably a reference to the mixed, metallic-looking pyrites of the Rammelsberg. The earthy brown-black nodules of cassiterite found in alluvial deposits would not fit the description given. *De min.* III, tr.1, c.1 (ed. Borgnet 5: 59a-60b; Wyckoff, p. 154).

[82] V. J. Koudelka gives the date for the founding of the chapter house of St. Michael at Litomerice in Bohemia as 1236, "Zur Geschichte der bohemischen Dominikanerprovinz im Mittelalter," *Archivum Fratrum Praedicatorum*, 25 (1956), 145-146. The founding of the cloister of Arndelhousen at Freiberg in 1234 is indicated in a manuscript footnote quoted in Heibert C. Scheeben, "Handschriften I," *Archiv der deutschen Dominkaner*, 1 (1937), 174-175.

[83] See Wyckoff's arguments on the "Date of Composition of the Book of Minerals" in introd. to her trans., pp. xxxv-xli, particularly p. xxxvi, where she argues that some observations made at Freiberg most probably date from his term as prior provincial.

Although incidental to his main purpose, Albert included several observations which do much to expand our knowledge of the state of thirteenth-century geology. One of these is his discussion of a formation later termed the *gossan* by Cornish miners or *Eisenhut* by the Germans: "If the metal is incorporated with the whole stone, the upper part is full of slag and useless, while the inside is better and more noble."[84] The passage accurately describes the weathered crust of oxides for a sulfide ore body. Whether Albert ever saw a formation is uncertain, but his passage shows that thirteenth-century miners recognized its importance. Finally, Albert recorded his personal observation of a formation peculiar to ore bodies, the pinching out of ore veins passing from one type of rock to another.

> As to natural processes, I have learned by what I have seen with my own eyes that a vein flowing from a single source was in one part pure gold, and in another silver having a stony *calx* mixed with it. And miners and smeltermen have told me that this very frequently happens; and therefore they are sorry when they have found gold, for the gold is near the source, and then the vein fails. Then I myself, making a careful examination, found that the vessel in which the mineral was converted into gold differed from that in which it was converted into silver. For the vessel containing gold was a very hard stone — one of the kind from which fire is struck with steel — and it had the gold pure and not incorporated [with the stone], but enclosed in a hollow within it; and there was a little burned earth between the stony part and the gold. And the stone opened out with a passage into the silver vein, traversing a black stone which was not very hard but earthy. And the black stone was fissile, the kind of stone from which slates are made for building houses. This proves, however, that from a single place which was the vessel of the mineral matter both [gold and silver] evaporated, and a difference in the purification and digestion had been responsible for the difference in the kind of metal.[85] (Wyckoff trans.)

While this passage is significant because it is the first apparent record of what now is recognized to be a common mineralogical phenomenon, it is important for a second reason. No passage in the *Minerals* is more indicative of Albert as scientist. There is the careful examination and accurate description of the formation uncolored by *a priori* assumptions about the nature of stones or ore formation. Yet the example is not one of random observation, for Albert has cited it

---

[84] *De min.* III, tr.1, c.10 (ed. Borgnet 5: 73b; Wyckoff, p. 183).
[85] *De min.* III, tr.2, c.6 (ed. Borgnet 5: 81a-82b; Wyckoff, pp. 200-201).

within the context of his theory of ore formation, thereby, in a sense, providing an explanation for the phenomenon while establishing greater credibility for the theory. Finally, Albert added to his own observation the corroboration of miners and sméltermen, expert testimony indeed. The juxtaposition of observation, hypothesis and authority constitutes the essence of scientific writing as we recognize it today; the same was no less true for Albert.

As the frequent references to "vessels" in the foregoing passage signify, throughout the treatment of metals and ores a second contemporary influence can be noted in the *Minerals*. For much of the discussion of the properties of metals and for the mechanisms of ore genesis Albert had recourse to the growing body of alchemical literature. In the work of the alchemists could be found artful processes analogous to the natural processes by which metals were generated in the earth. Since "art imitates nature," by studying the alchemical efforts to effect the transmutation of baser metals to silver and gold, one could better understand the way in which natural processes functioned. "For whatever the elemental and celestial powers produce in natural vessels they also produce in artificial vessels, provided the artificial [vessels] are formed just like the natural [ones]."[86] Hence, the genesis of ores could be likened to the alchemical operations of washing, boiling, sublimation and condensation, "because, of all the operations of alchemy, the best is that which begins in the same way as nature."[87]

While alchemical operations could be cited to help explain the way in which the natural mechanisms of ore generation functioned, Albert also found much information in the alchemical corpus concerning the properties of metals which could be used to support his theories. For a metal such as tin, of which he had little first hand knowledge, the alchemical corpus provided the primary source of information.

Tin, according to Albert, "has a 'stuttering' constitution;" hence, "it makes all metals with which it is mixed 'stuttering,'' too, and takes away their malleability, as Hermes says; and when it is itself drawn out, it is quickly and easily broken."[88] In one sense Albert is confused here, because pure tin is not, as the passage implies, brittle.

---

86 *De min.* III, tr.1, c.9 (ed. Borgnet 5: 71a; Wyckoff, p. 178).
87 *De min.* III, tr.1, c.9 (ed. Borgnet 5: 71b; Wyckoff, p. 179).
88 *De min.* IV, tr.1, c.4 (ed. Borgnet 5: 87b; Wyckoff, p. 215).

In the twelfth century Theophilus had given detailed directions on the manufacture of tin leaf by hammering.[89] Rather, it is more likely that Albert appears to refer to the embrittling effect on metals alloyed with tin, a fact well known to the alchemists, as indicated in this passage from the works of the Latin Geber:

> Therefore, not omitting to discourse of *Jupiter*, We signifie to the *Sons* of *Learning*, that *Tin* is a *Metallick Body*, white, not pure, livid, sounding little, partaking of little *Earthiness*; possessing in its *Roots Harshness, Softness*, and swiftness of *Liquefaction*, without *Ignition*, and not abiding the *Cupel*, or *Cement*, but Extensible under the *Hammer*. . . .yet its vice is, that it breaks every Body, but *Saturn* and most pure *Sol*.[90] (Russell trans.)

It is not surprising that Albert might confuse the effect of alloying with tin with the properties of the metal itself. Moreover, the source of the confusion between the nature of pure tin and its alloys appears to have originated in the unknown source, Hermes, which may not have been as explicit on the properties of tin as on its effects on other metals.[91] That Albert himself was not in error, but was accurately transcribing the opinions of the alchemists as he found them, may be illustrated by another example. In describing the origin of tutty (zinc oxide) Albert reported that "It is made from the smoke that rises upwards and solidifies by adhering to hard bodies, where copper is being purified from the stones and tin which are in it."[92] German copper ores are more commonly associated with zinc ores than with tin, and the tutty would result from the volatilization of the zinc, its oxidation and subsequent condensation. Yet the Latin Geber, drawing on the same alchemical tradition as Albert, gave a nearly identical explanation for its origin.

---

[89] Theophilus, *On Divers Arts*, trans. John G. Hawthorne and Cyril S. Smith (Chicago, 1963), pp. 180-182. Theophilus described several manufacturing operations using tin, but did not mention ores or tin mining.

[90] Geber, "Of the Sum of Perfection," tr.1, c.31, *The Works of Geber*, trans. Richard Russell (1678), introd. by E. J. Holmyard (London, 1928), p. 66. An early manuscript of *Summa perfecti* is from the thirteenth century (see, Dorothea Singer, *Cat. of Lat. & Vern. Alch. MSS in Gr. Brit. and Ireland*, 2 vols. (Brussels, 1928), 1: 94-96), which means that Albert may have seen the work despite Holmyard's dating the translation later.

[91] Albert made frequent reference to Hermes' *Book of Alchemy*, which neither Wyckoff nor the current writers can identify, although the same source apparently was used by the contemporary authors Arnold of Saxony and Bartholomeus Anglicus. As the quotation from Geber shows, however, Albert's citation accurately reflected the alchemical knowledge of metals such as tin.

[92] *De min*. I, tr.1, c.8 (ed. Borgnet 5: 102a; Wyckoff, p. 250).

> But *Tutia* is the fumes of *White Bodies*; and this is evidenced by manifest *Probation*. For the *Fume* of the *Mixtion* of *Jupiter* [Tin] and *Venus* [Copper], adhering to the *Sides* of the *Forges*, or *Furnaces* of *Artifices Working* in those *Metals*, makes the same impression as it.[93] (Russell trans.)

Throughout the *Minerals* the accuracy of Albert's citation is never in question. One can only regret that the scope of the project was so great as to preclude his firsthand observations of many such phenomena.

By drawing upon the alchemical tradition Albert, as he had done with miners, provided clues to the metallurgical knowledge and skill possessed by the artisans of the thirteenth century. Referring once again to the discussion of tutty, Albert reported that when mixed with copper by the alchemists it changed copper to the color of gold. This is a direct reference to the making of brass using zinc oxide instead of the traditional method of adding calamine (zinc carbonate) to copper, the method Albert had observed at Paris and Cologne.[94] Although it is probable that tutty had been used in this context since the Roman era, Albert may have been the first observer to distinguish clearly between the use of tutty and calamine. This is particularly noteworthy, since the commercial use of zinc oxide did not develop until the sixteenth century.[95]

The references to some metallurgical phenomena are not so easily interpreted, nor can they be assigned to the alchemical tradition with certainty. But they are of interest to historians of chemistry and of metals, because they constitute the earliest record we have on the subjects. One intriguing example is in the case of tin, where Albert wrote, "They say that cast tin quickly decays."[96] One could wish for a fuller explanation of what was occurring, but reference probably was being made to the phenomenon of "tin disease" or "tin pest," an

---

[93] Geber, "Of the Sum of Perfection," II, tr.1, c.4; p. 129.

[94] *De min.* IV, tr.1, c.6 (ed. Borgnet 5: 90b; Wyckoff, p. 224). Albert attributed the information that tutty gave copper the color of gold to Hermes.

[95] After Albert, Biringuccio may have been the next major writer on metals to note the use of tutty to make brass, in a passing reference: "In addition to calamine, copper is also colored yellow by tutty" (Biringuccio, *Pirotechnia*, p. 75). Smith's footnote to this quote gives the date of 1550 for the introduction of brass manufacture from zinc oxide at Rammelsberg.

[96] *De min.* IV, tr.1, c.5 (ed. Borgnet 5: 88a; Wyckoff, p. 216). "They," in this case, would seem to refer to smeltermen from the subsequent comment: "Now it has already been stated that tin is poorly mixed, and this is the reason it is damaged by fire; and if it is removed from the place where it originated, it is destroyed more rapidly than other metals."

allotropic transformation of malleable white tin to a brittle gray, powdery phase which takes place normally below 18°C. Such a transformation also would reinforce the belief that the metal itself was of an inherently brittle nature, as previously noted. The failure of tin plate by "tin disease" also is implied in the discussion of iron. According to Albert, "Tin poured over it [iron] penetrates into its substance. But after this penetration it becomes so brittle that it cannot be worked."[97] The significance of these passages is that the phenomena to which they apparently refer went unnoted in any of the later works on metals and were not explained in the technical literature before the start of the twentieth century.[98]

Some of the more perceptive observations concerning metals in the *Minerals* involve the effect of metals on health. The classification of stones in Tractate 2 followed the lapidary tradition of ascribing medical properties to minerals. Albert did not completely neglect medical properties in his discussion of metals, although, clearly, they were of secondary significance compared to the "accidental" or metallic properties of substances. For lead, Albert reiterated Pliny's claim that lead had a special power over lust and nocturnal emission.[99] "But," he continued, "care must be taken lest the lead, by its coldness contracting the material [below] too forcibly drive it upwards into the head, and cause madness or epilepsy; and care must also be taken lest it cause paralysis of the lower limbs and unconciousness."[100] The later passage is a clear reference to the symptoms of lead poisoning, resulting from the inhalation of lead fumes, as first described by Vitruvius.[101] Albert could not have seen Vitruvius but it is quite likely that Albert had knowledge of the noxi-

[97] *De min.* IV, tr.1, c.8 (ed. Borgnet 5: 94b; Wyckoff, p. 234). The plate would decay or become embrittled by tin disease, not the iron.

[98] Mantell, in discussing the allotropic forms, credits the first observation of the effect of extreme temperature change on tin to the pseudo-Aristotelian *De mirabilibus auscultationibus*. Modern observations of tin disease date from 1851 in tin objects, from 1908 for plated objects. The physical basis for tin disease was established in 1899. See C. L. Mantell, *Tin, Its Mining, Production, Technology and Application*, 2nd ed., American Chemical Society Monograph, 51, (New York, 1949), pp. 7-12.

[99] Pliny, *Natural History* XXXIV, c.50, 1. 166 (London, 1952) 9: 247.

[100] *De min.* IV, tr.1, c.3 (ed. Borgnet 5: 86a-b; Wyckoff, p. 210).

[101] Pliny warned of the dangers of breathing the "deadly vapour" of the lead furnace, but without describing symptoms. Vitruvius was more explicit: "For when lead is smelted in casting, the fumes from it settle upon their members, and day after day burn out and take away all the virtues of the blood from their limbs." Vitruvius, *The Ten Books on Architecture*, trans. Morris Hickey Morgan (Cambridge, Mass., 1914), pp. 246-247.

ous effects of lead from his acquaintance with both refineries and alchemists, where exposure to lead fumes in cupelation and assaying and in alchemical procedures might be expected to produce chronic lead poisoning with some regularity. In a similar vein Albert noted that quicksilver "is said to be a kind of poison. It is cold and moist to the second degree, and for this reason it causes loosening of the sinews and paralysis."[102] The passage appears to be the first description in Western literature referring to the affliction known as "hatters' shakes," a form of mercury poisoning characterized by trembling in the extremities resulting from inhalation of mercury vapors.[103]

While not directly affecting health, Albert also noted that metals have peculiar odors and tastes. In particular, he remarked on the ability of copper vessels to taint the taste of most liquids. Other authors, from Pliny onward, had made similar observations, but Albert added the perceptive distinction that the effect was more pronounced for brazen (*aeneus*) vessels.[104] Today, the greater solubility of copper ions from brass alloys in the presence of weak acids and bases is experimentally demonstrable.[105]

Throughout the consideration of metals Albert exhibited a sure instinct for the chemical basis for metallurgical processes. That instinct influenced his own observations and dictated the examples to be drawn from the blend of myth and fact which comprised the store of knowledge possessed by miners and alchemists. These observations together with his classification of minerals and stones gives Albert an important place in the history of the geological sciences.

---

[102] *De min.* IV, tr.1, c.2 (ed. Borgnet 5: 85a-b; Wyckoff, p. 207). There seems no question that Albert's information is drawn verbatim from some unidentified alchemical source. The reference to "degree" of cold and moist so indicates.

[103] Avicenna may have been the first person to describe hatter's shakes in his *Canon of Medicine*. However, this was not one of Albert's sources for compiling the *De mineralibus*. See discussion and citation in Leonard J. Goldwater, *Mercury, A History of Quicksilver* (Baltimore, 1972), p. 211.

[104] *De min.* III, tr.2, c.4 (ed. Borgnet 5: 79b; Wyckoff, pp. 195-196).

[105] Compare Albert's observation with the following quote from a modern metallurgical study of copper alloys: "In the presence of materials such as certain foodstuffs, sufficient copper may sometimes be dissolved, even though in traces, to effect the taste or flavor of the product. In such cases, tin coating of the copper alloys effectively overcomes the situation" (Henry L. Burghoff, "Corrosion of Copper Alloys," *Corrosion of Metals* [Cleveland, 1946], p. 127).

Appendix 1: Date for the Composition of *The Book of Minerals*

Estimates for the date of the composition of the *Minerals* has varied widely from 1248 to 1263. Dorothy Wyckoff suggested that it was probably not written until 1261-1262, or 1256-1257 at the earliest.[106] She thought that he might have started work on the project before 1254 while he was in Cologne where he was composing four treatises at about the same time, namely, *The Nature of Places, The Properties of the Elements*, the *Meteorology*, and *Minerals*. She argued that Albert delayed the final version of *Minerals* while travelling to find Pseudo-Aristotle's lapidary, about which Albert said he had "inquired assiduously in different parts of the world" to no avail.[107] She raised an objection to Paneth's theory concerning the short anonymous, fourteenth-century tract which bears resemblance to some sections in Albert's Books III and IV of the *Minerals*.[108] She wondered why, if Albert had written this unattributed tract in Bologna during his Italian trip as an early draft of the *Minerals*, a theory suggested by Paneth, did Albert not make reference to locations in Italy and Alpine regions of minerals as he did throughout the *Minerals* to places in Germany and France. Albert's reference to locations of mines is especially frequent in Books III and IV, the same section resembling the Paneth manuscript. Nonetheless, Wyckoff accepted Paneth's thesis because it supported her view of composition of the *Minerals* around 1258. She supposed that Albert's discussion of silver ores at Freiberg[109] and of alluvial gold in Westphalia,[110] a petrified bird's nest at Lubeck,[111] probably dated from Albert's trips when he was prior provincial in 1254-1256. The date 1248, as the earliest date that *Minerals* could have been written, is certain because Albert refers back to his time in Paris which he left in 1248 and mentions the recovery of "Moorish Seville, which is now returned to the

---

[106] Wyckoff, *Albertus*, pp. xxxv-xli.

[107] *De min.* III, tr.1, c.1; cf. also II, tr.3, c.6 (ed. Borgnet 5: 60a and 57; Wyckoff, p. 153, cf. p. 151).

[108] Wyckoff, *Albertus*, pp. xxxviii-xxxix; Fritz Paneth, "Ueber eine alchemistische Handschriften des 14. Jahrunderts und ihr Verhältnis zu Albertus Magnus' Buch 'De Mineralibus'," *Archiv für Geschichte der Mathematik der Naturwissenschaften und der Technik*, n.f. 3, 12 (1929), 35-45; 13 (1930), 408-413; and study of text by Karl Sudhoff, "Codex Fritz Paneth, Eine Untersuchung," *Arch. f. Gesch. der Math.*, n.f. 3, 12 (1929), 2-26.

[109] *De min.* III, tr.1, c.10 and probably IV, tr.1, c.5 (ed. Borgnet 5: 72a-b, 89b; Wyckoff, pp. 181, 220-221); cf. Wyckoff, p. xxxvii.

[110] *De min.* IV, tr.1, c.7 (ed. Borgnet 5: 93a; Wyckoff, pp. 230-231); cf. Wyckoff, p. xxxvii.

[111] *De min.* I, tr.1, c.7 (ed. Borgnet 5: 7a; Wyckoff, p. 28); cf. Wyckoff, intro., p. xxxvii.

Spaniards."[112] The Reconquista of Seville was in 1248. Thus, modern scholars have placed the writing of Albert's *Minerals* as between 1248 and 1263, with Wyckoff hypothesizing a date close to 1262 as most likely.[113]

As cogently argued as Wyckoff's thesis is, her later date seems incorrect in light of an explicit of Albert's *Minerals* in a fifteenth-century manuscript now at Krakow. The colophon states: "Here ends the Mineral Book written by Brother Albertus, of Teutonia at one time from Regensberg, professor of the Order of Preaching Friars, an excellent philosopher, [which was] written in the city of Cologne in the year 1250 of our Lord, under the distinguished guidance of Conrad, archbishop of the aforesaid city."[114] Certainly the Krakow text is copied, but it could hardly have been copied from a manuscript that did not trace back to a manuscript with the same colophon first composed in or near to Albert's lifetime. Albert was teaching in Cologne between 1248 and 1252 when Conrad of Hochstadt was archbishop.[115]

The date of 1250 seems likely when other evidence is considered. As stated above, Albert's knowledge of tin revealed no firsthand experience but, if he had written *Minerals* as late as 1258, he almost certainly would have come into contact with tin mines during this interval when he was travelling in the area. Wyckoff's belief that Albert's travels to Freiberg, Westphalia, and Lubeck were more likely after his Cologne post, is circumstantial when one considers Albert's statement that as a youth he travelled widely to learn of minerals.[116] His visit to Freiberg could have been earlier. Finally Paneth's thesis regarding the text which is connected to Albert's *Minerals* must be rejected out of hand. His thesis that the text is Albert's first draft (and Albert's missing *De alchimia*) written at or

---

[112] *De min.* II, tr.3, c.1; III, tr.1, c.4 (ed. Borgnet 5: 49a, 63b; Wyckoff, pp. 128, 163).

[113] James A. Weisheipl, "Albert the Great, St.," *New Catholic Encylopedia* (1967), 1: 257b ("before 1263").

[114] Kraków, Biblioteka Jagiellońska MS 6392 III, fol. 7-46v, ending: "Explicit liber mineralium editus a fratre Alberto quodam [*sic*] Ratisponense nacione theutonico, professione [*sic*] de ordine Fratrum Predicatorum precipuo philosopho editus a. D. MCCL in civitate Colonia Agrippina, presidente dicto Cum[ra]do archiepiscopo civitatis memorate. Amen." as reported by Anna Zabrzykowska, Zerzy Zathey, et al., *Inwentarz Rękópisow Biblioteki Jagiellońskie*, 7 vols. (Kraków, 1962), 2: 179. But see a more accurate view above in "Life and Works of St. Albert the Great," p. 35 and n. 75.

[115] Conrad was archbishop of Cologne between 31 May 1238 and 28 September 1261: U. Chevalier, *Répertoire des sources hist.*, 1220.

[116] *De min.* III, tr.1, c.1 (ed. Borgnet 5: 59a-b; Wyckoff, p. 153).

near Bologna is based on no greater evidence than that the text was in a north Italian hand, one of the early fourteenth century.[117] Since it is not an autograph, it is a copy and one made from a text which could have been written almost any place in Europe. Further, the evidence that it was Albert's work is no stronger than a counter hypothesis that it is a modification of sections from the *Minerals*. The possibility is, of course, present that Albert delayed his *Minerals* until he despaired of finding Pseudo-Aristotle's lapidary. However, when his search began, and how long his patience held before he wrote is conjectural. His search quite possibly could have succeeded because one of his source's for the *Minerals*, Arnold of Saxony whom Albert quoted extensively, had a copy of Gerard of Cremona's translation of the Pseudo-Aristotelian lapidary. There are two manuscripts of it.[118] Thus, there were in Albert's time manuscripts of the text. Within the time between 1250 and 1262 the chances of his locating the lapidary would have increased. But he did not know it except through other's works when he wrote the *Minerals*.[119] A date of 1250 for the composition of the *Minerals* keeps the time within the bracketed frame previously suggested but moves this creative interest in natural history closer to his tract on the *Physics*, composed between 1245 and 1248, and at the same time as his teaching of St. Thomas. Even without the evidence afforded by the Krakow manuscript, a 1250 date, or one no later than 1252, seems likely.

Appendix 2: Notes on Sources for *The Book of Minerals*

Professor Wyckoff identified most of Albert's sources. As was his usual practice, Albert frequently named his authorities. In the lapidary section (II tr.2) Albert relied on other writers, naming some fifteen authors and titles, more than he did, for instance, in Books III–V, where his outside authorities were more restricted. Some new

---

[117] Paneth "Ueber eine alt. Handschrift," *Arch. f. Gesch. der Math.*, n.f. 3, 12 (1929), 45, who based the location on K. Sudhoff's conclusion that the manuscript is *probably* copied in Northern Italy, perhaps Bologna or Padua ("Codex Fritz Paneth" *Arch. f. Gesch. der Math.*, n.f. 3, 12 [1929], 24).

[118] Liège, Bibl. del'Univ. MS 77 (s.xiv), fol. 146v-152v, and Montpellier, Ecole de Med., MS 277 (s.xv), fol. 127-130v. See discussion in Riddle, *Marbode*, pp. 11-12.

[119] See above, n. 118. Albert knew of Pseudo-Aristotle's lapidary through Arnold of Saxony, Marbode of Rennes, and Constantine's *De gradibus*.

evidence, however, has come to light which supplements Wyckoff's study.

Probably the largest unresolved questions regarding Albert's authorities are his use and relationship to the encyclopaedists, principally Thomas of Cantimpré and Arnold of Saxony, and the means of Albert's knowledge of Aristotle's lapidary. The question regarding Aristotle's lapidary was discussed above, p. 230. There can be no question as to the close relation, often word for word, between Albert's lapidary section (and in his section on sigils) and Thomas of Cantimpré's *The Nature of Things.* Since Thomas wrote before Albert, since he was a fellow Dominican, and since Albert normally cited his sources, why did Albert not cite Thomas? Wyckoff suggested either that Albert and Thomas used a mutual source which was anonymous, or perhaps that Albert had a copy of Thomas which lacked attribution.[120] We have confirmed the evidence of Thorndike and Rose that there are many copies of Thomas' encyclopaedia.[121] Thomas' lapidary section was often extracted and stood in manuscripts as an independent work, frequently without attribution.[122] Following the lapidary section of his encyclopaedia, Thomas of Cantimpré lifted Zael's (Thetel) tract on sigils and put it within his work almost intact.[123] This being the case, might not Thomas have bor-

---

[120] Wyckoff, *Albertus*, pp. 99, 269-270; see also, the older studies which noted the relationship between Thomas of Cantimpré and Albert, e.g., H. Stadler, "Albertus Magnus, Thomas von Cantimpré und Vinzenz von Beauvais," *Natur und Kultur*, 4 (1906), 86-90; F. Bormans, "Thomas de Cantimpré indiqué comme une des sources où Albert le Grand et surtout Maerlant ont puisé les materiaux de leurs écrites sur l'histoire naturelle," *Bulletin de l'Academie royales des sciences . . . de Belgique*, 19/1 (1852), 132-159.

[121] Thorndike, *A History of Magic and Experimental Science*, 2: 396-398; Valentin Rose, "Aristoteles *De lapidibus* und Arnoldus Saxo," *Zeitschrift für deutsches Altertums*, 18 (1875), 335-337.

[122] I have notes on the following MSS in addition to those noted in Thorndike and Kibre's *Incipits*, col. 582, and in Thorndike, *A History*, 2: 396-398, with the Inc.: "Generaliter primo dicendum est de lapidibus preciosis. . . ." This is the beginning of the lapidary section in Thomas of Cantimpré's *Liber de natura rerum*, e.g., in Brit. Libr., MS Egerton 1984 (s. xiii), fol. 126. But in many of these MSS the tract stands alone and is without attribution, e.g., Paris, Arsenal MS 1080 (anno 1343), fol. 206v-217; Bibl. Nat. MS lat. 523A, fol. 12; Erlangen, Bibl. Univ. MS 434 (s. xiii-xiv), fol. 152-156; Vatican, MSS Vat. lat. 724 (s. xiv), fol. 67-76; Vat. Pal. lat. 1144, fol. 154-161v; Vienna, Nat. Bibl. MSS lat. 1365 (s. xiv), fol. 81; lat. 2317 (s. xiv).

[123] Wyckoff, *Albertus*, p. 276. Zael's lapidary is in Thomas' *De natura rerum*, Brit. Libr., MS Egerton 1984, fol. 139-140. In addition to the MSS cited by Thorndike (*A History*, 2: 399-400), we have noted Zael's lapidary as a separate work in Milan, Ambrosiana, MS I 65 sup. (1), (s. xv), fol. 1-66 (cited by hand written catalogue); Oxford, Bodl. MS Ash. 1471 (s. xiv), fol. 65v-67v; Florence, Laurentian MS Ashburnham 1520 (s. xiv), fol. 51-55 (*Libellus sigillorum*); Naples, Bibl. Naz. MS XII.E.31 (s. xv), fol. 69v-81.

rowed fairly literally, at least not reworking his material to much extent, from an anonymous source? This unknown source Albert might also have used. The supposition is given support by the fact that manuscript texts without attribution of authorship exist which are parallel to Thomas' lapidary section. Interestingly there are two manuscripts of this tract, found in Thomas' encyclopaedia, which give Albert as the author.[124] An anonymous copy of this tract is found in another manuscript of the thirteenth century, Sloane MS 2428, which contains a text close to Albert's source, but which is not found in the manuscript version of Thomas of Cantimpré, cited as being most reliable, namely Egerton MS 1984; it is not found in the variant text of Thomas, in Bodleian MS Rawl. 545.[125] Specifically this anonymous lapidary manuscript adds the passage for the stone *isciscos* which is not found in Thomas' full encyclopaedia in Egerton MS 1984. Further the Sloane text adds to Thomas' encyclopaedia in the Egerton text the following stones: *karabre, kabrate, kacamon* and *liparia.*[126] They are not found in the variant Bodleian text, but the text on them seems to have been used by Albert for his entries on these stones. Finally Albert has an entry on the Jew Stone, which Wyckoff thought came from Avicenna's *Canon of Medicine*. The text, however, is not related to Avicenna, but it is related to the anonymous lapidary in Sloane MS 2428.[127] Although certainty cannot come until a thorough study of Thomas of Cantimpré's work has been completed the evidence cited here is enough to give Wyckoff support and even probability in her suspicion that Albert and Thomas were using a mutual source.

Albert was not beyond quoting an authority directly from an encyclopaedia without attribution. Albert used Arnold of Saxony but he never cited him by name. A recent study has added to our information of Arnold's souces, and, thereby, has given us a major source for Albert.[128] Wyckoff could not locate a work by "Dioscorides" whom both Arnold and Albert cite. It was not the well-known first-century Greek herbalist. Arnold of Saxony had two frequently

[124] Erlangen, Univ. MS 434 (s. xiii-xiv), fol. 152-156, and Vatican, MS Vat. lat. 724 (s. xiv), fol. 67-76.

[125] A Bodleian MS text is published by Joan Evans, *Magical Jewels of the Middle Ages and the Renaissance* (Oxford 1922), pp. 223-234, from MS Rawl. D.35A.

[126] Brit. Libr., MS Sloane 2428, fol. 5r-v.

[127] Ibid.; Wyckoff (*Albertus*, p. 100) gives Albert's reference to Avicenna as *Canon of Medicine* II, tr.2, c.394, but it should read c.404 (fol. 126, ed. Venice 1507).

[128] Riddle, *Marbode*, pp. 11-17.

repeated citations to Aristotle's lapidary, "Aristotle's lapidary translated by Gerard" and "Aristotle's lapidary translated by Dioscorides." There is no doubt but that the translation by Gerard was the text that Albert sought but could not find except through Arnold's fragments as well as fragments in Marbode, Constantine, and Costa ben Luca. On the other hand what Arnold cited as Aristotle's lapidary translated by Dioscorides is the same in content as that cited by Bartholomew the Englishman as being by "Dyascorides" without reference to Aristotle. The study of the context of these fragments revealed that the work allegedly by Dioscorides, whether as author or translator, was the work of Damigeron, a little known lapidarist, probably of the first century. Albert's source "Dioscorides" was Damigeron.[129]

Albert cites among the highest authorities on stones: "Hermes [Evax], king of the Arabs, and Dioscorides, Aaron, and Joseph."[130] In many manuscripts prefacing the lapidaries of both Damigeron and Marbode are two letters written by Evax, king of the Arabs to the Emperor Tiberius (14-37 AD) about the secrets of stones. Albert knew both Damigeron's and Marbode's works.[131] Damigeron's lapidary is in prose, Marbode's in verse. Probably either because the texts Albert used did not attribute correctly the authors or because Albert saw too close similarities between Damigeron and Marbode, he chose not to cite either except as "Evax" since Evax's letter preceded both works.

Albert's "Hermes" is more difficult for the modern researcher to trace. Dorothy Wyckoff noted the "bewildering number or books" ascribed to Hermes.[132] Although Wyckoff identified some of the Hermetic treatises employed by Albert, she was unable to determine all of Albert's Hermetic material, nor have we been able to add to Wyckoff's study.

Aaron's work escapes modern identification. Whereas Albert refers several times to Aaron in association with "Evax" and "Dioscorides," he three times cites Aaron for specific information on stones. In our study of Latin lapidary manuscripts, we did not find any lapidary text attributed to Aaron. Arnold of Saxony and Costa

---

129 Ibid., pp. 103-105.

130 *De min.* I, tr.1, c.1 (ed. Borgnet 5: 2a; Wyckoff, p. 10).

131 Riddle, *Marbode*, pp. 28-30.

132 Wyckoff *Albertus*, p. 273.

ben Luca cited Aaron, however.[133] On *amethysus*, and *hiena* Albert cites Aaron and the information is found in Arnold but without attribution. On the stone *iscustos*, Albert cites Aaron but the information is not in Arnold[134] but is found in the Sloane lapidary, MS 2428 which is related to Thomas of Cantimpré.[135] It is possible that Albert had a copy of a tract by Aaron, and it is equally possible that his knowledge of Aaron was indirect. For instance, Albert three times cited Isidore, but in the first case Albert's direct source was Thomas who named Isidore as his source[136] and, in the second and third instance, Albert's source may be found in the Sloane MS 2428 which names Isidore for the source.[137] It may be that Albert had no actual text of a lapidary by Aaron but instead employed him indirectly as an authority.

---

[133] Arnold, *De coelo et mundo*, 3 (ed. Emil Stange [Erfurt, 1905], p. 73), who begins the section: "Nam que utiliora, meliora et notabiliora ab Aristotele et Aaron et Evace, rege Arabum et Diascoride sparsim tradita sunt, excepi . . ." (3; ed. Stange, p. 67). Costa, *De physicis ligaturis*, in Brit. Libr., MS Add. 22,719, fol. 201: "Aaron dixit, stercus elefantum cum lacte. . . ." Noteworthy is the fact that Aaron's lapidary is not found cited in the Arabic lapidary tradition, viz. Al-Kitāb al-Muršid, *Über die Steine*. . ., trans. Jutta Schönfeld (Freiburg, 1976).

[134] *De min*. II, tr.2, c.1 and 8 (ed. Borgnet 5: 31b, 38b, 39a-b; Wyckoff, pp. 74, 96-100); Arnold, *De coelo*, 3 (ed. Stange, pp. 70, 73).

[135] Fol. 5.

[136] *De min*. II, tr.2, c.17, *syrus* (ed. Borgnet 5: 46b; Wyckoff, p. 122); cf. Thomas, London, Brit. Libr., MS Egerton 1984, fol. 136.

[137] *De min*. II, tr.2, c.8, *iscustos, judaicus lapis* (ed. Borgnet 5: 39b; Wyckoff, pp. 99-100); cf. Brit. Libr., MS Sloane 2428, fol. 5.

IX

Pseudo-Dioscorides' *Ex herbis femininis* and Early Medieval Medical Botany

> Actual social change is never so great as is apparent change. Ways of belief, of expectation, of judgment and attendant emotional dispositions of like and dislike, are not easily modified after they have once taken shape.
>
> – John Dewey, *Human Nature and Conduct*

Dewey's assessment of social change can readily be applied to scientific change in the early Middle Ages. The popular herbal of an unknown late fifth- or sixth-century author reveals that medical and botanical knowledge had only undergone apparent change. The Germanic barbarians brought (or continued?) political instability, but no radical change in medical practices. Although attributed to Dioscorides, the early medieval treatise *Ex herbis femininis* is largely a new work based on Dioscorides. It reflects a higher level of medical-botanical lore than currently attributed to the era, an uncommon linguistic skill in Greek and Latin, and some degree of originality, perhaps as much as can be expected in any herbal, whatever the time.

De materia medica by Dioscorides was fully translated into five Latin books probably by the sixth century. Likewise *Ex herbis femininis* was known in the West from the sixth century, and it was by far more popular than Dioscorides' own work. The popularity is measured by the number of extant copies. The Old Latin translation of Dioscorides is found in three complete, or nearly complete, manuscripts, two of the ninth century and one of the tenth.[1] *Ex herbis femininis*, which discussed some seventy-one herbal entries, is found in twenty-nine manuscripts, the majority lavishly illustrated.[2] By contrast, over 500

1. Munich Ms. 337, s. X; Paris BN Ms. lat. 12, 955, s. IX; Paris BN Ms. lat. 9,332, s. IX.

2. A complete listing and description of these manuscripts is forthcoming in my article on Dioscorides to be published in the Catalogus Translationum et Commentariorum series. In "The Medical Literature of the Early Middle Ages: A Program and a Report of a Summer of Research in Italy," *Bull. Inst. Hist. Med.*,

Journal of the History of Biology, vol. 14, no. 1 (Spring 1981), pp. 43–81.
Copyright © 1981 *by D. Reidel Publishing Co., Dordrecht, Holland, and Boston, Mass.*
Reprinted by permission of Kluwer Academic Publishers.

herbs were treated in Dioscorides' Greek text. Thirteen of the manuscripts of *Ex herbis femininis* are dated twelfth century or earlier. Seven are from the ninth century alone. Given the statistical probability of greater loss of earlier manuscripts than of later ones, these figures demonstrate the popularity of *Ex herbis femininis*. Its existence was known and referred to by some sixteenth-century botanists, such as Petrus Andreas Matthiolus and Johannes Sambucus, who used manuscript copies to help them identify plants in Dioscorides' Greek text. In 1896 Heinrich Kästner published a text of *Ex herbis*, its only printing, but he employed only three manuscripts and his version is defective.[3]

In some ways *Ex herbis* was superior to the Latin version of Dioscorides' work. Although shorter, it was easier to use, and the herbs *Ex herbis* discusses were more related to the flora of southern Europe; it often provides more detailed medicinal directions than *De materia medica*, and in many instances it reveals improved knowledge of pharmacy. Part of the reason for the popularity of *Ex herbis* was that it was illustrated, while the Latin Dioscorides was not. Nowadays the mention of Dioscorides' name invokes the notion of illustrated herbals. From the marvelously illuminated folios preserved in the complete Juliana Anicia Codex of about 512 A.D. to the wondrous woodcuts of Leonard Fuchs, Giorgio Liberale, and Jacob Cortusius in the sixteenth-century printed editions, Dioscorides was associated with botanical illustrations.[4] And yet during the Middle Ages the Latin text of Dioscorides was not illustrated except for some crude marginal sketches in Munich Manuscript 337 (s. IX), which may have derived from direct observation.[5]

2 (1934), 36, Henry Sigerist said he had located "nearly fifty manuscripts of this text," but unfortunately he never published his list. Having completed a search myself, I believe Sigerist overestimated his findings.

3. Heinrich Kästner, "Pseudo-Dioscorides *De herbis femininis*," *Hermes*, *31* (1896), 578-636, using Florence, Laur. Mss. Plut. 73.16 and Plut. 41.73, and Paris, BN Ms. lat. 6362; in this article, Kästner omitted two herbs that he later added in *Hermes*, *32* (1897), 160. Sigerist ("Medical Literature," p. 36) noted the need for another text.

4. Fuchs' woodcuts appear in *Historia stirpium* (Basel, 1542); Giorgio Liberale's drawings were cut by Wolfgang Meierpeck for Matthiolus' 1554 edition (Venice) of Dioscorides; and Jacob Cortusius' drawings were done for Matthiolus' 1583 edition (Venice).

5. Hermann Stadler, "Der lateinische Dioscorides der Münchener Hof-und Staatsbibliothek und die Bedeutung dieser Uebersetzung für einen Teil der mittelalterlichen Medicine," *Allgemeine medicinische Central-Zeitung*, *14* (1900), 1966, suggested that the drawings derive from textual descriptions, but this seems unreasonable to me. Those descriptions are far too sketchy to provide sufficient information except when supplemented by direct observations made from nature.

Still, the association of Dioscorides with illustrated herbals during the Middle Ages is not entirely unfounded. Medieval man thought *Ex herbis femininis* was by Dioscorides and it was beautifully illustrated in most manuscript copies.

Although I will not include here an iconographical analysis of the illuminations, a few general remarks are in order. Much is written disparaging the quality of illustrations in medieval herbals: they are said to be static, crude copies of copies, to have little resemblance to real plants, and so on. Like many generalizations, these descriptions contain elements of truth, but the case is overstated. The quality of illustration varies, of course, according to the manuscript. Limited individuality appears in each illustrator's depiction of the plant as a unit – root systems, stemmation, leaf structure, and appearance, flowers and/or seeds. A comparison of the illustrations in various *Ex herbis* manuscripts with the famous Juliana Anicia Codex of Constantinople reveals that the *Ex herbis* illustrations are not related to those in this version of the Greek text of Dioscorides. It must be left to others to determine whether the author of *Ex herbis* drew on a classical tradition for his drawings, as seems likely, or whether he caused the plants to be drawn for his own purpose. This much I feel some confidence in stating: if one already has some knowledge of plants, one can use many of the drawings in order to make a reasonable identification of some of the plants in the field. Since neither Dioscorides nor the author of *Ex herbis* gives detailed plant descriptions, the user must have had prior knowledge of plants. *Ex herbis* was no primer for a novice medical apprentice sent by his master to replenish the jars or for a monk on his initial assignment to infirmary duty. More to the purpose, *Ex herbis* probably extended knowledge and uses of plants on the part of medieval medical practitioners. When a generic name seems reasonably clear, one should not be unduly distressed by the difficulties of determining exactly which species is depicted in either the drawings or the text. The chemical compositions of various related species tend to have approximately the same pharmaceutical actions. The author's object was medical, not botanical.

The chapter on sage (*Ex herbis*, 4; see the table in the Appendix) demonstrates the difficulty in determining from the illustrations and text exactly what species, if any, was intended. Initially, the modern untrained eye might recognize sage even from the manuscript drawing.[6]

6. *Ex herbis* describes sage as "multos ex uno cespite stirpes mittit tetragonos et subalbidos. Folia habet mali cydonei [Greek: μηλέᾳ κυδωνίᾳ] similia, nisi quod angustiora et longiora et subaspera, odore suavi et gravi." Thus the leaves

But on closer inspection one can see a leaf arrangement impossible in nature. One stem has an alternate or spiral leaf arrangement that is characteristic of no species of sage. But the same stem also has parts of leaves arranged opposite each other, that is, two leaves at a node; this is characteristic of several species of sage, including *Salvia officinalis*, or common sage. The same stem also has three leaves on a single lobe, (See Figs. 1 and 2). Was the artist's intention to draw a composite of different species of sage? Probably. Still this does not explain the single, alternately arranged leaves on the one stem. Might it be that somebody brought the artist a plant from the garden that had had some of the leaves plucked off? If so, the artist would no doubt have seen, and depicted, these varieties of leaf arrangement on a single stem. There was no imperative, so far as I know, for the herbalist or artist to study only unaltered plants. He would know them as he encountered them. We have no means of knowing exactly what happened, of course; but we can be reasonably sure that this particular drawing, when included with the written description of the plant's appearance and uses, would enable a practitioner to identify and use the herb. Whether the user could distinguish among the species of sage is, in this case at least, unimportant. For medical botany, all the species would be used the same way.

Copies of *Ex herbis femininis* follow Pseudo-Apuleius' illustrated *Herbarius* in many manuscripts, and a few combine the two works by running the chapters continuously and without attribution to Dioscorides.[7] Sometimes a manuscript copyist selected chapters from *Ex herbis* and interspersed them with sections of Pseudo-Apuleius' work.[8] Pseudo-Apuleius' *Herbarius* illustrates some 130 herbs and

---

are described partly through analogy with the leaves of *Malus cydoneus*, but *Malus cydoneus* is otherwise not discussed by Dioscorides. The color description *subalbidus*, or "off-white," refers to the stem. Curiously, sage's purple or violet flowers are neither described nor drawn, although flowers are often described by both Dioscorides and *Ex herbis*.

7. Examples of *Ex herbis'* following Pseudo-Apuleius are: Cambridge, Trinity Col. Ms. 0.2.48, s. XIV; Florence, Laur. Ms. Plut. 73.41, s. IX; Florence, laur. Ms. Plut. 73.16, s. XIII; London, Brit. Lib. Ms. Add. 8928, s. X; London, Brit. Lib. Ms. Harley 5294, s. XII; London, Brit. Lib. Ms. Sloane 1975, s. XII; Vienna, NB Ms. 93, s. XIII. Those manuscripts that combine the two works continuously are: London, British Lib. Ms. Harley 5294, which has *Ex herbis* as chap's. 141–221, and Oxford, Bodl. Ms. 130, s. XI, fols. 57-66.

8. Paris, BN Ms. lat. 6862, s. IX; Leiden, Univ. Lib. Ms. B.P.L. 1283, s. XV (with material from other sources as well); Paris, BN Ms. lat. 13,955, s. IX; St. Gallen, Stiftsbibliothek Ms. 751, s. IX, pp. 339-340.

probably was produced in the fourth century.[9] *Ex herbis* probably was written a century or two later, as will be discussed below. There is some affinity between the illustrations in these two works, which may be expected whenever both were produced in the same scriptorium. Pseudo-Apuleius' procedure was to list headings under each herbal illustration by ailments, for example: "For stomach ache," "For wound," "For epilepsy." Both Pseudo-Apuleius' *Herbarius* and Pseudo-Dioscorides' *Ex herbis* discuss the same herb in some cases, but both the illustrations and medical uses are different. Rubrics and closings to some Pseudo-Apuleius manuscripts provide some evidence for associating the two tracts: Pseudo-Apuleius' *Herbarius* is referred to as being for masculine herbs.[10] Now undoubtedly the unknown authors of both herbals worked independently, at separate times, but later some man-scriptorium combined the two. The copyist, simplistically and incorrectly, said that one was an herbal of masculine herbs, the other of feminine herbs. In time, *male* was dropped from the title of Pseudo-Apuleius' herbal, but Pseudo-Dioscorides' work retained the designation female.

Is there any reason to call the herbs female? The ancients had a very loose classification system for ascribing sexual gender to plants and even to stones. In general, male plants were considered harder, rougher, drier, and more barren, whereas female plants were softer, smoother, moister, and more fruitful. Theophrastus, for instance, advanced reasons for ascribing sex to trees: female trees are usually fruit bearing, although some male trees also bear fruit;[11] and in some cases, he declared trees were male because of their hardiness.[12] Pliny

9. Charles Singer, "The Herbal in Antiquity and Its Transmission to Later Ages," *Hellenic Stud., 47* (1927), 38; Ernest Howald and Henry Sigerist, eds. of Pseudo-Apuleius in *Antonii Musae . . . , Pseudo-Apulei . . .* , Corpus Medicorum Latinorum, vol. IV (Leipzig: B. G. Teubner, 1927), pp. xvii-xxi. Singer's view that Pseudo-Apuleius is a Latin translation of a Greek prototype has not been generally acceptance. See Henry E. Sigerist, "Zum Herbarius Pseudo-Apulei," *Sudhoffs Archiv, 23* (1930), 197-204, esp. p. 200.

10. London, Brit. Lib. Ms. Add. 8928, s. X, fol. 19: *Ex herbis masculinis*; see Augusto Beccaria, *I codici di medicina del periodo presalernitano (secoli IX, X et XI)* (Rome: Edizioni di storia e letteratura, 1956), p. 270.

11. Theophrastus, *On Plants*, 1.13.5, 2.7.4, 3.8.9; Albertus Magnus, *On Plants*, I, tr. 1, chap. 7; see notes and references by Edward Grant, *A Source Book of Medieval Science* (Cambridge, Mass.: Harvard University Press, 1974), p. 691. An important new study is John Scarborough, "Theophrastus on Herbals and Herbal Remedies," *J. His. Biol., 11* (1978), 353-385.

12. Theophrastus, *On Plants*, 3.9.3.

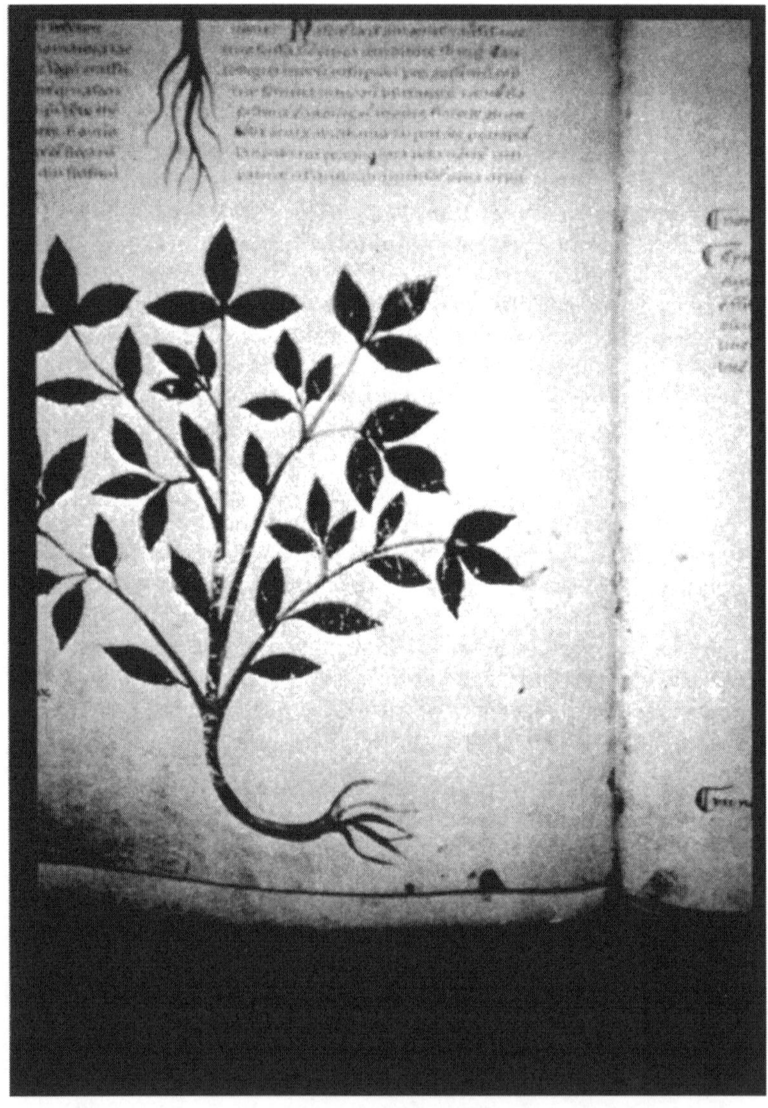

Fig. 1. The illustration of sage in the *Ex herbis femininis* manuscript in Vienna's Nationalibliothek (Ms. 93, s. XIII, fol. 137v).

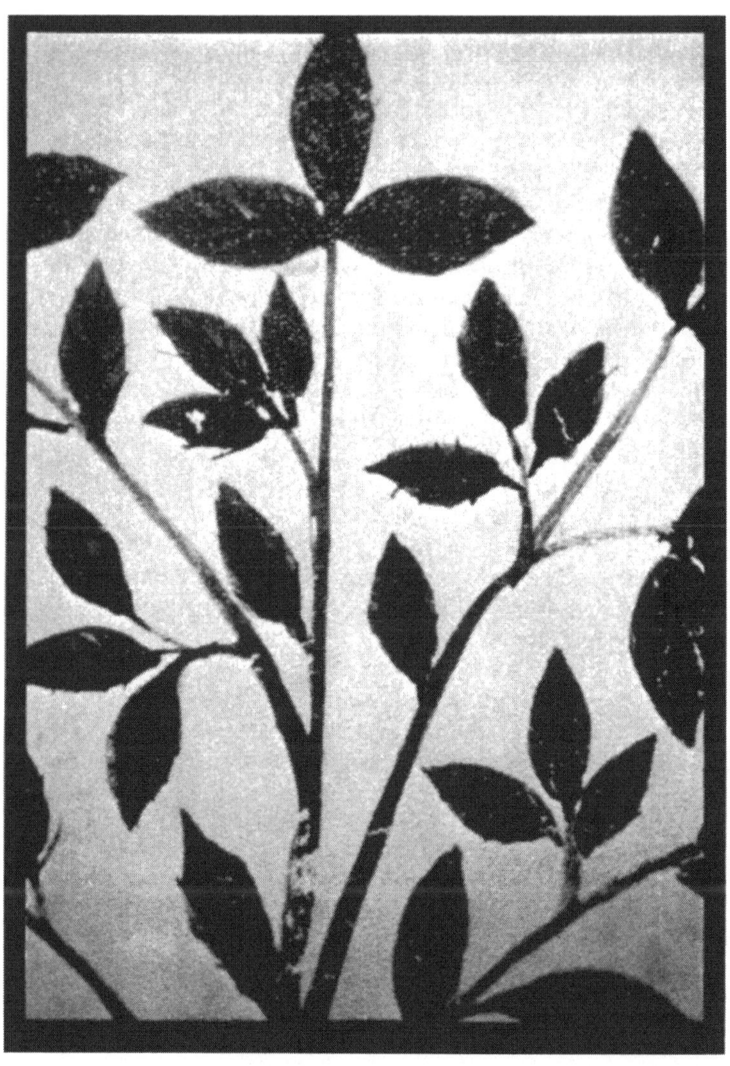

Fig. 2. Detail of Fig. 1.

used the terms loosely to distinguish varieties of the same plant family. He called a kind of knotgrass male because it has more seeds,[13] and called one kind of tarragon female because it is less hard than the male tarragon and is easier to cook.[14] Dioscorides occasionally attached sexual labels to plants, but without advancing reasons for them. Similarly *Ex herbis femininis* did not provide an explanation of plant gender. Among the seventy-one herbal entries, *Ex herbis femininis* has five (nos. 12, 21, 22, 23, and 70)[15] that name both male and female varieties, but often with the statement that both have the same medicinal strength. The female mercury plant (no. 22) has seeds growing in clusters, *Ex herbis* noted, while the male's seeds grow from the stem. In only two entries (nos. 15 and 45) are the plants listed as being female. In one of these, "*dracontea feminia*" (no. 45), Dioscorides distinguished both larger and smaller varieties, whereas *Ex herbis* borrowed Dioscorides' description of the smaller plant without mentioning the larger, and called the plant female.

One twelfth-century manuscript copy gave the title of Pseudo-Dioscorides' tract as *De herbis mulieribus* and included the colophon: "Explicit atque proficitur liber medicinarum Dioscoridis ex herbis masculinis atque de herbis femininis sive semininis. Feliciter."[16] Thus at least one copyist, at some time in or before the twelfth century, wanted the treatise's title to be "Women's Herbs" rather than "Female Herbs," but also he let it known, through design or error, that it was concerned with both male and female, or seed-producing, herbs. *Semininis* is presumably meant to be *seminariis*.

In other versions *Ex herbis femininis* has two separate chapters on Mediterranean mezereon: in the first (no. 34) the plant is designated female; the other chapter (no. 42) says there are seven kinds of mezereon, but it distinguishes only male and female forms. The drawings in each chapter show two different plants[17] and the texts list different usages.

13. Pliny, *Natural History*, 27.91.113-117.

14. Ibid., 24.92.143.

15. I have followed the manuscript numbering system, especially that in Vienna Ms. 93, rather than the numbering in Kästner's published text because of his omissions of two herbs and his slightly different arrangement. See the Appendix for herbs, with Dioscorides' chapter numbers included.

16. London, Brit. Lib. Ms. Sloane 1975, fol. 73.

17. The drawings in *Ex herbis* in Vienna, NB Ms. lat. 93, fol. 147, showing titmallos (no. 34), are similar to those in the Greek Dioscorides in Vienna, NB Ms. Gr. 1, fol. 350, showing *τιθυμαλλον ηλιωσκοπιος*; but there is less similarity between Ms. lat. 93, fol. 149, showing titmallos (no. 42), and Ms. Gr. 1, fol. 351, showing *τιθυμαλλον η οξυφυλλον*.

Pseudo-Dioscorides' *Ex herbis femininis*

There seems no adequate explanation of why *Ex herbis femininis* is so named. To say that the gender designation was employed occasionally to distinguish varieties is to ignore the numerous other instances when no attempt was made to differentiate varieties even among closely related herbs. Obviously, sexual labels were not systematically applied. One can only presume that the title was the product of a later copyist who sought to connect the herbals of Pseudo-Apuleius and Pseudo-Dioscorides by designating one male, the other female.

If we know then that the Pseudo-Apuleius and Pseudo-Dioscorides treatises were herbals falsely attributed to classical writers, what can we learn about when these attributions were first made? And, in the case of Pseudo-Dioscorides, was the authorship ascribed to Dioscorides at the period of the herbal's writing or later? Some manuscripts containing these herbals also include other tracts that may help answer these questions. These other tracts are Pseudo-Hippocrates' *Epistula ad Maecenatem*, Pseudo-Antonius Musa's *De herba vettonica*, (Pseudo-?) Sextus Placitus' *Liber medicinae ex animalibus, pecoribus et bestiis vel avibus*, and the anonymous *De taxone liber.*[18] In the case of each, except the last and possibly the obscure work by Sextus Placitus, the name of a known classical authority was attached. Probably this was done to lend authority and prestige and to forestall criticism. In our age, which extols uniqueness and novelty, it is difficult to imagine an age in which uniqueness was so undesirable that authors of original works scrupulously avoided claims of innovation and often went to the extent of obscuring their authorship. Just as the names of Hippocrates and Antonius Musa were attached to tracts to lend them authority, Dioscorides' name was no doubt added to *Ex herbis femininis* because he was the author of the largest work on materia medica written during antiquity. Similarly, Linda Voigts's recent argument is persuasive that Apuleius' name was attached to the *Herbarium Apulei* because of an association between Apuleius and the cult of Aesculapius.[19]

Gerhard Baader uses the term *Herbariencorpus* to describe these six treatises – *Ex herbis femininis* and the five mentioned above – associated in manuscripts, and places their association as a corpus "in and around

18. See the manuscripts described by Beccaria, *I codici*, index.

19. Linda Voigts's "The Significance of the Name Apuleius to the *Herbarium Apulei*," *Bull. Hist. Med.*, *52* (1978), 214-227, with excellent references to the controversy and related questions.

Ravenna" in the sixth and seventh centuries.[20] As Pierre Riché has observed, Ravenna in the sixth century was noted as a medical center – at least, it was where physicians were "particularly honored."[21] Possibly Dioscorides' name was attached then and there to *Ex herbis femininis*.

But this tells us nothing about the origin of *Ex herbis femininis*. It is uncertain when or where the unknown author lived, what sources other than Dioscorides he employed, when and by whom the drawings were made, and why the herbs were called female in the first place. These are an embarrassingly large number of unknowns for a work once so popular and highly influential. Varieties of evidence provide some tentative answers.

Several scholars have made suggestions about the time and place the writer lived. Hermann Stadler, for instance, postulated an African origin for the author on the basis of two African synonyms he added to Dioscorides' text: "Anchusae genera sunt duo; una quam Afri barbatam vocant est" and "Cynosbatos Latini zizfum agrestum dicunt, Punici didacholbat vocant."[22] Indeed, though I will later reject Stadler's argument, there are additional African synonyms in other chapters: "Colocinthis agria, id est cucurbita agrestis, quam Afri gelelam vocant" and "Eryngion quam Afri cherdan vocant."[23] I asked Gordon Newby, an Islamicist, for his advice on these allegedly "African" and Punic words, and I quote his reply:

> Re: "Colocinthis agria. id est cucurbita grestis, quam Afri gelelam vocant . . ."
>
> The problem of the identification of the African words in the *Ex herbis* is complicated by several factors. In the first instance, a distinction is apparently made between "Punic" and "African." It is

20. See Gerhard Baader, "Die Anfange der medizinischen Ausbildung in Abendland bis 1100," *La scuola nell' occidente latino dell' alto medioevo*, 2 vols. (Spoleto, 1972), II, 669-772, esp. 697; and also his earlier article, "Zur Überlieferung der lateinischen medizinischen Literatur des frühen Mittelalters," *Forschung, Praxis, Fortbildung. Organ für die gesamte praktische und theoretische Medizin, 17*, pt. 4 (1966), 139-141.

21. Pierre Riché, *Education and Culture in the Barbarian West from the Sixth through the Eighth Century*, trans. John J. Contreni (Columbia, S.C.: University of South Carolina Press, 1976), p. 70.

22. Hermann Stadler, "Dioscorides als Quelle Isidors," *Archiv für lateinische Lexikographie und Grammatik, 10* (1898), 411; Max Wellmann, "Dioskurides" (no. 12), in Pauly Wissowa, *Real-Encyclopädie der klassichen Altertumwissenschaft* (Stuttgart, 1903), V, pt. 1, 1134.

23. *Ex herbis*, nos. 47 and 54 (Kästner's nos. 46 and 53).

possible that this distinction is between the Northwest Semitic Phoenician dialect called Punic, but which varies little from its Mediterranean counterpart, and a dialect of one of the Hamitic Berber languages. If it is the case, as has been assumed, that the vocabulary designated "Punic" and "African" in *Ex herbis* derived through a literary source, then it is most probable that the distinction is artificial. Fifth century North African literate culture was primarily confined to the Mediterranean littoral with occasional incursions into the interior. We know that this population area was bilingual, at least, in Latin and Punic from Roman times and that the third major linguistic influence was Greek. Punic speakers survived in force into the fifth century as St. Augustine's Punic preferments demonstrate, so it is reasonable to assume that the term "African" could include Punic, as well as Latin, Greek, and, unlikely, Berber vocabulary, lacking evidence to the contrary. The second complication concerns the transmission of foreign words in a Latin textual tradition where it cannot be assumed that the original author or the subsequent transmitters were acquainted with the African language(s) in question. While we cannot be certain that the form of the words in our extant versions of *Ex herbis* is correct, any hypothetical etymology is subject to correction by a demonstration of a more valid textual tradition. The third difficulty involves our relative lack of knowledge of Punic, or Berber, for that matter, particularly in the realm of plant names. Most of our Punic vocabulary lists are derived from monumental inscriptions and from the Punic passages in Plautus. Decipherment of texts often rests on the ability of the scholar to find plausible analogs in other Semitic languages, relying on context to provide exact definitions.

In light of the above, it is possible to propose an etymology for one of the terms labeled "African" in *Ex herbis*, the term "*gelelam*." This is the "African equivalent of "*cucurbita*" gourd or cupping glass. If one assumes a root *GLL, a geminated form of *GL, one finds a Northwest Semitic analog, Aramaic *gelâl*, a lump, *gâlâl* (v.) to roll, *gâlâm* (v.) to roll up, and, in a reduplicative expansion of *GL, *galgêl* (v.) to roll. (M. Jastrow, *A Dictionary of the Targumim* . . ., New York, 1950, v. I). The semantic range of this root is paralleled in Arabic, cf. *jalla* and *juljul*. The semantic range of "roundness" parallels that of "*cucurbita*" and would seem to be apt in Semitic. If this be the case, it is possible that the terms "Punic" and "African" in *Ex herbis* overlap if not coincide, and it is probable that there was a genuine North African origin for the terms so named.

Under "red bulbs" (no. 44), however, the author of *Ex herbis* omitted Dioscorides' statement that they are "brought from Africa."[24] Under wild colocynth or bitter apple (no. 47), where *Ex herbis'* author gives the African synonym *gelelam*, he added that it has spread *per terram*, "throughout the earth."[25]

But the herbs listed in the treatise come from a southern European habitat, not an African one. Charles Singer, citing an apparently erroneous reference, reports that the author of *Ex herbis* may have lived in Ostrogothic Italy, but gives no reasons for this assertion.[26] Evidence presented in this paper supports the thesis that *Ex herbis'* author lived in Italy, southern France, or the Mediterranean littoral of Spain, probably in the fifth century, although an early sixth-century date seems possible. The 600 or so plants described by Dioscorides are preponderantly from the eastern Mediterranean regions.[27] The author of *Ex herbis* selected some seventy herbs (two chapters discuss the same plant). Difficult though it is to prove, the evidence suggests a southern European location for the plants described.

Botanical identification of the herbs according to modern classification is difficult. Descriptions are often vague or even lacking, and the drawings, as noted earlier, are often not accurate. Plants change their habitats and cultivation extends growth areas. Pilgrims, merchants, and traveling monks, especially those monks responsible for monastic herb gardens, could be expected to extend medicinal herbs to regions where the plants were not native.[28] Whereas the climate during Dioscorides'

24. *De materia medica*, 2.170 (vol. I, p. 236, Wellmann ed.).

25. *Per terram* might instead mean "on the ground," but the Old English version of *Ex herbis* (no. 185 in Thomas Oswalk Cockayne, *Leechdoms, Wortcunning, and Starcraft of Early England*, 3 vols. [London 1864-1866; repr. London: Holland Press, 1961], I, 325) translates the words *per terram* as "spreadth abroad its stems upon the earth." P. Font y Quer, *Plantes medicinales el Dioscorides renovado* (Barcelona: Editorial Labor, 1962), p. 770, says wild colocynth was not introduced to Europe until the Arabs brought it through Spain. My interpretation of *Ex herbis* would place the plant's introduction sooner.

26. Singer, "Herbal in Antiquity," p. 47, cites as his authority Max Wellmann, "Krateus," in *Abhandlungen der königlichen Gesellschaft der Wissenschaften zu Göttingen: Philologisch-Historische Klasse*, n.s. *2*, no. 1 (1900), but without pagination. I am unable to find Wellmann's statement.

27. C. Vaczy, "Nomenclature Dacica a plantelor la Dioscorides si Pseudo-Apuleius," *Acta Musei Napocensise* (Clui, Transylvania), *5* (1968), 59-73, esp. pp. 68-69; Jerry Stannard, "Medieval Herbals and their Development," *Clio Medica*, *9* (1974), 24.

28. Linda E. Voigts, "Anglo-Saxon Plant Remedies and the Anglo-Saxons," *Isis*, *70* (1979), 259-261.

time (first century A.D.) was approximately the same as today's climate, and the vegetation found in both periods is similar,[29] a variety of evidence points to the likelihood that climate was different in the late Roman and early medieval periods. From the second century A.D. to about 350 A.D. the climate in Italy was rather moist; there followed a drier period to about 450, with dry periods repeated around 800 and in the nine hundreds.[30] Evidence derived from the Fernau glacier, analyses of pollen indicating growth and recession of forests near peat bogs, changes in crop and vineyard growth areas, dendroclimatology, and other data suggest that from 300 to 500 A.D. there were warm summer periods accompanied by generally dry and cold winters in the area of Europe around near 50° N. Similar periods were repeated in the ninth and tenth centuries, and the years from 1000 to 1200 are associated with a moderate, warm climate and optimal growing conditions.[31] Linda Voigts has speculated on the basis of literary and climatological evidence that the erratic early medieval climate may have affected the kinds of crops and herbs cultivated in Anglo-Saxon England.[32] We may project similar patterns in vegetation changes throughout Europe. A further problem in botanical identification is that nomenclature shifts. The word used to refer to a plant in one era may not refer to the same plant in another.

But even with these problems, many identifications can be made with reasonable certitude. In the list of plants in *Ex herbis* there is no exception to this rule: where identification seems at least fairly certain the plants have southwestern Europe as a natural habitat. A few have wet, moist plains as their home, while some have mountains, for instance, the Alps or the Pyrenees. Proposing a north African origin for *Ex herbis* is therefore almost certainly incorrect. Its author was

29. Charles E. P. Brooks, *Climate through the Ages*, 2nd ed., rev. (New York: Dover, 1970), esp. pp. 300, 310ff; H. H. Lamb, *The English Climate*, 2nd ed. (London: English Universities. Press, 1964), p. 162; Robin Birley, "A Frontier Post in Roman Britain," *Sci. Amer.*, *236* (February 1977), 44.

30. H. H. Lamb, *Climate: Present, Past, and Future*, 2 vols., vol. II, *Climatic History and the Future* (London: Methuen, 1977), pp. 426-429; Brooks, *Climate through the Ages*, pp. 300-301.

31. Brooks, *Climate through the Ages*, pp. 310-311; Georges Duby, *The Early Growth of the European Economy*, trans. Howard B. Clarke (Ithaca: Cornell University Press, 1974), pp. 6-11; Jean Gimpel, *The Medieval Machine: The Industrial Revolution of the Middle Ages* (New York: Holt, Rinehart and Winston, 1976), pp. 30-32; Lamb, *Climatic History*, pp. 34-40, 426-429.

32. Voigts, "Anglo-Saxon Plant Remedies," pp. 261-263.

selecting herbs, those most readily available in his region, that were most useful in medicine.

Other evidence supports my contention. A copyist of Pseudo-Apuleius' *Herbarius* omitted some plants that were not grown in Central Europe, where he was copying the manuscript. For those plants he substituted plants locally grown.[33] Further, an eleventh-century copy of an Old English translation of selected chapters from *Ex herbis femininis* reveals that an unknown Old English author-translator altered his material and in some cases seems to be discussing plants different from those in *Ex herbis.*[34] Presumably, he made these changes to suit the botanical characteristics of his region.

If *Ex herbis* was written in southern Europe, when did the author live? Three pieces of evidence support the contention that the herbal was in existence by the sixth century: (1) a statement by Cassiodorus; (2) an anonymous letter, perhaps by Cassiodorus; (3) Isidore of Seville's use of *Ex herbis*.

Writing not later than 562 A.D., Cassiodorus advised some monks: "If you have not sufficient facility in reading Greek, then you can turn to the herbal of Dioscorides, which describes and draws the herbs of the field with wonderful faithfulness."[35] This quotation usually cited as evidence that the Old Latin translation of Dioscorides' full five books was completed by Cassiodorus' time; to this manuscript Cassiodorus allegedly advised the deplorably ill-trained monks to turn. More probably, however, Cassiodorus was referring them to Pseudo-Dioscorides' *Ex herbis femininis*. As observed earlier, manuscripts of Dioscorides' old translation are not normally illustrated, and Cassiodorous' reference was to work that was "drawn with wonderful faithfulness." Moreover,

33. Sigerist, "Medical Literature," p. 34; Erhard Landgraf, "Ein frühmittelalterlicher Botanicus," *Kyklos, 1* (1928), 3–36.

34. As shown in the Cockayne ed., and as noted in the Appendix. Hubert Jan de Vriend, *The Old English Medicina de quadrupedibus* (Tilburg: D. U. H. Gianotten, 1972), observes numerous instances of modifications and misunderstandings by the Old English translator(s) of this work attributed to Sextus Placitus. In the case of one manuscript, Oxford, Bodl. Ms. 130, which contains fragments of the Latin *Ex herbis femininis*, he sees evidence that the *Medicina de quadrupedibus* section may be a translation, at least in part, back into Latin from the Old English and one made by "a translator who did not know Old English very well" (p. xlv). I have compared the fragments of *Ex herbis* in Bodl. Ms. 130 with other texts and can report that they reveal no signs of being a Latin translation of the Old English.

35. Cassiodorus, *Institutiones divinarum et humanorum litterarum*, chap. 31.

he used the word for herbal. Dioscorides' text, usually called *De materia medica*, described items from all three kingdoms, animal, vegetable, and mineral, and thus was not restricted to herbs. This argument is not completely firm, however, because in rare instances during the Middle Ages Dioscorides' complete text was referred to as an herbal.[36] Nonetheless, Cassiodorus was probably referring to *Ex herbis femininis*.

An anonymous letter to Marcellinus is found in two manuscripts, one of the twelfth century, the other of the ninth. The letter reads:

> With you as I may say with all good art which has not been studied [in our age] in the old manner because it (that is, learning) is subject to change among us, Marcellinus, I send you the best known, little botanical book from Dioscorides' book, converted into Latin, and in which are drawn herbal figures. I commend not only the pleasing fidelity of the writing to you but also on both sides of the folios it is carefully described so that one may not make errors about what the herbs are, neither will they misjudge their healing qualities nor will they missidentify their varieties.[37]

In both manuscripts, the letter follows Pseudo-Apuleius's *Herbarius*. I observed above that in many other codices *Ex herbis femininis* follows Pseudo-Apuleius. Although the suggestion was made by Max Wellmann and Valentin Rose that Marcellinus is the same as Gargilius Martialis (flourished c. 222-235), the earliest-known Latin author to cite Dioscorides,[38] it seems too much to expect *Martialis* to become *Marcellinus*. I advance this possibility: The letter was written by Cassiodorus to Marcellinus (flourished c. 534), the secretary of the patrician Justinian who continued Eusebius' chronicles to the beginning

36. E.g., one copy of the Old Latin translation has the title *De virtutibus herbarum*. See Paris, BN MS lat. 12,995, s. IX, fol. 1.

37. The letter is found in London, Brit. Lib. Ms. Harley 4986, s. XII (variously dated from s. X), fol. 44v, and was published from this manuscript by Valentin Rose, "Ueber die Medicina Plinii," *Hermes, 8* (1874), 38; cf. Beccaria, *I codici*, pp. 252-254. The letter also appears in Lucca, Biblioteca Governative Ms. 296, fol. 18v, and published in part by P. Giacosa, *Magistri Salernitani nondum editi* (Turin, 1901), p. 351. Giacosa identifies part of the text as by Dioscorides, but it was not so identified by Beccaria (pp. 285-288). The letter is published from both manuscripts by de Vriend, *Old English Medicina*, pp. xlii-xliii, who verifies that Giacosa was correct in recognizing *Ex herbis* in the Lucca Ms.

38. Wellmann, "Dioskurides," pp. 1134-1135; Rose, "Medicina Plinii," p. 38.

of Emperor Justinian's rule.[39] The reference is to *Ex herbis femininis* because of (1) its location in the two manuscripts; (2) the words *libellum botanicon*, instead of *materia medica*; and (3) again the mention of illustrations. Finally from my interpretation of the other Cassiodorus quotation, I believe that Cassiodorus knew and appreciated *Ex herbis*.

Valentin Rose proposed that Isidore of Seville (c. 560-636) used *Ex herbis* as a direct source for his botanical discussions in *Origines*, Book 17, Chapters 7-11.[40] Rose compared the wording of Isidore's text for "bupthalmos" with the text for "bustalmon" in *Ex herbis* (no. 30). Herman Stadler pursued the suggestion by comparing other entries and noted the resemblance of the two texts in discussing "aristolochia" (no. 12), "celedonie" (no. 18), and "colocinthios" (no. 47). To the lists by Rose and Stadler can be added "buglossos" (no. 2; cf. Isidore 7.10.20). Stadler categorically rejected any assertion that *Ex herbis* is an extract of Isidore.[41] Even though Isidore based most of his botanical research on Pliny's *Natural History*,[42] the case is strong that Isidore knew the Pseudo-Dioscoridean text. Compared with Isidore's work, *Ex herbis* has much more information concerning the herbs, information that is known from no other identified source. Thus the author of *Ex herbis* did not use Isidore's *Origines* as his source; instead Isidore employed *Ex herbis* when he wrote early in the seventh century. Rose's suggestion is correct.

Ex herbis' language suggests late classical, early medieval Latin, that is, a date around the fifth century. The author unquestionably knew his languages well. There are a few examples of barbarisms, but far

39. Cassiodorus, *Letters*, 1.17.1-2 (L. W. Jones ed.); cf. Max Manitius, *Geschichte der lateinischen Literatur des Mittelalters*, 3 vols. (Munich, 1911-1931), I, pt. 2, pp. 79, 116-117. No other letter by Cassiodorus is addressed to Marcellinus, but it is clear that Cassiodorus held him in respect. About the time Marcellinus was writing his *Chronicum*, Cassiodorus was heading a Christian school in Rome that he had founded about 535 and that survived until it was destroyed in the fighting between Totila and Belisarius in the late 540's. See Pierre Paul Courcelle, *Late Latin Writers and Their Greek Sources*, trans. Harry E. Wedeck (Cambridge, Mass.: Harvard University Press, 1969), p. 334; for Cassiodorus' knowledge of Marcellinus' work, see pp. 261n, 374, 395, and 410.

40. Rose, "Medicina Plinii," p. 38; accepted by Singer, "Herbal in Antiquity," p. 47; Wellmann, "Dioskurides," p. 1134; and Lynn Thorndike, *A History of Magic and Experimental Science*, 8 vols. (New York: Macmillan, 1923-1941), I, 609.

41. Hermann Stadler, "Dioscorides als Quelle Isidors," *Archiv f. lat. Lex. u. Gram.*, *10* (1898), 403-412, esp. pp. 409-410.

42. Ernest H. F. Meyer, *Geschichte der Botanik*, 4 vols. (Königsberg, 1854-1857; repr. Amsterdam: A. Asher, 1965), II, 391.

fewer than are present in the Old Latin translation of Dioscorides, which was probably made in the sixth century.[43] And there are examples of new vocabulary words.[44] These qualities, in addition to the fact that no one earlier than Cassiodorus (c. 562 A.D.) refers to *Ex herbis* and no one earlier than Isidore (c. 560-636) quotes from it, are the principal factors in postulating a fifth-century date, or at any rate a date no later than early sixth century.

The translations from Dioscorides seem to be direcly from the Greek and in short, crisp Latin. The lexical skills were quite remarkable. The translation is free and frequently interspersed with additional comments either about the plants or about their medicinal uses. Most notably, the author added details about how to prepare and compound the herbs as medicines and how to administer them that Dioscorides had not included.

Ex herbis femininis is substantially a new botanical-medical treatise and contains new medical and botanical contributions; it added to, modified, and subtracted from the Dioscoridean core. Of the seventy-one chapters, only eighteen or nineteen are translated from Dioscorides with insignificant changes.[45] In no case is the translation a complete, unmodified Latin version of Dioscorides' Greek. In some twenty-nine chapters, the author has modified the Greek text and added medicinal uses of the plants not contained in Dioscorides' work.[46] In thirteen or fourteen, the text is completely new and totally unrelated to Dioscorides or, as will be shown later, to any other known literary

43. Hermann Stadler, "Der lateinisches Dioscorides der Münchener Hof-und Staatsbibliothek und die Bedeutung dieser Uebersetzung for einen Teil der mittelalterlichen Medicin," *Janus, 4* (1899), 548-550; and same title by Stadler but different text in *Allgemeine Medicinische Central-Zeitung, 14* (1900), 165-166; *15* (1900), 179-180; Vinzenz Bulhart, "Lexikalisches zum Spätlatein," *Wiener Studien: Zeitschrift für klassische Philologie, 67* (1954), 145-161; Max Niedermann, *Recueil Max Niedermann* (Neuchâtel: Secretariat de l'Université, 1954), pp. 39-43 and passim.; H. Mihaescu, "La versione latine di Dioscoride tradizione manoscritta, critica di testo, cenno linquistico," *Ephemeris Dacoromana, 8* (1938), 298-348; Hermann Stadler, Lateinische Pflanzennamen in Dioskorides," *Archiv für lateinische Lexikographie und Grammatik, 2* (1898), 83-114.

44. For a list of barbarisms and new vocabulary in *Ex herbis*, see Kästner, "Pseudo-Dioscorides," p. 579.

45. The chapter numbers are: 7, 11, 12, 14, 15, 16, 18, 20, 23, 26, 27, 28, 30, 33; 38, 41, 48, 51, 52 (maybe unrelated?), and 71. Throughout the chapter numbers are as they appear in most manuscripts, esp. Vienna Ms. 93, since Kästner's edition omits two chapters.

46. Nos. 1, 2, 3, 4, 5, 6, 8, 9, 10, 17, 19, 21, 22, 24, 25, 29, 32, 36, 37, 40, 42, 43, 45, 54, 56, 59 (?), and 70.

source.[47] Seventeen chapters significantly modify plant descriptions. In at least three chapters, differences in plant habitat are noted.[48] In one chapter (no. 31) the identification of the herb is uncertain because of an inability to find the equivalent chapter in Dioscorides.

The chapter on sweet marjoram (no. 10) is a good example of how the author modified his material. Dioscorides said marjoram's leaves are "rough and round like catmint [καταμίνθης]," but *Ex herbis*' author, showing some care in translating as well as botanical knowledge, said the leaves are "rough and round, similar to *nepeta.*" *Nepeta* is a variety of catmint known as Italian catmint. Rather than merely being content with transliterating the Greek to *cataminthus*, which is acceptable in Latin, the author-translator sought to identify the herb specifically by referring to a variety known in his locality. To Dioscorides' list of medicinal uses, *Ex herbis* added that the herb is useful in treating urinary complaints and a gripping pain of the intestine. Interestingly, a modern herbal by M. Grieves reports that sweet marjoram alleviates "spasms, colic, and . . . pain in dyspeptic complaints."[49] Where Dioscorides said it relieves swellings or tumors (*οἰδήματα*), *Ex herbis* was more specific: "eye tumor," *tumores oculorum. Ex herbis* follows Dioscorides in giving a synonym, *amaracon dicitur Cyzicenis*, but one eleventh-century copy omits this synonym and adds one of its own: *arabos dicitur herba ezuae.*[50] Perhaps even before the translations from Arabic to Latin, the copyist was adopting the text to his own time.[51]

In discussing sea holly's root (no. 54), the author said they "are collected at the summer solstice before the rising sun," material not in to Dioscorides' text, and omitted Dioscorides' claim that sea holly is a good amulet. *Ex herbis* directed that sea holly be cooked in oil until it is viscous, then placed in wax, then blended with three parts (?) of silver foam, and finally mixed with ashwood twigs. This recipe is "a wonderful aid against scorpion and all snake bites or mad dog bites if the wound is first opened by iron and it is applied locally so that the sick person does not perceive the smell. [At] this temperature [the

47. Nos. 35, 50, 57, 58, 59 (possibly), 60, 61, 62, 63, 64 (?), 65, 66, 67, and 69.

48. Nos. 8, 9, 10, 11, 23, 25, 27, 29, 33, 34, 37, 45, 51, 53, 59, 69, and 71, modify plant descriptions. Nos. 1, 5, and 11 give different plant habitats.

49. M. Grieves, *A Modern Herbal* (New York: Dover, 1971), p. 521.

50. Florence, Laur. Ms. Plut. 73.41, s. XI, fol. 91 (124).

51. John M. Riddle, "The Introduction and Use of Eastern Drugs in the Early Middle Ages," *Sudhoffs Archiv, 49* (1965), 185-198.

formula] also cools St. Anthony's fire, and it resists gout if applied at its inception."

More typical modifications are less drastic but have some medical significance. Under hawthorn (no. 1), *Ex herbis* translated Dioscorides' statement that applied locally it is good for swellings (*οἰδήματα*) with the phrase "applied locally it removes bruises [*livores*]." Thus *Ex herbis* refined the indefinite Greek word *οἰδήματα* to read "eye tumors" in the chapter on majoram and here to read "bruises." In five chapters *Ex herbis*' author came across Dioscorides' word *ἴκτερον*, meaning jaundice; twice (nos. 30 and 53) the author simply transliterated the word into *icterkon*, while in three chapters (nos. 29, 41, and 49) he inconsistently translated it *morbum regium*. In no. 41 he explained: "morbum regium id est icterikon." Examination of his free translation reveals that the author was no novice who dealt clumsily with Greek and Latin.

His linguistic knowledge was good but, more important, his medical and botanical knowledge was sufficiently sophisticated enough to allow him often to give more detailed analyses, more precisely and medically descriptive, than those recorded by his highly regarded classical authority, Dioscorides. For instance, still under hawthorn (no. 1), Dioscorides wrote, "Thus the root being drunk is good for hematosis [*ταύτης ἡ ῥίζα πινομένη ποιεῖ πρὸς αἱμοπτυικούς*]." The author of *Ex herbis* loosely translated this as: "Thus the root, beaten and grated, taken in two spoonfuls, drunk with water, is good for hematosis . . . [Huius radix tunsa et cribrata ad modum cocliaria duo cum aqua pota obduris, haemoptoicis . . .]."

We find examples of the author's knowledge throughout the herbal. To Dioscorides' assertion that burrage (no. 2) makes one happy at parties, the author of *Ex herbis* added that its leaves perforated are a good condiment when added to food. Dioscorides said that acantha (no. 3), or bear's breech, is "useful for convulsions and ruptures [*ῥήγματι* = in sense of fractures or breaks]," which *Ex herbis* rendered as it "heals inner veins which burst open" (that is internal hemorrhaging). Dioscorides asserted only that the root is drunk; *Ex herbis* added, "The root dried, beaten and grated, drunk with water." Sage (no. 4), Dioscorides said, is good "for wounds, staunching blood and as a cleanser of malignant humors [*καὶ τραυματικὴ καὶ ἴσχαιμος καὶ ἀποκαθαρτική τῶν θηριωδῶν*]." *Ex herbis* translated this as: "it stops blood from wounds, it cures old, festering bites of wild animals, and it joins together open wounds," which is really hardly a translation at all. And, to sample more at random, *Ex herbis* omitted Dioscorides' claims that if psyllium plantain (no. 25) is brought into the house, it prevents fleas from breeding, but added that it cures a protruding umbilicus. Whereas Dioscorides said horsetails (no. 32) stop bleeding, *Ex herbis* refined the statement to read, they are "good for ruptured veins within the body and on the eyes." A preparation of ground olive's leaves cleans filthy, festering wounds, wrote Dioscorides, while *Ex herbis* (no. 39) said their use should be continued until the wound has healed. Sorrel (no. 49), *Ex herbis* said, cures cysts on the breast; Dioscorides merely mentioned cysts without giving a location. Common teasle (no. 52), "beaten, chopped up, and drunk in warm water, cures one of worm disease most perfectly," *Ex herbis* added to Dioscorides' text in another place. Not all uses discussed are medicinal. Golden thistle (no. 36) was said by both Dioscorides and *Ex herbis* to remove bad smells from the armpits – indeed the entire body – and to reduce the smell of urine. Dioscorides noted that the herb is put in asparagus, presumably to counter the smell of urine, while *Ex herbis* simply said golden thistle is a healthy food.

The early medieval writer included a number of herbs used as abortifacients and one used as a contraceptive, but he said less about these uses than Dioscorides did for the same herbs. Shepherd's purse (no. 16) was said by both Dioscorides and *Ex herbis* to abort a fetus in pregnancy.[52] Likewise ploughman's spikenard (no. 28), friar's cowl (?, no. 45), and opoponax (no. 64) cause termination of pregnancies. Germander (?, no. 8), Dioscorides said, carried off the menses and embryo, while *Ex herbis* said, "it draws out the menses and expels a dead fetus." Both say that "aristolochia" (no. 12) "expels a retained fetus [*Ex herbis*: "herentes fetus discutit"]." Strictly speaking, these herbs are probably not intended as abortifacients. There is only one clear prescription of a contraceptive and this is suspect by modern judgment. Translating Dioscorides almost literally, *Ex herbis* reported of spleenwort (no. 41): "If it does not see the moon, collected by day or night, it is suspended [around the neck] with the spleen of a mule and it does not allow one to conceive." And the unidentified herb "isfieritis" (no. 31) was named by *Ex herbis* as an aid to conception. For three herbs (nos. 45, 56, and 59), however, *Ex herbis* omitted Dioscorides' claims about abortifacient qualities. The fact that there are fewer abortifacients in the later treatise than in its model is no certain indication that early medieval medicine was less inclined than classical medicine to abortions. Other early medieval medical writings are filled

52. The Old English version of *Ex herbis* states that it provokes menstruation – Cockayne ed., no. 150, I, 275.

with abortifacients. The author of *Ex herbis* was probably indicating by his omission his judgment on the herbs' effectiveness in causing abortions.

The old idea that early medieval medical works are replete with superstitions, clarms, amulets, and magic is shattered by *Ex herbis femininis*. Although it contains some instances of what today we call supernatural elements, they are few. Only three instances are noted among the hundreds of uses of herbs. In every case, the supernatural element is taken directly from Dioscorides. In four other places *Ex herbis*' author, even when translating from Dioscorides, has omitted superstitious elements from Dioscorides' text. In material added by *Ex herbis*' author, there is no mention of the supernatural. Snapdragon (no. 23) is worn as a suspension to keep away dangers, reported both Dioscorides and *Ex herbis*. Squill (no. 53), both stated, is suspended above doorways to keep out evil spirits. And, finally, there is the prophylactic use for spleenwort (no. 41), mentioned above. *Ex herbis* omitted Dioscorides' claim that friar's cowl (?, no. 45) emits a smell from its withering flowers that will destroy a newly conceived embryo; that sorrel's (no. 49) roots worn as an amulet around the neck alleviate *struma* (goiter or scrofula); that common plantain (no. 51) similarly worn dissolves *struma*; and that sea holly (no. 54) is worn as an amulet. One case is uncertain. *Ex herbis* added to Dioscorides' account that mayweed (no. 19) portends death. Accordingly, its juice is mixed with *aegrotus* oil to determine the imminence of death: if smeared on the body of a patient and he sweats, then death is coming; if the patient "sweats to a lesser degree," then he remains "longer." In the absence of modern experimentation, one must allow for the possibility that the mixture could have some physiological effect in inducing perspiration. Whatever may be the truth about mayweed, *Ex herbis* was definitely less superstitious and supernatural than comparable classical works.

Plant descriptions also are different in *Ex herbis* and Dioscorides' treatise. Generally, *Ex herbis* shortened Dioscorides' plant descriptions, occasionally completely omitting them. It may be noted again that *Ex herbis* had an accompanying picture of each plant, whereas the Latin Dioscorides had no such aid. Even so, *Ex herbis* often modified the description. One example is psyllium plantain (no. 25). Dioscorides reads:

> Psyllium has leaves similar to *coronopis*, hairy, twigs a thumb span long, and the whole plant grasslike. The leading part is the foliage from the middle of the stalk, two or three heads on the top twisted

up, in which seeds are like fleas, the black, hard kind. It grows in the countryside [φύεται ἐν αρούραις].

Ex herbis reads:

Psyllios. So-called because its seeds appear like fleas, the same as *cynomia*. In Latin they call the herb *pulicaria*, or fleawort. The leaf has small prickles, the stem branches, dry and fragile all over; from the middle of the stem it sends out stalks at the highest point, two or three heads in which the seed is black similar to fleas. It is found in cultivated places.

Thus *Ex herbis* says its habitat is cultivated places, while Dioscorides says its habitat is the countryside.

Elsewhere the author of *Ex herbis* also varied the habitat, presumably to suit better his time and place. Where Dioscorides mentioned Eastern habitats, *Ex herbis* omitted them (compare, for example no. 5 with Dioscorides, 3.60). Dioscorides said hawthorn (no. 1) "grows in mountainous and woody places," which *Ex herbis* rendered as "it grows in mountainous and rocky places and dry places." For cumin (no. 5) *Ex herbis* omitted Dioscorides' statement that "it grows in the hills [φύεται ἐν γεωλόφοις]"; but for houseleek (no. 11), Dioscorides' phrase "It grows in hilly places and places of broken pottery" is changed in *Ex herbis* to "in mountainous places ["in locis montuosis"]."

Most plant modifications are minor. In describing germander (no. 8), *Ex herbis* added this line to Dioscorides: "From one root many branches lead out into the turf." In describing annual mercury (no. 22), Dioscorides said there is a male and a female; the seed of the female grows in thick clusters and the male has small round stems longer than the female's. *Ex herbis* stated: "The seed of the female grows in clusters, the masculine on the stem itself." In this entry, *Ex herbis* added a synonym, *hermubotane*, for the herb.

For the color of flower *Ex herbis* sometimes changed hues slightly. Dioscorides reported knotgrass (no. 9) flowers as being white and purple (φοινικοῦν = purple toward red), while *Ex herbis* translated as white and ruddy, or rosy (*roseum*). Dioscorides said snapdragon's (no. 23) flowers are purple (πορφύρα), while *Ex herbis* has rose-colored (*colore roseo*), but for wall flower and/or mountain pansy (no. 59), where Dioscorides says its flowers are white, yellow, and purple (λευκὸν ἢ μήλινον ἢ πορφυροῦν εὑρίσκεται), *Ex herbis* accurately translates, "purple, white and yellow [*purpureum*, album et melinum]."[53]

Usually the author of *Ex herbis* transliterated Greek plant names into Latin letters, but sometimes this procedure changed the nomenclature. *Ex herbis*' "cestros" (no. 11) is not Dioscorides' κέστρον (4.1), but Dioscorides' ἀείζωον μέγα (4.88), or houseleek. To *sideritis* (no. 20), *Ex herbis* adds, "quam Afri cherdan vocant"; to *iera* (no. 55, or our vervain), *Ex herbis* adds, "quam Latini verbenam."

Fourteen or fifteen chapters in *Ex herbis* are completely different from anything in Dioscorides, even though for each of these herbs Dioscorides has a complete description of the plant and medicinal uses. The reason for this is unclear. The herbs are found throughout Dioscorides' text and in the same books as other entries from which the author of *Ex herbis* freely translated. Dioscorides included medicinal uses that were ignored in *Ex herbis*, but the sixth-century author added many new uses. Moreover, for many of the new entries the style changes. For many, not all, the style is to list ailments and then describe medicinal preparation. For heliotrope, which is either weber dandelion or chicory, *Ex herbis* has two separate, and separated, entries (nos. 35 and 50) with slightly different illustrations, but there are no descriptions to enable us to discern the differences between the plants. Entry no. 35 reads in *Ex herbis*:

> Heliotrope, so-called because its flowers turn to meet the course of the sun. By others it is called *helioscopion* and by the Romans *woods intybum*.
>
> For disease of the spleen. Take the juice of heliotrope with 17 grains of pepper for three days and you will marvel.
>
> For headache: Place the juice of the herb heliotrope with rose oil; anoint on the head and forehead.
>
> For heart-burn: Prepare it thus: ten drachmas of spice nard, thyme honey 4 drachma, 3 drachma casia, 4 drachma pepper, 4 *misces* with wine and with the juice of the aforesaid herb above, *cocliaria* 3, form in a round ball of 2 scrupula and administer in a drink in wine. It frees one.

And entry no. 50 reads in part:

53. Of course, *Ex herbis* could have employed another source here and not translated Dioscorides. Isidore (17.9.19) follows *Ex herbis*.

> Heliotrope – wheresoever it is found it is neither simple nor in rows.
> For warts: leaves from the highest parts and warts *inde fricabis*. With 3 parts . . . in vinegar, they suddenly fall away and they do not come back again.
> For scabies of the whole body . . .
> For disease of the bladder . . .

Pseudo-Apuleius's treatise has an entry on heliotrope and, although the same style of presentation is used, there is no similarity in texts.[54]

There are other examples of completely different material that *Ex herbis* added in the same style as Dioscorides, for example, "centimorbia," possibly yellow loosestrife or creeping Jenny (no. 58), and "cynosbatos," or dog rose (no. 62). It is possible in these cases that *Ex herbis*' author had an entirely different plant in mind than did Dioscorides, but Dioscorides' textual descriptions of other plants may have been his source. *Centimorbia* may be either a new plant introduced by *Ex herbis* or a new plant name. In the case of scarlet pimpernel (no. 63), the author omitted Dioscorides' description of the plant, translated two sentences from Dioscorides, and then added considerable new information. From Dioscorides he used: "Place in the nostrils, it drives away phlegm and all bad humors. It calms the toothache." He added:

> If the juice is mixed with rose oil and smeared on the face, one will look cheerfully on all things. It is effective for a light, smooth complexion on women. *Anagallis* juice, mixed with honey, Indian *lycium* and bitter vinegar, and anointed on a woman's face, makes the face clear and soft. For epileptics who have alien dispositions: The anagallis juice mixed with honey and injected in the nose by purging the head restores a balanced mental attitude to the epileptic. For removing blemishes from the head . . .

And so it goes, but where did the author get his material?

54. Pseudo-Apuleius no. 49 (pp. 99-100, Howald-Sigerist ed.): "Herba Heliotropia. 1. Ad omne venenum. Herba heliotropiae pulverem mollissimum ex ea aut sucum eius, cum vino veteri optimo potui datum mire venena discutit. 2. Ad luxum herba heliotropia contusa et adposita efficaciter sanare dicitur." There follows a nomenclature section that is thought to be a later addition: "A Graecis dicitur heliotropia, alii heliotropos. alii heliopun, aii adialiton, alii scorpion, alii Heraclea, profetae gonos scorpiu, alii ema titanu, alii ura scorpio, Pythagoras parmoron, Aegyptii nisene, Itali vertumnum, alii mulcetram, alii intibum silvaticum. Nascitur ubique locis cultis et mundis et in pratis. Huius herbae divinae ad solis cursum floscelli si vertunt, et cum sol occidit, flosceli se cludeunt; rursum cum sol oritur, flosceli se aperiunt. Facit ad remedia multa."

Determining the extent of *Ex herbis*' originality depends largely on discovering whether the author employed literary sources other than Dioscorides' text. Heinrich Kästner and Charles Singer said that the author used Pliny's *Natural History* and Pseudo-Apuleius' *Herbarius.*[55] Kästner added Galen's *On Simple Medicines.*[56] Max Wellmann rejected Pseudo-Apuleius' *Herbarius*, and his judgment is vindicated by a close comparison of texts.[57] Although Pseudo-Apuleius is earlier, probably dating from the fourth century, the author of *Ex herbis* probably was unaware of the work. Certainly, he wrote about some of the same herbs discussed by Pseudo-Apuleius, but the text, iconography, plant descriptions, and uses do not resemble one another. In attempting to demonstrate Pseudo-Apuleius as a source for *Ex herbis*, Kästner used a text of Pseudo-Apuleius that differs from the critical edition prepared by Ernest Howard and Henry Sigerist.[58] Kästner's claim must be rejected in favor of Wellmann's arguments.

Galen was also not a source for *Ex herbis femininis*. Galen's *On Simple Medicines* was not known to the early Middle Ages in Latin. There exist Latin Pseudo-Galenic works on simples (drugs from a single plant), called *Ad Paternianum* and *De dynamidiis* and known during the early Middle Ages, but these tracts were not sources for *Ex herbis.*[59] Of course, since *Ex herbis*' author knew Greek and was using Dioscorides' Greek text, he could have used Galen's *On Simple Medicines* in Greek, but the new information in *Ex herbis* does not relate to Galen's account.

Although the case for Pliny as a possible source is more difficult to assess, Pliny is an unlikely candidate. The problem is compounded by the fact that both Dioscorides and Pliny drew on a common source, Sextius Niger, for some of their material on herbs.[60] In isolated instances

55. Kästner, "Pseudo-Dioscorides," p. 582; Singer, "Herbal in Antiquity," p. 47.

56. Kästner, "Pseudo-Dioscorides," p. 582.

57. Wellmann, "Dioskurides," p. 1134.

58. Cf. Kästner's text, p. 588, on the herb *buglossa* with the Howald-Sigerist ed. of Pseudo-Apuleius, p. 89, no. 41.

59. *De simplicibus medicamentis ad Paternianum* and *De dynamidiis* (and *Alter liber de dynamidiis, magna ex parte ex Aetio desumptus, plurimis in locis correctus*) as published in Galen, *Omnia, quae extant in Latinum sermonem conversa . . .*, 11 vols. (Basel, 1561) III, 18-36, 79-92.

60. Max Wellmann, "Sextius Niger. Eine Quellenuntersuchung zu Dioscorides," *Hermes, 23* (1888), 530-569; cf. W. H. S. Jones, *Pliny: Natural History*, 10 vols. (Cambridge, Mass.: Harvard University Press, 1951), vols. VI, VII. An example of similarity between Pliny and Dioscorides is seen in their treatment of wild astaphis – Dioscorides, 4.152; Pliny, *Natural History*, 23.13.17-18.

Ex herbis' added material is somewhat similar to the same medicinal uses in Pliny; but the instances are rare and one would expect some similar but coincidental uses. The fact that Pliny lists numerous medicinal uses that *Ex herbis* does not give for the same herb mitigates against the possibility that the author of *Ex herbis* used Pliny. The near certainty is that he did not.

A study of other ancient writers on materia medica and plants fails to identify the source of *Ex herbis*' new material. The author did not use Aetius of Amida, Theophrastus, Gargilius Martialis, Solinus, Oribasius, Caelius Aurelianus, Aretaeus, Pseudo-Hippocrates, Scribonius Largus, Cassius Felix, Quintus Serenus, Alexander of Tralles, Theodorus Priscianus, Marcellus, or the Pseudo-Pliny.[61]

In the absence of evidence to the contrary, I proposed that the author of *Ex herbis femininis* added new material largely from his own medical and botanical knowledge and experience. Certainly his free translations, his interspersing of new material, and his medically and botanically reasonable omissions suggest that he was sufficiently capable and knowledgeable to have composed the new material. Nonetheless,

61. Aetius of Amida, *Libri medicinales*, ed. Alexander Olivieri, Corpus Medicorum Graecorum, 8, 1-2 (Leipzig: B. G. Teubner, 1935-1950); Theophrastus, *Enquiry into Plants*, ed. Arthur Hort, 2 vols. Cambridge, Mass.: Harvard University Press, 1948); Gargilius Martialis, *Medicinae ex oleribus et pomis*, ed. Valentin Rose, in *Plinii secundi* ... (Leipzig, 1875); Oribasius, *Collectionum medicarum reliquiae*, ed. Johannes Raeder, Corpus Medicorum Graecorum, 6, 1, 1 (Leipzig and Berlin: B. G. Teubner, 1924); Pseudo-Oribasius, *Apla urivasii de herbarum virtutem (Euporistes)*, in vol. VI of *Oeuvres d' Oribase*, ed. C. Bussemaker and Charles Daremberg (Paris, 1876); Pseudo-Hippocrates, *Dynamidia*, ed. Valentin Rose, in Rose, *Anecdota Graeca et Graecolatine* (Berlin, 1870; repr. Amsterdam: Hakkert, 1963); Scribonius Largus, *De compositionibus medicamentorum liber unus* ... (Paris, 1528), and *Compositiones*, ed. G. Helmreich (Leipzig, 1887); Cassius Felix, *De medicina*, ed. Valentin Rose (Leipzig, 1879); Paulus Aegineta, *The Seven Books of* ... , trans. Francis Adams, 3 vols. (London: Sydenhan Society, 1844-1847); Quintus Serenus, *Liber medicinalis*, ed. R. Pépin (Paris: Presses Universitaires de France, 1950); Alexander Trallianus, *Practica* (Venice, 1522), also in *Original-Text und Uebersetzung* ... , ed. Theodor Puschmann, 2 vols. (Vienna: W. Baumüller, 1879); Marcellus, *De medicamentis liber*, in *Ueber Heilmittel*, ed. Max Niederman, 2 vols., Corpus Medicorum Graecorum, 5 (Berlin: Akademie-Verlag, 1968); Caelius Aurelianus, *On Acute Diseases and On Chronic Diseases*, ed. and trans. I. E. Drabkin (Chicago: University of Chicago Press, 1950); Celsus, *De medicina*, ed. and trans. W. G. Spencer, 3 vols. (Cambridge, Mass: Harvard University Press, 1948-1953); Theodorus Priscianus, *Euporiston Libri III*, and Pseudo-Theodorus, *De simplici medicina*, ed. Valentin Rose (Leipzig: B. G. Teubner, 1894).

there is the evidence to the contrary, because often, when he used completely new material for a whole entry, not relying on Dioscorides at all, the style changes. This fact suggests that he was copying from another literary source. This may be a lost herbal or more probably, given the style of listing ailments and then prescriptions, a *receptarius.*[62] We can speculate that the unknown source, or one of the sources, was African, and thus explain the African synonyms that may have confused Hermann Stadler. Newby's suggestion that the African synonyms may have a factual basis would support this possibility. Probably *Ex herbis*' author used an unidentified source or sources in addition to Dioscorides *and* employed his own medical-botanical judgments and information in managing his material.

Since the author relied demonstrably on Dioscorides and perhaps on other sources, can this treatise still be called original? Even if we judge by modern standards, the answer is surely yes. The modifications of information about herbs are not small or trivial contributions. Nowadays, when a researcher "discovers" a "new" curative or beneficial use of some organic or inorganic chemical, the work is hailed as a contribution to knowledge. By the same token, when the author of *Ex herbis* said, for instance, annual mercury (no. 22) relaxes the stomach when taken as an elixir with oil, that statement itself may be a claim for originality, since it was not in the works of his known authority. When a scientist or a historian writes a journal article or book, he does not reauthenticate every item of information he handles; mostly he reviews previous work before advancing the limited new data or consideration. If anyone today were to publish a medical herbal with so many changes in previously conventional factual knowledge, the work would immediately be hailed as a significant contribution. And so it should be with *Ex herbis femininis*.

Beginning with the first manuscript copy in the ninth century, abbreviated chapter headings, called *capitula*, were added to *Ex herbis*. In each chapter heading the herb was named and its medicinal uses indicated. This served as a brief guide for easy reference by a physician.[63] At some time during the twelve century or earlier, as revealed in

62. Some herbals, e.g., Felix Cassius' *De medicina*, Alexander Trallianus' *Practica*, and Scribonius Largus' *Compositiones*, do, however, use the format of listing afflictions and then giving recipes.

63. Florence, Laur. Ms. Plut. 73.41, s. XI, fols. 84-86v; London, Brit. Lib. Ms. Add. 8928, s. X, fols. 62v-65; Vatican, Ms. Barberiniano lat. 160, s. IX, fols. 38-39v.

seven manuscripts, three written in the twelfth century, some unknown author expanded the *capitula* by increasing the textual discussion of the medicinal uses of herbs, while at the same time he dropped eight herbs from the text: "centimorbia," "purpurea," "zamalentition," "zamalentition masculum," "sion," "lycanis," "abrothonum," and "aperine."[64] In rare instances the author added new medicinal uses found neither in the regular text of *Ex herbis* nor in the earlier *capitula.*[65] This work constituted a separate book and always preceded the full version of *Ex herbis*. Wherever and whenever he lived, whoever he was, the unknown author of Book I made a small attempt to make medical knowledge of plants more readily and easily accessible and added some new medical and pharmaceutical discoveries. As contributions go, however, it was small.

The Old English translation of *Ex herbis* is found in three manuscripts, of the ninth, tenth, and eleventh centuries. This translation is still another indication of the adaptiveness of the copyists/translators.[66]

64. Florence, Laur. Ms. Plut. 73. 16, s. XIII, fols. 179r-v; Florence, Strozz. Ms. lat. 73, s. XIII, fols. 39v-44v; London, Brit. Lib. Ms. Harley 1585, s. XII, fols. 79-82v (specifically calling this material a separate book); London, Brit. Lib. Ms. Royal App. 3, s. XIV, fols. 18-20v; London Brit. Lib. Ms. Sloane 1975, s. XII, fols. 49v-52v; Oxford, Bodl. Ms. Ashmole 1462, s. XIII, fols. 61-63v; Vienna, NB Ms. lat. 93, s. XIII, fols. 133-135v. See the description in John M. Riddle, "Dioscorides," *Catalogus, 4* (1980), 132-133.

65. For instance, Book I adds to the entry for the herb camelleon, or pine-thistle, that it sharpens vision ("visum exacuit"). Where *Ex herbis* says of *adiantos*, or maidenhair (no. 14), that "capillos cadentes continent," Book I has "Alopiectias vastat," or "it destroys fox-sickness." Fox-sickness, or fox mange, causes baldness. For *cameleuca*, or common teazle (no. 52), Book I adds to *Ex herbis*' advice on preparation by stating that the herb is beaten into a pliant powder and strained. The italicized words are those added to the text: Tunsa et *pulverem mollissimum redacta* et cribata et in aqua calida data."

66. London, Brit. Lib. Ms. Cotton Vitellius C III, s. XI, fols. 58/14b-74v/11b, 316; London, Brit. Lib. Ms. Harley 585, s. X, fols. 66v/11-101v/114; Ms. Harley 6258b, s. XI, fols. 110a/20a-124/29b; Oxford, Bodl. Ms. Hatton 76, s. XI, fols. 110a/20a-124/29b, published in *Rerum Britannicarum medii aevi scriptoris* (London 1864-1866), vol. I: Cockayne, *Leechdoms, Wortcunning, and Starcraft*, vol. I, and reprinted with Cockayne's Introduction with discussion of texts omitted and Charles Singer's Introduction substituted in London, 1961. The Cotton Vitellius Ms., which was the principal manuscript followed by Cockayne, has many of the leaves for the *Ex herbis* section disarranged in the binding. The correct order is 11-61, 64, 63, 74, 65-67, 62, 71, 70, 68, 73, 72, 69, 75-82. See George T. Flom, "On the Old English Herbal of Apuleius Vitellius C III," *J. Eng. Ger. Phil., 40* (1941), 29-37, esp. p. 32; and the more recent discussion of all manuscripts in de Vriend, *Old English Medicina*, p. xii, which notes the

Chapters numbered from 134 through 175 are mostly derived from *Ex herbis*, often freely translated and modified. Although this paper does not encompass an analysis of the Old English version, I note several examples of changes. To the medical uses of acanthus (no. 1), the Old English version adds that it promotes milk in the breast;[67] for shepherds' pure (no. 16), it changes *Ex herbis*' apparent claim of an abortative quality to that of a provoker of menstruation.[68] New herbs are added.[69] In one case, even where the same herb is in *Ex herbis*, the Old English version has an entirely different text.[70] Plants habitats are modified.[71] In a few cases the author of the Old English version probably had in mind plants different from those in *Ex herbis*, probably because he was treating a few herbs prevalent in the British Isles but not well-known in southern Europe, where most of *Ex herbis*' plants came from.

The influence *Ex herbis* diminished in the high and late Middle Ages. The enlarged Alphabetical Dioscorides Latin Recension, providing some competition, was produced by the late eleventh or early twelfth century.[72] More competitive yet were the *Circa instans* of Matthews Platearius and the *Herbal* of Macer. *Ex herbis* was still used, but mainly as a resource authority for new herbals. Copyists occasionally lifted entire chapters together with the illustrations for their herbals when *Ex herbis* had information that fit some particular need. Simon of Genoa (flourished in the late thirteenth century), referred to *Ex herbis* as "librum antiquum istoriatum."[73] By the late Middle Ages *Ex herbis*

disarrangement. The most recent study of Cotton Vitellius C III is admirably done by Linda E. Voigts, "A New Look at a Manuscript Containing the Old English Translation of the *Herbarium Apulei*," *Manuscripta, 20* (1976), 40-60, where Voigts accepts Ker's eleventh-century dating and adds new evidence; see also Voigts' new study, "One Anglo-Saxon View of the Classical Gods," *Stud. Icon., 3* (1977), 3-16. I am indebted to Dr. Voigts for her assistance in helping me with the Old English Texts.

67. No. 161, I, 288-290, Cockayne ed.

68. No. 150, I, 276-6, Cockayne ed.

69. E.g., nos. 140, 146, and 151.

70. Cf. no. 35 in *Ex herbis* with Old English no. 137, I, 254-257, Cockayne ed.

71. Cf. no. 11 in *Ex herbis* with Old English no. 139, I, 257-258, Cockayne ed.

72. John M. Riddle, "The Latin Alphabetical Dioscorides," *Proc. 13th Int. Cong. Hist. Sci.* (Moscow, 1974), secs. 3, 4, pp. 204-209.

73. Montpellier, École de médicine Ms. H 127, s. XV, fols. 101v-111: "Incipit liber Apuliensis Platonis De herbis femininis quem Simon Januensis vocat Librum Antiquum Istoriatum." The text is Pseudo-Dioscorides' *Ex herbis*. The rubric and colophon in the Montpellier Ms. are the same.

femininis was virtually forgotten, but its influence surpassed its memory. It is a good example of early medieval medical literature in which an unknown author, appropriating the name of a classical authority, sought to record in pictures and words the herbs of the field and their uses for man. The effort was important, influential, and meritorious. Flaws there are, but fewer than previously noted. There is no reason to relegate this work to the margins of history as an example of poor botany and poor medicine in a poor age that cared about neither field. The author of *Ex herbis femininis* wrote a praiseworthy herbal.

Acknowledgments

I gratefully acknowledge the many helpful suggestions of Dr. Linda Voigts, Dr. Karen Reeds, and Professor John Scarborough, who read drafts of this paper. Their knowledge and assistance were invaluable. Also, I am grateful to Dr. Gordon Newby, whose extensive reply to a question regarding African languages is quoted in this article. An earlier version of this article was read before the American Society for the History of Science, Philadelphia, December 1976.

APPENDIX. TABLE OF HERBS

Key

André	Jacques André, *Lexique des termes de botaniques en latin* (Paris: C. Klincksieck, 1956)
Bierbaumer	Peter Bierbaumer, *Der botanische Wortschatz des Altenglischen*, Part 2, *Lacnunga, Herbarium Apuleii, Peri Didaxeon* (Frankfurt: Peter Lang, 1976)
Carnoy	Albert Carnoy, *Dictionnaire, ètymologique des noms grecs de plantes* (Louvain: Publications Unviersitaries, 1959)
Cockayne	Thomas Oswald Cockayne, *Leechdoms, Wortcunning, and Starcraft of Early England*, 3 vols. (London 1864-1866; repr. London: Holland Press, 1961)
Daubeny	Charles Daubeny, *Lectures on Roman Husbandry* (Oxford, 1857)
D.	Dioscorides, *De materia medica libri quinque*, ed. Max Wellmann, 3 vols. (Berlin: Weidmann, 1958)
Font y Quer	P. Font y Quer, *Plantas medicinales el Dioscórides renovado* (Barcelona: Editorial Labor, 1962)
Grieves	Maud Grieves, *A Modern Herbal* (New York: Dover, 1971)
Gunther	Robert T. Gunther, *The Greek Herbal of Dioscorides* (New York: Hafner, 1959)
Hort	Arthur Hort, *Theophrastus: Enquiry into Plants*, 2 vols. (Cambridge Mass.: Harvard University Press, 1949)
Jones	W. H. S. Jones, *Pliny: Natural History*, in 10 vols., vols. 6-7 (Cambridge, Mass.: Harvard University Press, 1951, 1956)
Kraemer	Henry Kraemer, *A Textbook of Botany and Pharmacognosy*, 4th ed. (Phildadelphia: Lippincott, 1910)
Leek	Sybil Leek, *Herbs, Medicine, and Mysticism* (Chicago: H. Regnery, 1975)
Polunin	Oleg Polunin, *Flowers of Europe* (London: Oxford University Press, 1969)
Pseudo-Apuleius	*Herbarius*, in *Antonii Musae . . . Pseudo-Apulei . . .*, ed. Ernest Howald and H. E. Sigerist, Corpus Medicorum Latinorum, vol. IV (Leipzig: B. G. Teubner, 1927)
Pushmann	Theodor Puschmann, *Alexander von Trallus*, 2 vols. (Vienna: W. Braumüller, 1879)
Schneider	Wolfgang Schneider, *Lexikon zur Arzneimittelgeschichte*, 7 vols., vol. V in 3 parts., *Pflanzliche Drogen* (Frankfurt: Govi-Verlag, 1974)

Ex herbis	Dioscorides	Probable scientific name	Common name	Old English (nos. to Cockayne ed.)
1. Acantha leuca; hecynum	3.12: 'ἀκανθα λευκή (citations to Wellmann ed.)	*Crataegus oxyacantha* L., *Crataegus monogyna* Jacq.	Hawthorn, whitethorn, etc. (Grieves, p. 385; Polunin, no. 461)	Beowyrt, or becwort no. 154 (Bierbaumer, 2, p. 11)
	Bierbaumer believes the Old English text comes from Dios., 3.19, which concerns *Acanthus mollis* L., or bear's breech. The Old English text, however, has some material, e.g., a use for lung disease, not found in either *Ex herbis* or Dioscorides.			
2. Buglossos	4.127: βούλγωσσον	*Borago officinalis* L. (Font y Quer, no. 389); *Lingua bubula* (André, p. 188)	Burrage (Grieves, pp. 119-20)	
3. Acantus	3.17: 'ἀκανθος	*Acanthus mollis* L. (Font y Quer, no. 99a, or, possibly, *Acanthus spinosus* L. (Schneider, V, 1, 34-35)	Bear's breech (*A. Mollis*) or spiny bear's breech (*A. Mollis*) (Polunin, nos. 1266-1267)	
4. Helylosfacos; Salvia	3.33: ἐλελίσφακον	*Salvia officinalis* L. (Font y Quer, no. 474); *Salvia triloba* (Poulnin, no. 1143)	Common sage (Grieves, pp. 700-705)	
5. Cyminum	3.60: κύμινον ἄγριον	*Cuminum cyminum* L. (Font y Quer, no. 342; Schneider, V, 1, 398-399) *Cuminum agreste* (André, p. 180)	Cumin (Grieves, pp. 242-243)	Cymen, no. 155 (Bierbaumer, pp. 3, 31)
6. Camelleon	3.8: χαμαιλέωη λευκός	*Atractylis gummifera* (Font y Quer, no. 599; cf. Carnoy, p. 75); *Chamaeleon albus* (André, p. 84)	Pine-thistle (Polunin, no. 1471)	
	Hort (II, 483) identifies camelleon as *Atractylis gummifera*. Cockayne (I, 283) says that in the Old English version what is probably described is wolfs' teazle – *Carlina acaulis* or *Acarna gummifera*. Jones (Pliny, 22.21.45) agrees with Hort's identification in translating Pliny. The description in *Ex herbis* might also fit European ground pine or yellow bugle (*Ajuga chamaepitys*, Schreb.) – see Grieves, p. 141. *Ex herbis* modifies Dioscorides' plant description.			
7. Erpullos	3.38: 'ἑρπυλλος	*Thymus serpyllum* L. (Font y Quer, no. 493; Schneider, V, 3, 340; Carnoy, pp. 143-144)	Wild thyme (Grieves, pp. 813-815; Polunin, no. 1164)	

Ex herbis	Dioscorides	Probable scientific name	Common name	Old English (nos. to Cockayne ed.)
8. Camedrios	3.98: χαμαίρωψ	*Teucrium chamaedrys* L. (Font y Quer, no. 445; André, pp. 85, 322); *Buisson epineux* (Carnoy, p. 76)	Wall germander (Grieves, p. 760)	
	It is possibly *Veronica chamaedrys* L. or speedwell, germander; Polunin, no. 1228.			
9. Polygonos	4.4: πολύγονον 'άρρεν	*Polygonum aviculare* L. (Font y Quer, no. 71; Carnoy, p. 221; André, p. 257)	Knotgrass (Grieves, pp. 457-458; Polunin, no. 80)	
	Dioscorides has two chapters: 4.4, πολύγονον 'άρρεη, which he says is male, and 4.5, πυλύλονον θῆλυ, which is female. *Ex herbis* uses the description of the male plant, although D. says that both plants have about the same medicinal virtues. D. says the plant has many seeds, and therefore it is called male. *Ex herbis* omits the statements of D. that the plant is male but does note that it has many seeds. Pliny (27.41.113-117: *sanguinaria*) says there are four kinds, two being male and female.			
10. Samsucon	3.39: σάμψουχον	*Origanum majorana* L. (Font y Quer, no. 491; Carnoy, p. 234; Schneider, V, 2, 283-284)	Sweet marjoram (Grieves, pp. 519-521)	
	There is also marjoram (*Origanum vulgare* L.), which may be the plant described, but both species have the same medicinal action.			
11. Cestros, sive Stergestros vel Sempervivum (in various mss)	4.88: ἀειζῳον μέλα	*Sempervivum tectorum* L. (Font y Quer, no. 183; Carnoy, p. 11; André, p. 289)	Houseleek (Grieves, pp. 422-423; Polunin, no. 383)	Aizos (?), no. 139
	D. has "larger Aeizôon" (4.88) and "smaller Aeizôon" (4.89), and Sprengler believes the larger one is *Sempervivum arboreum* and the smaller *S. tectorum*. Houseleek is suggested in the *Ex herbis* description. See also no. 33 below. *Cestros*, presumably from κέστρον (D., 4.1), means betony (Pliny, 26.46.84), but the author of *Ex herbis* took the text and description from D.'s entry ἀειζωον μέγα, which refers to houseleek. The Old English text refers to *Aizus minor* (see *Ex herbis*, no. 33) and seems to distinguish it from aizos without further description.			
12. Aristolochia	3.4: ἀριστολοχέια			
	D. says there are three kinds: female (round leaves, sweet-smelling, etc.), male (round leaves but longer ones, purple flowers, etc.), and *Aristolochis clematitis*. *Ex herbis* says there are two kinds, male and female, thereby omitting *A. clematitis*. Pliny (25.54.97-98) names four kinds: male, female, clematis, and pistolochia. Font y Quer (pp. 193-197) says that there are around 400 species of plants in the genus of *Aristolochia*. For D., he distinguishes: 101: *Aristolochia rotunda* L; 102: *A. longa* L; 104: *A. pistolochia* L; 105: *A. baetica*. What *Ex herbis* describes is uncertain because the description is even sketchier than D.'s text, but it would appear to be Font y Quer's no. 101 as the female and no. 102 as the male. The drawing in Vienna Ms. 93 appears closest to *A. longa*, or the male variety; cf. Carnoy, p. 37, and André, pp. 40-41.			
13. Sticas	3.26: στοιχάς	*Lavandula stoechas* L. (Font y Quer, no. 454; André, p. 304; Carnoy, p. 354)	French lavender (Grieves, pp. 468-473; Polunin, no. 1110)	Stecas, no. 149
14. Adiantos; polytichos; callistrichos	4.134: ἀδίαντον	*Adiantum capillus-Veneris* L. (Font y Quer, no. 34; André, p. 18; Carnoy, p.9)	Maidenhair, or maiden spleenwort (Kraemer, pp. 61ff; Leek, p. 219)	
15. Mandragora	4.75: μανδραγόρας	(?) *Mandragora officinarum* L.	Mandrake	
	D. says there is a female and a male variety but also a third kind called *morion*. The text appears to give the medicinal virtues of the male variety. *Ex herbis* gives the male and female varieties and says both have the same medicinal action. Font y Quer (pp. 590-595) and André (p. 199) say that the male and female varieties described in D. may be *M. officinarum* and *M. vernalis* or *M. autumnalis*. Grieves (pp. 510-512) reports that the mandrake contains two mydriatic alkaloids and is therefore akin to belladonna and identical with			

Ex herbis	Dioscorides	Probable scientific name	Common name	Old English (nos. to Cockayne ed.)
	atropine, or hyoscyamine. Polunin (no. 1185) reports *M. officinarum* as having a European habit. There may be some confusion between *M. officinarum* and *M. autumnalis*.			
16. Thlaspis; mia	2.156: θλάσπι	*Thapsia garganica* L. (Font y Quer, no. 362) *Capsella bursa pastoria*	Shepherd's purse (Grieves, pp. 738-739; Polunin, no. 340)	Lombes cyrse, no. 150 (Bierbaumer, p. 75)
	André (p. 315) and Carnoy (p. 264) identify D.'s *thlaspis* with *Capsella bursa pastoris*. *Ex herbis* gives *mia*, as a synonym, and André (p. 208) believes *mia* in *The Old Latin Dioscorides* (2.156) is probably μυίτις. Bierbaumer (p. 75) identifies the Old English "Lombes cyrse" as (1) *Cardamine hirsuta* L.? (2) *Capsella bursa-pastoris* L., or shepherd purse, or (3) *Thlaspi arvense* L., or field pennycress.			
17. Sisimbrium	2.128: σισύμβριον	*Sisymbrium sophia* L. (Font y Quer, no. 166) *Nasturtium offinale* R. Br. (Carnoy, p. 296) *Mentha sativa* (André, p. 296; Carnoy, p. 246)	Flixweed (Polunin, no. 288) Watercress (Polunin, no. 307) Wild mint	
	The picture in Vienna Ms. 93 suggests that what *Ex herbis* is describing is *Mentha sativa*, or wild mint. Flixweed is in the mustard family, but according to Grieves (p. 570) has almost the same medicinal action as wild mint. Carnoy (p. 246) believes that *sisimbrium* applies to a variety of aquatic plants, specifically *Mentha aquatica* and/or *Nasturtium officinale*.			
18. Celedonie	2.180: χελιδόνιον μέγα	*Chelidonium majus* L. (Font y Quer, no. 135, cf. André, p. 86, who has a broader list of possibilities, but the pictures in *Ex herbis* seem to go with greater celandine)	Greater celandine, or common celandine (Grieves, pp. 178-179; Polunin, no. 274)	
19. Camemelos	3.137: ἀνθεμίς	*Anthemis arvensis* (?) (Font y Quer, no. 575, cf. André, p. 84; Carnoy, p. 75)	Mayweed (Grieves, p. 523); corn chamomile (Polunin, no. 1411)	
	D. says that there are three kinds. The description of the first approximates *A. arvensis*, and the other two are probably *A. tinctoria* and *A. cotula*, all varieties of mayweed. The *Ex herbis* description is taken from D.'s first type. André and Carnoy say the D. entry could refer to a variety of plants.			
20. Sideritis	4.33: σιδηρῖτις	*Sideritis hirsuta* L. (?) (Font y Quer, nos. 458, 460)	Heracules panaces (?) Polunin, no. 1115; cf. no. 1114)	
	Daubeny (p. 313) believes D.'s entry to be *Sideritis romana*; Gunther (p. 428) has *Sideritis remota*. The illustration in Vienna Ms. 93 is closest to *Sideritis hirsuta*. André (p. 292) identifies D.'s entry with millefolium and Carnoy (p. 243) says the entry particularly applies to *Sideritis romana*.			
21. Flommos	4.103: θλόμος	*Verbascum thapsus* L., but possibly *V. sinuatum* (Font y Quer, no. 416; cf. André, pp. 326-327)	Great mullein / golden / rod / foxglove / Aaron's rod, etc. (Grieves, p. 562; Polunin, no. 1193)	
	There are about 210 species, and certainty is therefore difficult.			
22. Lynozostis; lingostes	4.189: λινόζωστις	*Mercurialis annua* L. (Font y Quer, no. 95) *Mercurialis perennis* L. (André, p. 188)	Annual mercury (Grieves p. 530; Polunin, no. 667) Dogs mercury (Polunin, no. 666)	
	Both D. and *Ex herbis* speak of a male and a female variety.			
23. Antirenon	4.130: ἀντίρρινον	*Antirrhinum majus* L. (Font y Quer, no. 419); *Antirrhinum orontium* L. (André, p. 33)	Snapdragon (Grieves, p. 746; Polunin, no. 1197); Weasel's snout (Polunin, no. 1199)	

Ex herbis	Dioscorides	Probable scientific name	Common name	Old English (nos. to Cockayne ed.)
24. Britannica	4.2: *βρεττανική*	Veronica chamaedrys (?)	Germander speedwell (?) (Polunin, no. 1228)	
	The *Notha*, a later addendum to some Greek D.'s Mss, say that the British plant is the same as vettonica (*ρυμαῖοι βεττονῖκαμ*), which Paul of Aegina (7.3) has as Paul's betony and which is listed by Grieves (p. 759) as *Veronica chamaedrys*, or Germander speedwell. Font y Quer has no identification. *Ex herbis* has: "Brittanica sive damasonion." Pliny (25.77.124) says *damasonion* is the same as *lyron*, which is today called purple loosetrife (*Lythrum salicaria* – Grieves, p. 496). The description given by D. seems closest to *Veronica chamaedrys*. André (p. 58) suggests it might be a kind of *rumex*, whereas Carnoy (pp. 49– 50) associates it with betony. The picture in *Ex herbis* corresponds to Germander's speedwell.			
25. Psillios	4.69: *ψύλλιον*	*Plantago psyllium* L. (Font y Quer, no. 507; André, p. 263)	Psyllium plantain (Grieves, pp. 643-644)	No. 169
26. Melena	4.183: *ἄμπελος μέλαινα*	*Tamus communis* L. (Font y Quer, no. 653); *Tamus viridis* (Carnoy, p. 23)	Poison black bryony / blackeye root (Grieves, pp. 130-131; Polunin, no. 1674)	
27. Tribulenta	4.15: *τρίβολος*	*Tribulus terrestris* L. (Font y Quer, no. 300)	Land caltrop / Small caltrops / Maltese cross (Polunin, no. 655)	Gorst, no. 142 (Bierbaumer, p. 54)
	D. and Pliny (22.13.17) say that there are two kinds – one that grows on land and another in water, probably water caltrop (*Traba natans*). *Ex herbis* says that there are two kinds: "one which is found in gardens, the other is wild." *Ex herbis'* description seems to be only of land caltrop; why the author says that there are to kinds is unclear. The Old English version says *tribulus* is gorst.			
28. Coniza	3.121: *κόνυζα*	*Inula conyza DC* (Font y Quer, no. 559); *Inula vis cosa* for male and *graveolen* for female variety (André, p. 100)	Ploughman's spikenard / great fleabane / and little fleabane (Grieves, pp. 760-761; Polunin, no. 1387)	Conize,
	D. describes three kinds, two of which Gunther (p. 366) lists as *Inula viscosa* and *I. saxatilits*. *Ex herbis* describes two kinds, which are probably great fleabane and little fleabane.			
29. Strygnos	4.70: *στρύχνον κηπαῖον*	*Solanum nigrum* L. (Font y Quer, no. 407; André, p. 305; Carnoy, p. 255)	Black nightshade (Grieves, pp. 582-583; Polunin, no. 1182)	Foxglove (?), no. 144 (Bierbaumer, p. 49)
	A synonym given by *Ex herbis* is *manicos*. D. has an entry (4.73) that the Old English version took to mean foxglove. The entry of *στρύχνον μανικόν* in *Ex herbis* is clearly from D., 4.70, while the Old English seems to be giving the medicinal uses for foxglove, *Digitalis purpurea*.			
30. Bustalmon	3.139: *βούφθαλμον*	*Anthemis tinctoria* L. (Schneider, V, 1, 102) *Anthemis valentina* (?) = *Chrysanthemum coronarium* L. (André, p. 61)	Yellow chamomile (Polunin, no. 1409) Mayweed (?)	Buoptalmon, no. 141
	Pliny (25.102.160) says *buphthalmos* is a kind of *aizoōm*, or houseleek. *Buphthalmos* means "bull's eye." There is a plant today called bull's eye, but it is marsh marigold (*Clatha paulstris*). The description in *Ex herbis* does not fit (see Grieves, p. 519). Probably, *buphtholomos* is a variety of *anthemis*, or mayweed, but Dioscorides, *Ex herbis*, and the Old English Text are unclear as to the plant described.			

Pseudo-Dioscorides' *Ex herbis femininis*

Ex herbis	Dioscorides	Probable scientific name	Common name	Old English (nos. to Cockayne ed.)
31. Isfieritis				Spreritis, no. 138
	Identification is uncertain, this being the only plant in *Ex herbis* for which a corresponding chapter in D. cannot be found. The Old English version's entry (Cockayne, I, 256-257) identifies it as D.'s ἀναγαλλίς (2.178). The Old English word is *spreritis*, of which Cockayne said: "Σ πυρίτις is a medieval synonym of the ἀνάγαλλις ἡ φοινικῆ, the scarlet pimpernel," on the basis of marginal notes to D., 2.209. The text is *Ex herbis* does not relate to the D. entry. There are two drawings of *anagallis* found in the Greek Dioscorides, Vienna Ms. Gr. 1, fols. 39-40, but despite some similarities there is a different leaf arrangement on the stems, when one compares the drawings in *Ex herbis* to those in Vienna, Ms. 93, and Florence, Laur. Ms. Plut. 41.73. Further, I could find no such synonym as that referred to by Cockayne in Vienna, Ms. Gr. 1, fol. 40. André (p. 299; cf. p. 66) lists *spieritis* in *Ex herbis* (no. 31) as possibly "caltha" (*Calendula arvensis L.*), or marigold, but the illustrations in the *Ex herbis*' manuscripts do not resemble marigold. André cross-lists *spieritis* with caltha and cites the entry on λευκόϊον in George Goetz, *Corpus Glossariorum Latinorum*, 7 vols. (Leipzig, 1888-1923), index, VI, 170, but Goetz does not identify *spieritis* with caltha (*caltha*, however = λευκόϊον). Bierbaumer does not identify the Old English herb *spreritis*. The picture in *Ex herbis* has two different structures of flowers, which makes identification even more difficult.			
32. Hyppypres	4.47: ἑτέρα ἵππουρις	*Equisetum telmateia* (Font y Quer, no. 23; André, p. 163; Carnoy, p. 146)	Horsetails	
	Gunther (p. 438) believes that D.'s horsetails may be either *Equisetum sylvaticum* or *E. fluviatile*. Grieves (pp. 419-421) reports four species of horsetails common in Europe.			
33. Aizos	4.89: ἀειζωον τὸ μικρόν and	*Sempervivum tectorum* L. (Font y Quer, no. 183; cf. André, p. 289; Carnoy, p. 11)	Houseleek (Polunin, no. 383)	Aizos minor, no. 139
	4.88: ἀεζωον τὸ μέγα			
	See no. 11 above. Gunther (p. 487), lists *Sempervivum ochroleucum*; Cockayne (I, 257) gives *S. sediforme*, for Old English descriptions. *Ex herbis* modified D.'s description and combines two chapters in D. (89 and 88), "major" and "minor" houseleeks, but D. says the medicinal virtues of both are the same.			
34. Tytimallos	4.164: τιθυμάλλου	*Daphne gnidium* L.	Mediterranean mezereon (Polunin, no. 758)	
	εἴδη ἑπτά	or *Euphorbia characias* (Font y Quer, pp. 388-389; cf. André, pp. 317-318; Carnoy, p. 268)	Large Mediterranean spurge (Polunin, no. 678)	
35. Eliotropios	[4.190: ἡλιοτρόπιον τὸ μέγα]	*Taraxcum offinale*	Weber dandelion	[Sigilhweorfa. no. 137 – text not related to *Ex herbis*] (Bierbaumer, p. 104)
	[4.191: ἡλιοτρόπιον τὸ μικόν]	*Cichorium intybus* L.	Chicory (Polunin, no. 1512)	
	Ex herbis has two entries, no. 35 and 50, but neither correspond to D.'s chapters. Moreover, the pictures of the two plants in *Ex herbis* are different. And the drawings of plant 35 in *Ex herbis* show an impossible arrangement of leaves. The drawings show large, broad, serrated leaves coming from a fleshy rhizome, while from the nodes come stems from which branch narrow, long, smooth-edged leaves in alternate arrangement and small flowers on stems, some of which branch from leaf nodes while others come from stems without foliation. Font y Quer (nos. 335 and 921) identifies the two entries in D. as *Heliotropium europaeum* (heliotrope, no. 1045 in Polunin) and *Chrozophora tinctoria* (turnsole, no. 665 in Polunin), but these appear impossible in *Ex herbis*. The Old English entry *sigilhweorfa*, with synonym *heliotropus*, does not relate textually to either *Ex herbis* or D. Bierbaumer (p. 104) lists for *sigilhweorfa* five possibilities: *Calendula officinalis* L.; *Cichorium intybus* L.; *Taraxacum officinale* L.; *Hypochoeris glaba* L.; or, least likely, *Heliotropium*			

Ex herbis	Dioscorides	Probable scientific name	Common name	Old English (nos. to Cockayne ed.)
	europaeum L. Of these, the picture in *Ex herbis* is closest to *Taraxacum officinale*, or dandelion, with the exception of the troublesome smooth long leaves on some stems. The medicinal usages listed also make this identification more likely. The *Ex herbis* text has: "ideo alii helioscopion vocant, Romani intybut sylvaticum." *Cichorium intybus* is chicory. Dandelion is sometimes substituted for chicory in coffee. It would appear that *Ex herbis* refers here to dandelion and possibly also to chicory.			
36. Scolymbos	3.14: *σκόλυμος*	*Scolymus hispanicus* L. (Font y Quer, no. 615; André, pp. 285-286; Carnoy, p. 238); or, *S. maculatus* (André, pp. 285-286)	Golden thistle / Spanish oyster plant (Polunin, no. 1510)	Scolimbos, no. 157
37. Achilleia	4.36: Ἀχίλλειος	*Cynara cardunculus* L.	Cardoon (Polunin, no. 1491)	Achillea, no. 175
	The *Notha* (D. 4, 36 RV) gives a synonym as *μιλλεφόλλιουμ*, or *millefolium*, and the drawing in Vienna, Ms. Gr. 1, suggests *Achillea millefolium* L. (Font y Quer, no. 577), which is also D.'s 4.114: *μύριοφυλλον* (see Carnoy, p. 5). The drawing in *Ex herbis*, esp. in Vienna Ms. 93, suggests artichoke. *Ex herbis* may be describing *Scolymus cardunculus*, or Cardoon artichoke. The drawing in *Ex herbis* is close to Pseudo-Apuleius' no. 89, *Millefolium*. Grieves (p. 863) and Polunin (no. 1417) identify *Achillea millefolium*, or yarrow or milfoil. The Old English version has *Achillea*, which Cockayne suggests may be *Archillea magna*, *A. tanacetifolia*, *A. abtotanifolie*, or *A. tomentosa*. André (p. 15) identifies *Ex herbis' Achilleia* with *millefolium*. Polunin (no. 1491) distinguishes *Cynara cardunculus*, or cardoon, from *C. scolymus*, or globe artichoke, by the fact that globe artichoke is unknown in the wild.			
38. Stafis agria	4.152: *σταφὶς ἀγρία*	*Delphinium staphisagria* L. (Font y Quer, no. 117; André, p. 303; Carnoy, p. 252)	Stavesacre / lousewort (Leek, p. 220; Polunin, no. 212)	Stavis agria, no. 171
39. Cameleia; turbiscon	4.171: *χαμελαία*	*Daphne oleoides* (Gunther, p. 572) *Daphne gnidium* L. (André, p. 315)	Ground olive (Polunin, no. 757) Mediterranean mezereon (Polunin, no. 758)	
	Although the picture in *Ex herbis* bears little resemblance to the *Daphne* family, the text says the plant has a fruit like an olive. This probably is the ground olive.			
40. Ficios; hecios; alcidiabios	4.27: *ἔχιον*	*Echium vulgare* L. (Font y Quer, no. 398; cf. André, p. 123; Carnoy, p. 115)	Viper's bugloss (Polunin, no. 1082)	Acius, no. 161
	Cockayne (I, 288-291) gives the Old English version plant as *Echium rubrum*.			
41. Splenios	3.134: *ἄσπληνος*	*Ceterach officinarum* Candolle (Font y Quer, no. 32; André, p. 45; Carnoy, p. 41) *Asplenium ceterach* L. (Grieves, pp. 302-303)	Spleewort, common	
	Ceterach is not in Polunin, but is listed in H. Gilbert Carter, *Glossary of The British Flora* (Cambridge, 1950), p. 18.			
42. Titmallos	4.164: *τιθύμαλλον*	See no. 34.		
43. Glisirisa	3.5: *γλυκύρριζα*	*Glycyrrhiza glabra* L. (Font y Quer, no. 251; Carnoy, p. 132)	Licorice (Grieves, pp. 487-492; Polunin, no. 536)	Glycyridam, no. 145
44. Bulbus rufus	2.170: *βολβὸς ἐδώδιμος*	*Hyacinthus comosum*, Sibthrop or *Muscari comosum* L. (Gunther, p. 211; Cockayne I, 321; André, p. 60)	Red bulbs or Tassel hyacinth (Polunin, no. 1645)	Bulbus, no. 184
45. Dracontea	2.166: *δρακόντιον*	*Arisarum vulgare* L. (Font y Quer, no. 677), or	Friar's cowl (Polunin, no. 1821)	

IX

Pseudo-Dioscorides' *Ex herbis femininis*

Ex herbis	Dioscorides	Probable scientific name	Common name	Old English (nos. to Cockayne ed.)
		Arum dracunculus L. (Font y Quer, no. 677; André, p. 120)	Arum arrowroot	
46. Moecon	4.64: μήκων	*Papaver somniferum* L. *Papaver rhoeas* L. (Font y Quer, nos. 132, 133: Carnoy, p. 172; cf. André, p. 202)	White poppy Red poppy or corn poppy (Grieves, p. 651; Polunin, nos. 264, 265)	
47. Colocinthios agria	4.176: κολόκυνθα ἀγρία	*Citrullus colocynthis* Schrader, or *Cucurbitam silvestrem*, or *C. caprariam*, or *C. agrestis* (Font y Quer, no. 547; André, p. 97)	Bitter apple (Grieves, pp. 45-50; Polunin, no. 812) Colocynth Pulp Bitter cucumber (Grieves, pp. 49-50)	
48. Ypericon; corion	3.154: ὑπερικόν	*Hypericum perforatum* L.; *H. coris, H. crispum*; or *H. barbatum* (Font y Quer, pp. 292-294; Cockayne, I, p. 277; Gunther, p. 394) *H. Crispum* André, p. 166)	Common St. John's wort (Grieves, p. 707; Polunin, no. 768)	Hypericon, no. 152 (Bierbaumer, p. 143)
49. Lapatium	2.114: λαπάθον	*Rumex patienta* (Gunther, p. 151)	Sorrel	
	Font y Quer (no. 601) identifies D.'s entry as *Arctium lappa*, but the description fits sorrel more closely. *Ex herbis* and D. said there are four kinds: possibly, *Rumex patienta, Oxyria reniformis* (mountian sorrel), *Rumex acetosa* (common sorrel) and *Oxalis acetosella* (wood sorrel). See André, pp. 178-179; Carnoy, p. 157. It is difficult to judge the species, if any, that *Ex herbis* intended. The drawing is closest to *Rumex sanquineus*, which is widespread in Europe. See Polunin, no. 98.			
50. Heliotropium	See no. 35, above.			
51. Arnoglossa	2.126: ἀρνόγλωσσον	*Plantago major* L. or *P. lagopus* (Font y Quer, no. 511; cf. André, p. 41, who identifies it only as plantain). *Alisma plantago-aquatica* L.	Common plantain, or snakeweed; or water plantain (Grieves, pp. 640-642)	
	D. says that there are two kinds, one larger and the other smaller. Gunther (p. 165) identifies the smaller as *Plantago lagopus*, while Font y Quer identifies the larger as *P. major*. *Ex herbis* discusses only one kind, and says it grows in wet places, a comment not recorded in D. This is more descriptive of water plantain (*Alisma plantago*); see Grieves, p. 645, and Polunin, nos. 1294, 1291, and 1560.			
52. Cameleuca	3.8: χαμαιλέων λευκός	*Dipsacus fullonum* L., *D. laciniatus* L., *D. silvestris*, *Atractylis gummifera* (Font y Quer, pp. 836-837; Jones, VI, 323; Gunther, p. 243; André, p. 84, gives *A. gummifera*)	Common teasle or (Polunin, nos. 1318-1319), or Pine thistle (?)	Wolfes camb, no. 156 (Bierbaumer, p. 135)
	Ex herbis' cameleuca may not be the same plant as D. was describing. The picture in Vienna, Ms. 93, does not appear to be *Atractylis gummifera*, and it resembles teasle, but *Ex herbis* gives no plant description. The Old English version gives a description and a picture that do not correspond to D.'s. Cockayne (I, 283) says the Old English version is probably describing wolf's teasle or common teasle. André identifies *Ex herbis*' entry as chamaccissos = *glechoma hederacea*; see Carnoy, p. 74.			
53. Scylla	2.171: σκίλλα	*Scilla maritima* L. (André, p. 284)	Sea squill (Grieves, pp. 766-769; Polunin, no. 1630)	

Ex herbis	Dioscorides	Probable scientific name	Common name	Old English (nos. to Cockayne ed.)
		Urginea maritima Baker; (Font y Quer, no. 639)		
54. Erigion	3.21: ἠρύγγη	*Eryngium campestre* L. or *E. maritimum* L. (Font y Quer, nos. 334-335) André, p. 129; Carnoy, p. 123)	Sea holly (Grieves, pp. 407-409)	Eryngius, no. 173 (Bierbaumer, p. 142)
55. Iera	4.60: ἱερὰ βοτάνη	*Verbena officinalis* L. (Font y Quer, no. 438; cf. André, p. 162)	Vervain (Grieves, pp. 431-433; Polunin, no. 1084)	
	4.60RV: περιστέρεων ὕπτιος			
56. Strutios	2.163: στρούθιον	*Saponaria officinalis* L. (Font y Quer, no. 90; cf. André, p. 305; Carnoy, p. 254)	Soapwort (Grieves, p. 748; Polunin, no. 181)	
57. Delfion	[3.73: δελφίνιον; *Ex herbis* text unrelated]	*Delphinium consolida*	Field larkspur (Grieves, p. 464)	Delfinion, no. 160 (Bierbaumer, p. 142)
	Gunther (p. 316) says D.'s entry is *Delphinium peregrinum* L. and *D. consolida*, but the picture in *Ex herbis* indicates *D. consolida*. The drawing in Vienna, Ms. Gr. 1, does not resemble the drawings in various *Ex herbis* mss. André identifies *Ex herbis*' entry as *Bucinus, B. minor* (p. 117) and Cockayne (p. 289) gives *Delphinium consolida*.			
58. Centimorbia	[4.3: λυσιμάχειο; *Ex herbis* unrelated]	*Lysimachia vulgaris* L.	Yellow loosestrife (Polunin, no. 963)	Centimorbia (Bierbaumer, p. 141), no. 162
		L. nummerleria	Moneywort, or creeping Jenny (Polunin, no. 96)	
	Ex herbis' text and picture (cf. Vienna, Ms. Gr. 1) and various *Ex herbis* mss. do not resemble D.'s. Font y Quer (no. 368) and Gunther (p. 400) say D.'s entry is *Lysimachia vulgaris*. The drawings are closest to *L. nummuleria* (see Cockayne, I, 291), but the description of the habitat does not fit. *Ex herbis* says *Centimorbia* is "found in cultivated places and rocky places, that is, in mountains and fields." According to Grieves (pp. 549-550, 497-498) *L. nummuleria*, or moneywort, grows in damp places and *L. vulgaris*, or yellow loosestrife, beside streams. André (p. 80) identifies *Ex herbis*' entry as *L. nummuleria*. The plant is in *Ex herbis*, and its name may be new and introduced by *Ex herbis*.			
59. Viola; viola aurosa	3.123: λευκόιον γνώριμον	*Cheiranthus cheiri* L. (Font y Quer, no. 150)	Wall flower (Polunin, no. 299)	Bānwyrt, nos. 165 and 166 (Bierbaumer, p. 8)
		Viola lutea (André, pp. 330-331)	Mountain pansy (Polunin, no. 785)	
	The picture in *Ex herbis* seems to be *Cheiranthus cheiri*, but the text says there are three kinds, with purple, white, and honey-colored flowers, and the best kind for medicine is the yellow, which is wall flower. Perhaps another kind is *Viola odorata*, but it is also *Ex herbis*' no. 65. Bierbaumer identifies four plants described in the Old English Text: (1) *Bellis perennis* L., (2) *Centaurium umbellatum* Gilibert, (3) *Symphytum officinale* L., (4) a *viola*.			
60. Capparra	[2.173: κάππαρις; *Ex herbis* unrelated]	*Capparis spinosa* L. (Font y Quer, no. 137, André, p. 70)	Caper (Polunin, no. 283)	Wudubend, no. 172 (Bierbaumer, p. 130)
		Lonicera periclymenum L.	Honeysuckle (Polunin, no. 1304)	
	The drawing in *Ex herbis* is close to *Capparis spinosa*, but the text is completely unrelated to D.'s. The common caper, or wood caper, is a different plant described in D.'s 4.166 as spurge. Bierbaumer identifies the Old English woodbind as *Lonicera periclymenum* L. The picture in *Ex herbis* resembles both caper and honeysuckle.			

IX

Pseudo-Dioscorides' *Ex herbis femininis*

Ex herbis	Dioscorides	Probable scientific name	Common name	Old English (nos. to Cockayne ed.)
61. Ancusa	[4.23: ἄγχουσα; *Ex herbis* text unrelated]	*Anchusa tinctoria* L., or *Anchusa officinalis* (Font y Quer, no. 392); *Alanna tinctoria* Tausch (André, p. 30)	Anchuse, or true alkanet (Grieves, pp. 18-19)	Ancusa, no. 168 (Bierbaumer, p. 140)
	The illustrations in *Ex herbis* do not appear to be alkanet. In the text, however, *Ex herbis* describes two kinds: the first fits the description of *Anchusa tinctoria* and the second that of *A. officinalis*.			
62. Cynosbatos	[1.94: κυνόσβατος; *Ex herbis* text unrelated]	*Rosa canina L.*, or *Rose sempervirem* (cf. André, p. 112)	Dog rose or Wild briar (Polunin, no. 432)	Cynosbastos, no. 170 (Bierbaumer, p. 142)
	Drawings in *Ex herbis* resemble *R. canina*. Cockayne (I, 300-301) believes that the Old English version describes and draws *R. sempervirens* L., which Kraemer (p. 289) says is found only in Asia and Africa, but Polunin (no. 430) observes is located in the Mediterranean and south western Europe.			
63. Anagallis	[2.178: ἀναγαλλίς; *Ex herbis* text unrelated]	*Anagallis arvensis* L. (André, p. 30)	Scarlet pimpernel (Polunin, no. 967)	Spreritis, no. 138 (?) (Bierbaumer, p. 146)
	Gunther (p. 223) says D. is describing two plants, *A. arvensis* and *A. coerulea*, or blue pimpernel. Cockayne (I, 257) identifies the Old English no. 138 – spreritis – as scarlet pimpernel, but the text does not relate to *Ex herbis*.			
64. Panacia	3.48: πάνακες Ἡράκλειον	*Gladitsia farnesiana* L., or *Opopanax chironium* Koch (Font y Quer, no. 356; cf. André, p. 236)	Opoponax (Grieves, pp. 600-601; Polunin, no. 491)	
65. Purpurea	4.121: ἴον	*Viola odorata* L. (Font y Quer, no. 175); *Viola purpurea* (André, p. 170)	Sweet violet (Grieves, pp. 834-839; Polunin, no. 774)	Viola purpurea, no. 166 (Bierbaumer, p. 147)
66. Camalention; zamalention	[3.8: χαμαιλεὼν λευκός, *Ex herbis* unrelated; entry already in *Ex herbis*, no. 8]			
	The drawing in Vienna, Ms. 93, does not resemble *Chamaileon leuka* or *Atractylis gumnifera*, pine thistle, which drawings in nos. 66 and 67 are close to one another; see entry in no. 8; André (p. 340) noted *Zamalention* in *Ex herbis* but could be identify it.			
67. Camalention masculis; Zamalention masc.	[3.9: χαμαιλέων μέλας; *Ex herbis* unrelated]			
	Pliny (22.21.47) says that the male variety is darker in color. It is possibly *Cardopatium corymbosum* L. Pers. (Polunin, no. 1463).			
68. Sion	2.127: σίον	*Sium latifolium* L.	Water parsnip (Polunin, no. 870)	*Sion* = *laber* no. 136 (Bierbaumer, p. 74)
	D.'s entry is probably *Sium nodiflorum* (Gunther, p. 167), but sium is now water parsnip. The Old English version gives the name as *laber*, which is *Porphyra laciniata* and *Ulva latissma* (see Cockayne, I, 255). Bierbaumer identifies it as *Sium latifolium*, or water parsnip. The description in *Ex herbis* seems closest to water parsnip although it could possibly be *Stratiotes aloides*, or water soldier (Polunin, no. 1565). Puschmann (II, 564-565) believes *Sion* in Alexander Trallianus may be *Sium latifolium*. André does not enter it, whereas Carnoy (p. 245) identifies Theophratus' *Sion* as *Sion qraecum*.			
69. Lichnis	[3.100: λυχνὶς στεφανωματική; *Ex herbis* text unrelated]	*Lychis coronaria* L. Dest. (André, p. 192)	Rose campion (Polunin, no. 158)	
70. Abrotonum	3.24: ἀβρότονον	*Artemisia arborescens* L. (Font y Quer, p. 824; Carnoy, p. 1)	Southernwood; shrubby wormwood (Grieves, pp. 754-755; Polunin, no. 1438)	Abrotanum, no. 135 (Bierbaumer p. 140)
71. Aparine; filantropos	3.90: ἀπάρινη	*Galium aparine* L. (Font y Quer, no. 531; Carnoy, p. 30, cf. André, p. 3)	Cleavers goosegrass (Polunin, no. 1023)	

X

Gargilius Martialis as a Medical Writer

THE late Roman writers on medicine suffer in comparison to their more renowned predecessors who lived in the early Empire, such as Galen and Dioscorides, or those of the Hellenistic and the Classical Ages of Greece. A number of these medical and scientific authors, who lived and wrote from the third through the sixth centuries, were learned individuals in their own right and they were quoted as authoritative during the Middle Ages. Although these Latin works are not frequently listed in the "great writings" of Latin literature, the following formed a major bridge between Classical and Medieval medicine and they became authorities for medicine in the early Latin Middle Ages: Quintus Serenus Sammonicus (d. A.D. 212), the anonymous work we call Pseudo-Pliny and the text termed *De medicina*, Pseudo-Apuleius (probably 4th cent. A.D.), Theodorus Priscianus (*fl.* A.D. 390), Marcellus Empiricus (*fl.* A.D. 410), Cassius Felix (*fl.* 450), Caelius Aurelianus (?*fl.* 450), and Anthimus (*fl.* 500).[1] Rose,

1. The best currently available editions of these late Roman Latin authors are: Serenus Sammonicus: R. Pépin, ed. and trans. *Quintus Serenus (Serenus Sammonicus): Liber Medicinalis*, Paris, Presses Universitaires de France, 1950; Pseudo-Pliny: Alf Önnerfors, ed., *Plinii Secundi Iunioris qui feruntur De medicina libri tres*, Corpus Medicorum Latinarium (CML) III, Berlin, Academiae Scientiarum, 1964; Pseudo-Apuleius: [in] Ernest Howald and Henry Sigerist, eds., *Antonii Musae De herba vettonica liber. PseudoApulei Herbarius. Anonymi De taxone liber. Sexti Placiti Liber medicinae ex animalibus etc.*, CML, IV, Leipzig, Teubner, 1927, pp. 13–225; Marcellus Empiricus: Max Niedermann, ed., 2nd ed. rev. Eduard Liechtenhan, trans. by Jutta Kollesch and Diethard Nickel,

Professor John Scarborough read and made many and always good suggestions. Also, I have called upon a number of specialists who have assisted me in developing answers to some technical questions: Charles Apperson (Entomology), Richard Axtell (Entomology), Robert E. Brackett (Food Science), Guido Majno (Pathology), Vivian Nutton (Medical History), Joanne Phillips (Classics), and David Walker (Pathology). Each of these people has patiently given his or her time while helping me understand, interpret and relate some vexing questions. They can not, of course, be held responsible for how I received their advice but the reader may be assured that each of these scholars contributed immeasureably to this attempt to understand why Gargilius was considered a medical writer for so long.

Niedermann, Howell, and Sigerist labored to produce reliable texts of several of these authors, but they did little with the analysis and evaluation of the medical content, in part because of the arduous task of providing good, modern texts. More recently, Drabkin, Kollesch, Nickel, and Liechtenhan have advanced our understanding of three of these authors through their excellent editions and translations, Caelius into English and Marcellus and Anthimus into German.[2]

Quintus Gargilius Martialis (*fl.* 220–260) was an author for whom the early Middle Ages had a high regard as judged by medieval testimonials and the number of modern survivals of his manuscript texts. For one example of a medieval testimony, there are the words of Cassiodorus (*c.* 480–*c.* 575):

> Gargilius Martialis has written most excellently on gardens and has carefully explained the raising of vegetables and the virtues of the latter, so that under the Lord's guidance by a reading of his treatise everyone may be filled and restored to health.[3]

Palladius (4th cent.), Servius (4th cent.), Isidore of Seville (d. *c.* 636), Macer or Marbode (11th cent.), the anonymous eleventh century editor of the Latin Alphabetical Dioscorides, ʾIbn-Hedijadi (11th cent.), and ʾIbn ʾAḥmad ʾibnᶜ al-Awwâm (12th cent.) used Martialis' works.[4] Two new studies with texts, both published in 1978 in Italy, have appeared with new texts of fragments of Martialis' work, one by Sebastian Condorelli[5] and another by Innocenzo Mazzini.[6] In the United

---

Marcelli De medicamentis liber, 2 vols., CML v, Berlin, Akademie-Verlag, 1968; Theodorus Priscianus: Valentin Rose, ed., *Theodori Prisciani Euporiston*, Leipzig, Teubner, 1894; also the trans. by Theodor Meyer, *Theodorus Priscianus und die römische Medizin*, Jena, Gustav Fischer, 1909; rptd. Wiesbaden, Martin Sandig, 1927, pp. 79–304; Cassius Felix: Valentin Rose, ed., *Cassii Felicis De medicina*, Leipzig, Teubner, 1879; Caelius Aurelianus: I. E. Drabkin, ed. and trans. *Caelius Aurelianus On Acute Diseases and On Chronic Diseases*, Chicago, University of Chicago Press, 1950; Anthimus: Eduard Liechtenhan, ed. and trans. *Anthimi De observatione ciborum ad Theordoricum regem Francorum epistula*, CML VIII 1, Berlin, Academiae Scientiarum, 1963.

2. Drabkin, (n.1) *Caelius*; Kollesch and Nickel, (n.1) *Marcelli*; Liechtenhan, (n.1) *Anthimus*.

3. Cassiodorus. *Institutiones*. 1. 28. 6, trans. by Leslie Webber Jones, New York, Columbia University Press, 1946. When citing ancient authors, I will follow the convention of citation by book, chapter, and paragraph or line, which are constant for all editions, rather than a particular page number, which varies from edition to edition.

4. Sebastian Condorelli, *Gargilii Martialis quae exstant* vol. 1: *Fragmenta Ad holera arboresque pomiferas pertinentia*, Biblioteca di Helikon, Testi e Studi, 11, Rome, L'erma di Bretschneider, 1978, pp. xi–xiv, 3–5; John M. Riddle, "Dioscorides," *Catalogus Translationum et Commentariorum*, Paul O. Kristeller and Edward Crantz, eds., 4 vols. to date. Washington, Catholic University Press, 1960–1981, 4, 1–143.

5. Condorelli, (n.4) *Gargilii*.

6. Innocenzo Mazzini, ed., Q. *Gargilii Martialis. De hortis*, Opuscula Philologa, 1, Bologna,

States, Ruth M. Tapper translated and annotated Gargilius' works.[7] Both Condorelli's and Mazzini's works assist our evaluation but, even so, each one was concerned primarily with textual, source, and philological problems and neither has addressed in detail the science and medical contents. Tapper's excellent doctoral dissertation is concerned with Martialis' materia medica, but her work does not evaluate why Gargilius was regarded as a medical writer, nor does it deal with his originality.

Gargilius is an author about whom some biographical information is found in various sources—an uncommon occurrence with late classical writers. Two tombstones are associated with him: one belonged to his parents which was found north of the Roman colony of Auzia in Mauretania, North Africa; another a stone dedicated by the citizens of Auzia to Q. Gargilius Martialis as their *patronus*.[8] Although doubt is expressed by some scholars,[9] Innocenzo Mazzini's exhaustive study proves that the two tombstones belonged to the author and his family.[10] The second inscription commemorates a soldier and local politician in the north African province of Mauretania, modern Morocco. A member of the equestrian class as was his father, Gargilius served as a prefect of a cohort in Britain and as a tribune of a cohort of Spanish troops in Mauretania Caesariensis. He received the usual titles for a provincial official and he was a *decurion* of two colonies, Auzia and Rusgunia, *patronus* of the province, and victor over a rebel named Faraxen. He died in a local Berber uprising and his benefactors, the

---

Patron Editore, 1978.

7. Ruth M. Tapper, "The Materia Medica of Gargilius Martialis," Ph.D. dissertation, Madison, University of Wisconsin, 1980.

8. *Corpus Inscriptionum Latinarum* (Berlin, 1863–) VIII. 9047 and *C.I.L.* VIII. 20751, reprinted and discussed by Innocenzo Mazzini, "Dati biografici ed opera di un minore: Quinto Gargilio Marziali," *Atti Mem. Arcadia*, Ser.3a, *7*: 99–121, 1977; Condorelli, (n. 4) *Gargilii*, p. 4; Tapper, (n. 7) "Materia Medica," pp. 3–5; see discussions by Hermann Stadler, "Gargilius," *Real Encylopaedie der classischen Altertumswissenschaft*, Stuttgart, 1910, 7, pt. 1, cols. 760–2, and Ludwig Schwabe, ed., *Teuffel's History of Roman Literature*, 5th ed., trans. by George C. W. Warr, 2 vols., London, Bell, 1900, rptd. New York, B. Franklin, 1967, 2, 276–78; M. Schanz, C. Hosius, G. Kruger, *Geschichte der römischen Literatur*, 4 vols., Munich, Beck, 1927–59; reissue, 1969, 3, 222–3.

9. Alfred von Domaszewski, *Die Personennamen bei den Scriptores Historiae Augustae*, Heidelberg, C. Winter, 1918, p. 54, n. 3; H. Barton, *La littérature latine inconnue*, 2 vols., Paris, 1956, 2, 261; Ludwig Edelstein, "Gargilius," *Oxford Classical Dictionary*, 2nd ed., Oxford, Clarendon Press, 1970, p. 458; and, finally, the early article by Conrad Cichorius, "Gargilius Martialis und die Maurenkriege unter Gallienus," *Leip. Stud. Clas. Philol.*, *10*: 319–27, 1887, who argued that the inscription belonged to the author.

10. Mazzini, (n. 8).

citizens of Auzia, erected at public expense the tombstone with the date of 7 April 260. The Emperor Alexander Severus (222–235 A.D.) raised the *municipium* of Auzia to a colony.[11] The *Historia Augusta* author of Alexander Severus' life spoke of Gargilius as a contemporary (*quae Gargilius eius temporis scriptor singillatim persecutus est*), who had written a description of the Emperor's diet.[12] Another *Historia Augusta* writer, the author of *Probus* (emperor in 271–2), included "Gargilius Martialis" among those more recent authors whose writings "have handed down to memory those and other details not so much with eloquence as with truthfulness."[13] These literary notices and the two inscriptions all support a reasonable conclusion that the Gargilius of these sources is the same person as the author for whom the Middle Ages had such high regard. To this evidence Mazzini has tied various circumstantial factors to support a connection between Martialis, the Roman soldier in Africa, and the Emperor Alexander Severus.[14] Finally, several autobiographical details in his works show that he was married, once wounded, and had a farm in Africa. (*vide infra*) Nothing in his biography as we know it indicates that he was a physician (*medicus*), not even a military physician. And yet, history has known him as a medical writer.

Considering his accomplished career as a soldier, Gargilius' writings were extensive—at least they were larger than what is now extant. There are many manuscripts with fragments from his works, many

11. Ibid.

12. *Historia Augusta: Severus Alexander*. XXXVII. 9. Ronald Syme, *Ammianus and the Historia Augusta*, Oxford, Clarendon Press, 1968, pp. 99–100, 200, and 203, takes an iconoclastic and critical approach to the biographers of the emperors, known as the *Historiae Augustae*, specifically raising a question whether the authors mentioned by Severus' biographer were real; however, Syme's position has not found universal acceptance. Those who have studied Gargilius accept this passage as pointing to the agricultural writer whose tombstone we have, viz. Mazzini, (n. 8); Condorelli, (n. 4) *Gargilii*, pp. 3–5. Mazzini (pp. 104–5) proposes that the Severus' biographer was referring to Gargilius' *Medicinae ex oleribus et pomis* when he spoke of an author on the Emperor's eating habits. Gargilius' work does have some dietetic items. In Mazzini's judgment, the Emperor may have been guided in his diet by Gargilius, who was, after all, from the same region of Africa as the Severi family; Alexander was born near Carthage. In contrast, Syme (*Emperors and Biography*, Oxford, Clarendon Press, 1971, p. 47) assumes that the author of *Severus* meant that Gargilius was a biographer of the emperor when Gargilius wrote of the imperial eating habits. See, David Magie, ed. and trans., *Scriptores Historiae Augustae*, 3 vols. Loeb Classical Library, London, Heinemann; Cambridge, Harvard University Press, 1921–32, 2, 251.

13. *Historia Augusta: Probus*, II. 8 in Magie, (n. 12) *Scriptores*. Mazzini, (n. 8), believes that the author of *Probus* (whom he accepted as being Flavius Vopiscus) referred to the same work by Gargilius as had the author of Alexander's life; cf. Syme, (n. 12) *Emperors*, pp. 47, 258, and 278, who rejects Vopiscus as the author's name.

14. Mazzini, (n. 8).

dating from the early Middle Ages. Originally one work was much larger than the fragments which remain: *Gardens* (*De hortis*) or *Vegetables and Fruit Trees* (*De holera arboresque pomiferas*).[15] From it Innocenzo Mazzini published the texts on the quince, peach, almond, and chestnut trees, each one of which has an extensive chapter devoted to each tree's botany and horticulture with nutritional and medicinal components. With the aid of a sixth century Bobbio manuscript, now in Naples, Sebastian Condorelli added fragments of the text on the cucumber, basil, pomegranate, quince, citron, fig, cherry, almond, pistachio, and chestnut.[16]

We know that Gargilius' *Gardens* once covered many more plants, herbs and trees because, among other evidence, Palladius[17] (*fl.* 4th cent.) cited Gargilius thirteen times with information from plants not presently extant in the manuscript texts.[18] Gargilius' only work on medicine was titled *Medicines from Vegetables and Fruits* (*Medicinae ex oleribus et pomis*). Although it is generally regarded as a separate work, it may have been a part of the large work, *Gardens*.[19] Mazzini proves on linguistic grounds that the same person wrote both works.[20] This text is to be distinguished from another treatise, known either by the title *De oleribus Martialis* or by *De virtutes herbarum*, published last by Valentin Rose in 1870. This text is not an authentic Gargilius work, but it is related to a Latin translation of the second book of the Hippocratic tract, *peri diaitēs*.[21] There is also a small veterinary tract attributed to

15. Mazzini, (n. 6) *De hortis*, pp. 86–125; for full listing of printed editions see Mazzini, (n. 6) *De hortis*, p. 11 and S. Condorelli, (n. 4) *Gargilii*, pp. xlv–xlvii.

16. Condorelli, (n. 4) *Gargilii*, pp. 9–53, also using fragments found in the works of: Palladius and 'Ibn 'al-Awwâm, with a doubtful fragment from Pseudo-Apuleius.

17. Palladius. *Opus agriculturae*, ed. J. C. Schmitt, Leipzig, B. G. Teubner, 1898.

18. Mazzini, (n. 6) *De hortis*, pp. 34–5; Condorelli, (n. 4) *Gargilii*, pp. x, xxii–xxiv; and earlier studies by Max Wellmann, "Palladius und Gargilius Martialis," *Hermes*, *43*: 3–15, 1908; J. Svennung, "De auctoribus Palladii," *Eranos*, *25*: 123–78, 1927. Portions of *Geoponica*, ed. H. Beckh, Leipzig, 1895, a Byzantine agricultural collection of various earlier writers, are also helpful in some reconstructions, *e.g.*, lines 80–6 and 132–5 on the peach, Mazzini, (n. 6) *De hortis*, pp. 96, 100.

19. Valentin Rose, ed., *Plinii Secundi quae fertur una cum Gargilii Martialis Medicina*, Leipzig, B. G. Teubner, 1875, pp. (129)–208.

20. Mazzini, (n. 8); Mazzini, (n. 6) *De hortis*, p. 10.

21. V. Rose, *Anecdota Graeca et Graecolatina*, 2 pts., Berlin, Ferd. Duemmler, 1870, pt. 2, 131–50, from text found in St. Gallen, Stiftsbibliothek Ms 762, s. IX, pp. 25–71, described by Augusto Beccaria, *I codici di medicina del periodo presalernitano (secoli IX, X e XI)*, Rome, Edizioni di Storia e Letteratura, 1956, pp. 388–90. Innocenzo Mazzini, "De observantia ciborum. Un 'antica traduzione latina del *peri diaitēs* pseudoippocratico I. II (editio princeps)," *Romanobarbarica*, *2*: 286–357, 1977. The Hippocratic treatise is also known as *Regimen*.

Gargilius called *Curae boum*.[22] The concern of this paper will be principally with the text known as *Medicines from Vegetables and Fruits*.

As it now exists the tract discusses the medicinal usages of about sixty field and garden plants with a chapter devoted to each. There is no description of the plant, presumably because the tract is the lifted section of the larger work, *De hortis*, which has a full botanical description. Also Cassidorus referred to one work by Gargilius which told both of "the raising of vegetables" *and* their medicinal values. In its entirety, the first chapter reads:

Radish. On the good authority of all medical people, a radish has a warming property [*virtus*], and yet it is proper for us to appreciate its value through experience [*de usu*]. Why, when it is mixed with other foods, it alone causes the stomach to belch, unless first it is cooked first? With three parts honey, it restores the hair destroyed by the injury from *alopecia* [probably, "fox-mange"]. Dropped in the ears, its juice truly improves earache [*gravitas aurium*].[23] It is an extraordinary antidote if it is taken by someone with an empty stomach. Against the "lice disease" [*phthiriasis*] its juice, which alone can penetrate because of its rarefied nature to the internal parts [*liniamenta*] of the body, is applied. Egyptian kings, whose concern it was to study the bodies of the dead and, when proof was exposed to view in order to examine the causes of illnesses, have reported that this kind of weakness is found in the very heart itself. With three parts honey, radish seed taken calms deep breathing [*suspirium*] and coughing is prevented. Taken alone with salt, it kills the living creatures of the stomach, stimulates sexual desire, promotes urination, and adds plenty of milk at [the time of] childbirth.[24]

In his critical text, Rose lists Pliny as Gargilius' source on the radish. In parts of two books, Pliny discussed all of the medicinal uses for the radish that Gargilius listed, much as Rose says.[25] Gargilius wrote that all doctors (*medici*) agree on the warming property and uses. Galen, Dioscorides, Scribonius Largus, Celsus, Nicander, and Theophras-

22. The most recent edition is published in *P. Vegeti Renati digestorum artis mulomedicinae libri*, ed. Ernest Lommatzsch, Leipzig, B. G. Teubner, 1903 and in English translation by Tapper, (n. 7) "Materia Medica," pp. 109–14 (notes and index, 115–23).

23. W. H. Jones in *Pliny Natural History*, 10 vols. Loeb Classical Library, London, Heinemann; Cambridge, Harvard University Press, 1938–63, 6 (1951), 19, translates the affliction as "deafness" but I favor a broader meaning.

24. Rose, (n. 19) *Medicina*, no. 1, pp. 133–4. John Scarborough assisted me in the translation, and Vivian Nutton and Joanne Phillips assisted me in the section pertaining to post-mortem examinations to be discussed below.

25. Pliny, (n. 23) *Natural History* (hereafter abbreviated *N.H.*), XIX. 26.85–7, XX. 13. 23–8.

tus,[26] to name some earlier authorities, have similar uses. Just as Gargilius said, there was little controversy in antiquity about radishes as a medicine. Moschion wrote an entire book on the plant according to Pliny.[27] When Gargilius said that there was a consensus about radish, he was being fair (although it is likely that he was employing Pliny in this chapter as his principal source).

Gargilius noted that radishes have a warming property, but here and in his other chapters, he was not employing the high learning of the writers on pharmacology who sought to determine two actions to redress humoral imbalance according to whether the drug's property (*dynamis* in Greek or *virtus* in Latin) was either warming or cooling *and* drying or moistening. According to what we now believe was the prevailing theory about drugs in the medicine of the Roman Empire, these actions were quantified up to four possible degrees of intensity.[28] Gargilius had apparently rejected the contemporary theoretical pharmacology, because we know that he had read Galen's works which explicated those ideas.[29] Gargilius said that radishes have a warming property while neglecting to specify the degree or its passive quality—that is, whether it is moistening or drying. Moreover, he was not administering the radish juice to rectify an imbalance produced by disorders which were cooling by their nature. He signalled his attitude towards the humoral balance theory for drug administration, when after his reference to a radish's warming quality, he wrote, "*and yet* it is proper for us to appreciate its value through experience." Galen and others, who accepted and expounded on what Dioscorides called the *logos* of *pharmaca* or pharmacology,[30] would have said, "warming *there-*

26. Galen, *De simplicium medicamentorum temperamentis ac facultatibus*. VIII. 17, C. G. Kühn, ed., *Galenus opera omnia*, 20 vols. in 22, 1821–33, rpt. Hildesheim, 1965, (hereafter abbreviated K) *12*, 111–2; Dioscorides. *De materia medica*. II. 112, Wellmann, ed., 3 vols., Berlin, Weidmann, 1906–14, repr. Berlin, 1958; Scribonius. *Compositiones*. 60, 133, 195–6, S. Sconocchia, ed. Leipzig, Teubner, 1983; Celsus. *De medicina*. II. 33 et passim., W. G. Spencer, ed., 3 vols. Loeb Classical Library, London, Heinemann; Cambridge, Harvard University Press, 1935–38; Nicander. *Alexipharmaca*. 430, A. S. F. Gow and A. F. Scholfield, eds. Cambridge, University Press, 1953; Theophrastus. *Enquiry into Plants*. IX. 9. 1 and 12. 1, Arthur Hort, ed., 2 vols. Loeb Classical Library, London, Heinemann; Cambridge, Harvard University Press, 1916.

27. Pliny, (n. 23) *N.H.* XIX. 26. 87.

28. On Galenic pharmacology, see Georg Harig, *Bestimmung der Intensität im medizinischen System Galens*, Berlin, Akademie Verlag, 1974; and Harig, "Der Begrift der lauen Warme in der theoretischen Pharmakologie Galens." *NTM*, *10*: 64–81, 1973.

29. Especially in Galen's treatise, (n. 26) *De simplicium medicamentorum temperamentis ac facultatibus*.

30. Dioscorides, (n. 26) *Materia Medica*, Preface. 5; see John Scarborough and Vivian Nutton, "The Preface of Dioscorides' *Materia Medica*: Introduction, Translation, Commentary," *Transac-*

fore it is proper for medicinal uses for. . . ." Gargilius' proof of its warming property was a rhetorical question that raw radishes cause one to belch. This clue provides an interesting insight into the means by which the ancients derived properties from empirical evidence. Some of the pharmaceutical properties must have been postulated through sense perception, despite Galen's caution that the senses are faulty. In fact, taste and smell are useful in identifying many alkaloids, tannins, oils and other compounds which are usually the pharmaceutically active ingredients in plant chemistries.[31]

For the most part, the medicinal uses that Gargilius prescribed for the radish were common afflictions such as we would treat in the home by over-the-counter remedies. One of the more sophisticated usages might be *alopecia* or "fox-mange," which may be our alopecia, a progressive natural or abnormal baldness. Exactly what the Greeks and Romans meant by it is uncertain.[32]

One means of evaluating Gargilius' medical remedies is to observe what remedies were in his sources but which he chose to omit in his account. Pliny said that radishes expel kidney stones (*eiciunt calculos*), reduce the size of the spleen, are beneficial for dropsy, lethargy, epilepsy, melancholia, ileocolitis, colicotis, intestinal ulcers and suppurations of the diaphram (*praecordia*). Radishes rubbed on the hands, Pliny reported, enable one to handle horned vipers (*cerastes*) without harm, and a radish placed on a scorpion kills it.[33] Gargilius chose not to include these usages, nor does he include other usages in his sources, such as Dioscorides who recommended radishes as a diuretic, emetic, and of assistance in treating growths, ulcers, or boils known as *nomas* and *gaggrainai*. Dioscorides incidentally wrote that radishes taken internally with wine help those bitten by the horned viper. Dioscorides'

---

tions and Studies of the College of Physicians of Philadelphia, *4*: 187–227, 1982; and the discussion in John M. Riddle, *Dioscorides and Medicine*, Austin, Texas University Press, 1984 (forthcoming).

31. R. W. Moncrieff, *The Chemical Senses*, 3rd ed., London, Wiley, 1967.

32. In the *De materia medica* of Dioscorides, *alopecia* is treated some thirty-five times (Antoine DuPinet, *Historia plantarum earum imagines*, Lyons, G. Coter, 1561, no. 320. Onions, garlic and white mustard ([n. 26] *De materia medica*. II. 151–4) were favorite remedies. In the pseudo-Galen, *Definitiones medicae*, 314, K. *19*, 431, *alopecia* is defined as baldness produced by a disease called by that name (see Aristotle, *Problemata*. X. 27 [893b. 38], W. S. Hett, trans., Loeb Classical Library, London, Heinemann; Cambridge, Mass., Harvard University Press, 1970, and Celsus, [n. 26] *De medicina*. VI. 4.2–3), but in the Galenic work, *Introductio seu medicus*, XIII, K. *14*, 757, alopecia is described as a type of *elephantiasis*. Cf. Pliny, (n. 23) *N.H.* XXIII. 54. 101.

33. Pliny, (n. 23) *N.H.* XX. 13. 25–6.

use of it as an emetic is in contrast to Pliny's more magical use.[34] Some of these afflictions required sophisticated diagnoses, such as "the enlargement of the spleen,"[35] and in distinguishing the *nomas* and *gaggrainae* from other dermatological and subcutaneous growths and ulcers.[36] Gargilius deliberately omitted these afflictions: he employed not only Pliny but Galen, Dioscorides, and Celsus, therefore Gargilius chose to omit almost all usages of the radish where a sophisticated diagnosis was required.

Gargilius' most intriguing comment is about the "Egyptian kings" sponsoring research which proved through post-mortem examinations that radish juice, alone among the drugs, was effective in penetrating deep within the body and successfully treats *phthiriasis*. Gargilius was simply copying Pliny's similar statement which reads in translation:

> They also say that radish juice is a necessary [*necessarius*] [drug in the treatment] for the disease of the diaphragm [*praecordia*], inasmuch as in Egypt, when the kings ordered *post mortem* dissections to be made for the purpose of research into the nature of diseases, it was discovered that radish juice alone was capable of removing *phtheiriasis* attacking the internal parts of the heart [*cor*].[37]

Phthiriasis (alt., *phtheiriasis*) meant in Greek "the lice disease." In a rare example in medical terminology, the ancient and modern words are apparently the same for similar distinctions: *phthiriasis* was and is a chronic lice infestation in distinction from *pediculosus* which is simply a lice infestation.[38] The disease is mentioned a number of times in ancient

34. Dioscorides, (n. 26) *De materia medica*. II. 112.

35. According to Galen, the spleen's purpose was to "eliminate the thick, earthy, atrabilious humors formed in the liver." See, Galen, *On the Usefulness of the Parts*, IV. 15, trans. Margaret T. May, 2 vols. Ithaca, Cornell University Press, 1968, I, 232, and Galen, *De naturalibus facultatibus*. II. 50, K. 2, 131 ff. On the diseases whose symptom is the enlargment of the spleen, see the Hippocratic work, *De internis affectionibus*, in Émile Littré, ed., *Œuvres complètes d' Hippocrate*, 10 vols., Paris, 1839–61; repr. Amsterdam, A. M. Hakkert, 1962, 7, 166–303, and Paulos Aegineta, *Seven Books of*, 3 vols., Francis Adams trans., London, Sydenham Society, 1844, I, 577. And the study by Robert Herrlinger, "Die Milz in der Antike," *Ciba Z.*, *8*: 2982–3012, 1958.

36. Jeremiah Reedy, "Galen on Cancer and Related Diseases," *Clio Medica*, *10*: 227–38, 1975; and Riddle, (n. 30) *Dioscorides*.

37. Pliny, (n. 23) *N.H.* XIX. 26. 86. My translation was guided by the translation by H. Rackham in (n. 23) *Natural History* vol. 5, p. 477.

38. Caelius Aurelianus, (n. 1) *Chronic Diseases*. IV. 2. 14: "It [phthiriasis] takes its name not from the basic nature of the disease, but from the large number of lice present." Latin writers considered *morbus pedicularis* as the same as *phtheiriasis*, *viz*. Celsus, (n. 26) *De medicina*. VI. 6. 15. For a modern discussion of lice, see Robert Matheson, *Medical Entomology*, 2nd ed., Ithaca, Cornell, 1950, pp. 194–217.

sources, but Thomas Africa observes that "the lice disease" was often used and misused by literary sources to denote a horrible death, often reserved for evil rulers who meet their just end in misery.[39] Doubts are expressed that any precise medical diagnosis could be made on the basis of these literary descriptions.[40] People do not die from lice, no matter how much they itch. Lice infestations on humans cause surface symptoms, such as eczema, infections from scratching, and disgusting odors —symptoms which do not readily apply to the internal corruption, sometimes with "worms," as described in the ancient accounts. Scabies together with other, and various, illnesses may be what are described in some of literary accounts according to a recent study by Keaveney and Madden.[41] Galen described phthiriasis as a serious illness and among its remedies were strong alkaloids, such as stavesacre (*Delphinium staphisagria* L.)and white hellebore (*Veratrum album* L.), in prescriptions for external application.[42] Caelius Aurelianus describes *phthiriasis*:

The signs of the disease are sleeplessness, itching of the body, pallor, loss of appetite, weakness of the esophagus, and loss of hair. The affection is one which involves a state of looseness. For a considerable discharge of reddish bile appears through the thin pores, and it is from this matter that the animals are generated.[43]

39. Thomas Africa, "Worms and the Death of Kings: A Cautionary Note on Disease and History," *Classical Antiquity*, *1*: 1–17, 1982. Africa states: "What is common in all accounts [in the writings of ancient historians] is a fatal corruption of tissue in the lower abdomen, swarming with worms or 'lice' and emitting a terrible stench." While undoubtedly this is true with many of the literary accounts in the histories [although Africa's citation to Herodotus. *Histories*. *4*. 205 is not to phthiriasis or connected with lice], the medical writings do not mention "worms" nor do they describe phthiriasis as a lower abdominal disease. Part of the confusion arises because modern translators confuse *skōlēkobrōtos*, "eaten by worms" (from *skōlekosis*) with *phtheir* which is sometimes incorrectly translated as "worm," as observed by Arthur Keaveney and John A. Madden, "Phthiriasis and its Victims," *Symbolae Osloenses*, *58*: 87–99, 1982.

40. Africa, (n. 39); Rackham, (n. 37) *N.H.*, 5, 476; Reinhard Hoeppli, *Parasites and Parasitic Infections in Early Medicine and Science*, Singapore, University of Malaya Press, 1959, pp. 342–59, refers to the numerous classical descriptions and assumes that, at best, what was being described was phthiriasis with subcutaneous and, perhaps, muscular infection; J. R. Busvine, *Insects, Hygiene, and History*, London, Athlona, 1976, pp. 195–203; A. T. Sandison, "Parasitic Diseases," in Don Brothwell and A. T. Sandison, eds. *Diseases in Antiquity*, Springfield, Charles C. Thomas, 1967, p. 181, has no mention of *phthiriasis* (a striking omission!) but he identifies pediculosis as appearing in Assyro-Babylonian documents. Galen's description is suggestive of a type of dermatitis in connection with the eyelids (*Introductio seu medicus*. 15, K. *14*, 771; cf. Celsus, (n. 26) *De medicina*. VI. 6. 15) and in the Pseudo Galen, *Definitiones medicae*. 353, K. *19*, 437, *phtheiriasis* is defined as a scabies (*lepidas*).

41. Keaveney and Madden, (n. 39).

42. Galen. *De compositione medicamentorum secundum locos*. I. 7, K. *12*, 462–3; cf. *De remediis parabilibus*. I. 1, K. *14*, 323, and other discussions in *Introductio seu medicus*. 14, K. *14*, 771; *De probis pravisque alimentorum succis*. 8, K. *6*, 793 and *De theriaca ad Pison*. 18, K. *14*, 290. Caelius ([n. 1] *Chronic Diseases*. IV. 2. 16–8) also employed these drugs in much the same prescriptions as Galen.

43. Caelius, (n. 1) *Chronic Diseases*. IV. 2. 15.

In another section of his work on the spleen, Caelius said that diseases of the spleen are sometimes accompanied with lice infestations.[44] (To be noted, Gargilius recommended radish juice both for spleen diseases and *phthiriasis*.) Morbidity is not mentioned by Caelius as a possible outcome of phthiriasis but Aristotle said: "Some people get this disease when there is a great deal of moisture in the body; some indeed have been killed by it."[45] Neither Caelius nor Aristotle give enough details for judgment about a disease we might recognize in our terms.

While phthiriasis today is not fatal, there is a possibility that what Gargilius, Pliny and some of the other ancients were describing is epidemic (louse-borne) typhus which is an acute infectious disease caused by *Rickettsia prowazeki* and transmitted by the human louse, *Pediculus humanus*. Rickettsiae are inoculated into the skin by a person scratching the skin. Once inside the skin, rickettsiae spread throughout the bloodstream and enter endothelial cells where they proliferate. During the course of the disease, various progressive neurological symptoms appear ranging from apathy through mental confusion, disorientation, twitching, delirium and convulsions to stupor and coma, a course which is roughly compatible with ancient literary accounts of phthiriasis. Vascular lesions are produced which lead to hemorrhaging; the cells of the brain, liver and kidneys in particular become heavily infected and will rupture, allowing the organism to escape; in the circulatory system the progressive developments can lead to myocarditis. Cardiac arrest is sometimes the cause of death.[46] The literary accounts which described worms swarming inside the victim could not be a proper description of such an infection.

It is important information which Martialis and Pliny related—that "Egyptian kings" sponsored experimental post-mortem examinations by autopsy in order to determine not only the cause of death but, in this case, to verify the proper drug therapy. Historians agree on the evi-

44. Ibid., III. 4. 52.

45. Aristotle. *Historia animalium*. V. 30. 557a, A. L. Peck, trans. Loeb Classical Library, London, Heinemann; Cambridge, Mass., Harvard University Press, 1965.

46. See, Theodore E. Woodward and Edward F. Bland, "Clinical Observations in Typhus Fever," *J. Am. Med. Assoc.*, *126*: 287–93, 1944; *Epidemic (Louse Borne) Typhus*, Department of the Army Technical Bulletin, TB MED 218 / NAVMED P-5052-3 / AFP 160-5-17 (6 December 1956), pp. 1–2, 5–7; Alfred J. Saah and Richard B. Hornick, "Ricksettsia prowazeki," in Gerald L. Mandell, R. Gordon Douglas, Jr., and John E. Bennett, eds., *Principles and Practices of Infectious Diseases*, 2 vols., New York, Wiley, 1979, 2, 1520–23; Matheson, (n. 38) *Medical Entomology*, pp. 205–8.

dence that the Ptolemaic kings supported human dissections for anatomical research and, more a matter of controversy, vivisection for physiological investigations.[47] Postmortem examinations to determine the cause of death are less well known but are documented in various papyri. The earliest one extant is from 173 A.D. where a physician certifies in writing that a man's death was by strangulation.[48] In another papyrus from 182 A.D. a physician certified the cause of death in the case of a slave boy who fell from a window while leaning out "to see the dancers."[49] Cases of violent or abnormal death required official examinations, often by physicians.[50] Inasmuch as most of the legal and administrative practices of Roman Egypt were a continuation of Ptolemaic procedures, we can be reasonably sure that these second century testimonials are evidences of earlier practices.[51] Galen said that two kings, Mithridates VI and Attalus II, tested antidotes of poisons on condemned criminals,[52] but this practice is different from testing correct drug therapy through a post-mortem autopsy.

In attempting to make modern medical sense out of Gargilius' passage, one is faced with a number of perplexing problems. In modern post-mortem examinations of victims of rickettsial infection, the left ventricle is contracted, the right moderately dilated, the atria are distended with blood, and the myocardium shows pallor, loss of consistency and yellowish streaks and points.[53] This suggests that Gargilius' passage may have been a reference to epidemic typhus with post-mortem discoveries confirming correct drug therapy by sophisticated tissue examinations. However, modern pathologists report that the gross changes in cardiac tissue are slight or even negligible.[54] Clinically the

47. For general accounts of dissections and anatomical research, see G. E. R. Lloyd, *Greek Science After Aristotle*, New York, Norton, 1973, pp. 75–90; Lloyd, *Science, Folklore and Ideology*, Cambridge, University Press, 1983; Peter Marshall Fraser, *Ptolemaic Alexandria*, 3 vols. Oxford, Clarendon, 1972, 1, 338–60; for a rejection of vivisection, see, John Scarborough, "Celsus on Human Vivisection at Ptolemaic Alexandria," *Clio Medica*, *11*: 25–38, 1976.

48. Darrel W. Amundsen and Gary B. Ferngren, "The Forensic Role of Physicians in Ptolemaic and Roman Egypt," *Bull. Hist. Med.*, *52*: 336–353, 1978, from *Oxyrhynchus Papyri* 51.

49. Ibid., p. 344, from *Oxy. Pap.* 475, and discussed more recently with a full translation by Naphtali Lewis, *Life in Egypt under Roman Rule*, Oxford, Clarendon, 1983, p. 106.

50. Amundsen and Ferngren, (n. 48).

51. Lewis, (n. 49) *Life in Egypt*, pp. 14–7.

52. Galen. *De antidotis*. 1. 1, K. *14*, 2.

53. S. B. Wolbach, J. L. Todd, and F. W. Palfrey, *The Etiology and Pathology of Typhus*, Cambridge, Mass., Harvard University Press, 1922, pp. 153–4.

54. David H. Walker, Christian E. Paletta, "Pathogenesis of Myocarditis in Rocky Mountain Spotted Fever," *Arch. Path. Lab. Med.*, *104*: 171–4, 1980.

most important organ affected is the brain, with a rickettsial encephalitis. It is questionable, therefore, that gross observation by Ptolemaic physicians of typhus victims could have detected the myocardial changes.[55]

Still, there is the consideration of radish juice. It contains sufficient saponins and other constituents that topical application in lice-infected body areas would in reasonable likelihood reduce the population.[56] Assuming, first of all, that typhus was a disease afflicting the ancients, would they have connected lice infestation with the symptoms of a louse transmitted disease, such as typhus? The answer must be speculative: perhaps, because Aristotle, Pliny, Celsus, and Caelius Aurelianus clearly made a connection between lice infestation and phthiriasis, which they described as having *some* typhus type symptoms. Certainty is illusive and doubt must remain. Possibly Gargilius and Pliny preserved a significant detail about Alexandrian science which escaped notice except by these two Romans who probably little understood what they said. North Africa, Gargilius' home, is the region where epidemic (louse-borne) typhus has been reported as recently as World War II.[57] Most likely neither Gargilius nor Pliny were aware of the actual pathology of the disease because each was copying from his source(s) and neither had likely experienced an autopsy. Perhaps Gargilius' motive in relating this story was similar to Pooh's words, written by W. S. Gilbert in *The Mikado*: "Merely corroborative detail, intended to give artistic verisimilitude to an otherwise bald and unconvincing narrative."[58] Regardless of how much he knew about what he related, the fact remains that his words and those of Pliny indicated that Ptolemaic physicians conducted post-mortem examinations to determine the cause of death and to test proper drug therapy. Whether real

55. I am grateful to David H. Walker and Guido Majno, pathologists, who have assisted me in this trying to understand the pathology of typhus as the Greeks may have seen it.

56. According to James A. Duke, "Phytotoxin Tables," *C.R.C. Crit. Rev. Toxicol.*, 5: 232, 1977, *Raphanus* contains: acetaldehyde, acetone, butyraldehyde, ethyl alcohol, isobutyraldehyde, isovaleraldehyde, methanethiol, methanol, oxalic acid, propionaldehyde, pyrocatechol, and saponins. Soybean and alfalfa saponins interfere with midgut proteases of *tribolium* larvae (J. R. Whitaker and R. E. Feeney, "Enzyme Inhibitors in Foods," *Toxicants Occurring Naturally in Foods*, 2nd ed., Washington, National Academy of Sciences, 1973, p. 292). I acknowledge the assistance of Richard Axtell and Robert Brackett in forming this judgment. While both Martialis and Pliny employed radish juice as an applicant, Caelius Aurelianus recommended it as an emetic in the treatment of phthiriasis.

57. Matheson, (n. 38) *Medical Entomology*, p. 206; (n. 46) *Epidemic Typhus*, p. 5.

58. *Complete Plays of Gilbert and Sullivan*, New York, Modern Library, 1936, p. 390.

or not, the concept is there. What phthiriasis was in antiquity remains uncertain; typhus appears a possibility, albeit a small one.

Throughout *Medicines from Vegetables and Fruits*, Gargilius usually gave general information without attribution where there was general agreement and cited his source when the information appeared unique or controversial. He named some twenty authorities, some of whose works are no longer extant (except as preserved by quotations in later works), including Olympia Thebena, Sextius Niger, and Diocles of Carystos.[59] Probably most of the authorities that he cited actually were taken from Pliny as an intermediate source.[60] Most of the authorities Gargilius named, whether as direct or indirect sources, wrote in Greek. Dioscorides (*fl.* 40–79 A.D.) and Galen were most frequently cited, Dioscorides in fifteen chapters and Galen in thirteen.

Gargilius' discussion of the pomegranate affords an example of how he dealt directly with Greek sources.[61] Dioscorides' chapter on *rhoa*[62] was translated by Gargilius into Latin as *malus granatus* ("grainy apple"), the fruit of the *punicus arbor* ("Punic tree"). Citrons, cherries, quinces, apples, pomegranates, and, eventually, lemons and oranges were all called *mala* or "apples." Differentiation came from the adjectives.[63] An apple meant a fruit with a fleshy outside and a hard kernel, seed or core. In Latin, *malus* for "apple" was often interchanged with *pomum* meaning "fruit." Thus, a pomegranate was called *malus grana-*

59. For fragments, see, Max Wellmann, "Sextius Niger: Eine Quellenuntersuchung zu Dioscorides," *Hermes, 24*: 530–69, 1889; and Max Wellmann, "Die Fragmente der sikelischen Ärtze Akron, Philistion und des Diokles von Karystos," *Fragmentsammlung der greichischen Ärzte, 1* Berlin, Weidmann, 1901, 117 ff.

60. In order of encounter and with Rose's chapter number, Heras Cappadox (2), Diospoliticus (3), Galen (4–7, 23, 27, 30, 40, 42, 44, 46, 51–2), Xenocrates (4—via Pliny. *N.H.* xx. 82. 218), Olympia Thebana (5 via Pliny *N.H.* xx. 84. 226), Sextius Niger (5 via Pliny. *N.H.* xx. 84. 226), Dioscorides (5–6, 11, 21, 27 [?], 30, 40–3, 46–7, 53, 56, 60 [?]), Hippocrates (9, 18, 21), Glaucia (17 via Pliny. *N.H.* xx. 99. 263), Diocles [of Carystos?] (18, 35), Praxagoras (18), Chrysippus (19, 22 via Pliny. *N.H.* xx. 48. 119, and 30), Asclepiades (27 via Pliny. *N.H.* xx. 20. 42), Pythagoras (29 via Pliny. *N.H.* xx. 87. 236, and 49 via Pliny. *N.H.* XXIII. 63. 122), Pliny (29, 49), Cato (30 via Pliny. *N.H.* xx. 33. 78, 34. 84), Cornelius Celsus (30), Melitus (30), Democritus (35 via Pliny. *N.H.* xx. 9. 19) and Dionysius (35 via Pliny. *N.H.* xx. 9. 19). For a discussion of Gargilius sources, see I. Mazzini, (n. 6) *De hortis*, pp. 41–4, and compare those in the large tract of *De hortis* on pp. 35–41.

61. (n. 19) *Medicina*, No. 41, p. 179, Rose ed. In the new reconstruction of fragments of the work, Martialis discussed the arbor culture of the pomegranate, *viz*. it flowers beginning in May; its fruits ripen in the Autumn and proper fertilizer procedures. See Condorelli, (n. 4) *Gargilii*, pp. 11–2.

62. Dioscorides, (n. 26) *De materia medica*. I. 110.

63. Jacques André, *Lexique des termes de botanique en latin*, Paris, C. Klincksieck, 1956, pp. 196–9; Hermann Fischer, *Mittelalterliche Pflanzenkunde*, Munich, Münicher Drucke, 1929, p. 280.

tus, *malus punicus*, *pomum granatum*, and *pomum punicum*. There was much confusion; for an example, Pliny's *malus granatus* is a citron, also called the Assyrian apple (*malus Assyria*) and the Median apple (*malus media*/ alt., *medicus*). This misled later writers to use the term "Medical apple" for the citron and, when it was discovered in the Middle Ages, the lemon.[64] The English "pomegranate" retains the Latin base for "grainy fruit," thus showing a gradual resolution in distinctions between lemons and pomegranates. Also the modern scientific name for pomegranate, given by Linnaeus, is *Punica granatum*, and for citron is *Citrus medica*. Translating Dioscorides for botanical identification and medicine requires knowledge which Gargilius displayed when he correctly took Dioscorides' *rhoa* to mean "grainy apple" or pomegranate. The modern phrase "comparing apples with oranges" obscures the history that once oranges were apples.

A general consensus exists among authorities, Gargilius wrote, that pomegranates have an astringent property.[65] Modern science agrees about their quality because pomegranates have a tannin and an alkaloid called pelletierine.[66] We now recognize the crude drug from pomegranate as effective against the tapeworm, a use noted by Dioscorides,[67] but Gargilius did not include its anthelmintic use. Modern use of it as an anthelmintic is restricted because it is toxic. Possibly seeing the requirement to control carefully the dosage, Gargilius preferred not to recommend this use in his simple cures. We have seen, however,

64. Pliny, (n. 23) *N.H.* XII. 7. 15–6. Most authorities agree that the lemon was either not known or not employed in Graeco-Roman medicine; see Friedrich A. Flueckiger and Daniel Hanburg, *Pharmacographia*, 2nd. ed., London, MacMillan, 1879, pp. 114–5; F. Adams in Paulos, (n. 35) *Seven Books*, vol. 3, pp. 472–3; Wolfgang Schneider, *Lexikon Zur Arzneimittelgeschichte*, 7 vols. Frankfurt a. M., Govi, 1974, 3, pt. 2, 321–4. But some scholars, such as Max Meyerhof, (*Moses Maimonides. Glossary of Drug Names*, Trans. from French by Fred Rosner, Philadelphia, American Philosophical Society, 1979) say that Dioscorides' *melea persica* ([n. 26] *De materia medica*. I. 115) is a lemon but this is not accepted by J. Berendes, *Des Pedanius Dioskurides aus Anazarbos Arneimittellehre*, Stuttgart, Ferdinand Enke, 1902, pp. 137–8. For references which support a medieval discovery of the lemon, see H. Fischer, (n. 63) *Pflanzenkunde*, p. 265. The lemon is seen drawn in a medieval madonna and child painting where Jesus is seen holding a lemon; see Reay Tannahill, *Food in History*, New York, Stein and Day, 1973, p. 180. The ancients' *malus medica* was the fruit of the *Citrus medica* Risso which we call citron, which is related to the lemon. See William Thiselton-Dyer's identification of the Greek term in *Theophrastus. Enquiry into Plants*. 2 vols., trans. Arthur Hort. London, Heinemann; Cambridge, Harvard University Press, 1948. I, 311.

65. Rose, (n. 19) *Medicina*, No. 41, p. 179.

66. Henry Kraemer, *A Textbook of Botany and Pharmacognosy*, 4th ed., rev., Philadelphia and London, Lippincott, 1910, pp. 534–6; George Edward Trease and William Charles Evans, *Pharmacognosy*, 11th ed., London, Bailliere Tindall, 1978, p. 120.

67. *The Dispensatory of the United States of America*. 25th ed., Philadelphia, Lippincott, 1950, pp. 1797–8.

that Gargilius recommended the radish against "living things" in the intestinal tract, doubtlessly tapeworms. Radish was employed as an anthelmintic up until the eighteenth century when it fell out of favor. As a drug, it was less dangerous than pomegranate. Gargilius' practice was to recommend mild drugs for simple medical problems.

Gargilius began the chapter on pomegranates as he did with the one on radishes. In an unattributed quotation possibly from Dioscorides, Gargilius noted that the sweet kind of pomegranates was warming and good for the stomach against flatulency, but it ought not be given for fevers. In contrast, Galen listed pomegranate fruits as having a cooling property, hence implicitly suitable as a possible antipyretic remedy.[68] Dioscorides had only referred to the sweet pomegranate without giving its properties. Pliny noted that there were at least five kinds of pomegranates.[69] Gargilius was critically evaluating his material to clarify at least a potential for a mistake by making sure that he did not cite the contradictory testimony of his sources, as between Dioscorides and Galen, nor the unnecessarily complicating information that was in Pliny.

Continuing his discussion, Gargilius cited Dioscorides by name about pomegranate flowers but his translation and understanding were truly imperfect:

> A remedy from pomegranate flowers is believed to be effective for all eye afflictions. Dioscorides simply reports that, when there begins a bursting of the loosening action [i.e., when the flower calyxes break open in blooming], the flowers, three in number, are swallowed without touching any tooth.[70]

This is a purported translation for what Dioscorides had written:

> Pomegranate flowers, which are also called *kytinoi*, are astringent, drying, checking, and drawing together bloody wounds—the same purposes as those drugs from [the other parts of] the tree. The flowers serve in a mouthwash for moistening rotten gums and for making strong teeth and in an applicant they have an adhesive quality for hernias. It is reported that one who has as much as three small flowers does not have eye trouble for a year.[71]

68. Galen, (n. 26) *De simpl. med. temp. ac fac.* IV. 3, but in VIII. 17, Galen did not give cooling as the fruit's property.

69. Pliny, (n. 23) *N.H.* XIII. 33. 113, cf. *N.H.* XXIII. 57. 107, where Pliny said that the Sweet pomegranates are strictly forbidden for fevers.

70. Rose, (n. 19) *Medicina*, No. 41, p. 181: Ex cytinis fit remedium quod creditur tutos ab oculorum dolore praestare. Dioscorides simplicius in hunc modum tradit ut cum primum cytini erumpere incipiunt, tres numero additi sine contactu dentium transvorentur.

71. Discorides, (n. 26) *De materia medica*. I. 110. 2–3.

Gargilius' citation of Dioscorides is very muddled. Pliny, not Dioscorides, referred to swallowing pomegranate flowers without touching the teeth but Pliny's use was for the purpose of preventing eye trouble.[72] Although Gargilius displayed some knowledge and critical skill about pomegranates, overall, he was careless with his information in contrast to his chapter on radishes.

Gargilius' citations are usually straightforward. "A cooking of celery and its roots boiled in drinking water effectively combats dangerous poisons,"[73] Gargilius wrote in what was or could have been a literal translation of Dioscorides, but he did not name his source. At times, Gargilius was less precise in his citations even when he was combining sources:

Both Sextius Niger and Dioscorides believe that *malva* [*Hibiscus sylvestris* or *Alcea rosea*[74]] is useless for the stomach. Dioscorides and Galen complain that *malva* is only slightly nourishing to the body but quickly it runs through the bowels and is evacuated.[75]

As earlier noted, the full text of Sextius Niger's work is now lost, but it is not apparent that Gargilius had seen it either. Likely Gargilius received the citation from Pliny, who named Sextius but was not named by Gargilius.[76] Dioscorides said that the plant was bad for the stomach (upper tract), good for the lower digestive tract, and that its roots given in a broth was an antidote by causing vomiting.[77] Galen, not Dioscorides, said that *malva* was only slightly nourishing but he gave no purgative or emetic qualities to it.[78]

Rue is pharmaceutically a strong plant, containing a volatile oil, which is a powerful local irritant,[79] and rutin, which is a vasopressor agent.[80] Dioscorides said that mountain rue is fatal, if too much is ingested. Carefully he prescribed its use for a number of things from headaches and earaches to such hard to diagnose and treat problems as *erysipilis*, *herpes*, *achor*, and *exanthema*,[81] which are various subcutane-

72. Pliny, (n. 23) *N.H.* XXIII. 59. 110.
73. Rose, (n. 19) *Medicina*, No. 2, p. 135.
74. André, (n. 63) *Lexique*, p. 195.
75. Rose, (n. 19) *Medicina*, No. 5, p. 139.
76. Pliny, (n. 23) *N.H.* XX. 84. 226.
77. Dioscorides, (n. 26) *De materia medica*. II. 118. 1.
78. Galen, *De alimentorum facultatibus*. II. 42, K. 6, 629.
79. (n. 67) *Dispensatory*, p. 1832. Gargilius' *ruta* is *Ruta graveolens* L. + sp.
80. Walter H. Lewis and Memory P. F. Elvin-Lewis, *Medical Botany. Plants Affecting Man's Health*, New York, Wiley, 1977, p. 190.
81. Dioscorides, (n. 26) *De materia medica*. III. 45. 4–5.

ous eruptions and growths whose specific etiologies are not known to moderns. In the area of dermatological afflictions in general, we are unsure of precisely the distinctions the Greeks were making. Uncharacteristically Gargilius included rue among his plants,[82] most of which were mild drugs,[83] and Gargilius employed Dioscorides as a source for information on rue. Gargilius warned of the plant's harmful potentialities and related only the mild, simpler uses—totally omitting the difficult dermatological usages as well as the employment of rue as an abortifacient which Dioscorides gave as well.[84]

Occasionally Gargilius was critical of his authorities. He said that Dioscorides believed that dried Damson plums or prunes would impede bowel movements but Gargilius noted that Galen thought Dioscorides to be incorrect about this.[85] While Gargilius did not express his opinion directly, at least he put the correction in his text, without explaining Dioscorides' inexplicable error about prunes.

The study of Gargilius' use of Dioscorides as an authority begins what will be a long, complex series of problems. It appears that he had a text that he believed to be Dioscorides but one which differs from the texts we attribute to him. On the *castanea* or Sardian acorn, Gargilius wrote, "Dioscorides thought it to be a purgative," but no statement of this sort is found in any copy known of Dioscorides' Greek text in the chapter on *castanea*.[86] Similarly Dioscorides' opinion is cited for *hypomelidius* but that statement is not found in Dioscorides.[87]

82. Rose, (n. 19) *Medicina*, No. 3, pp. 136–7.

83. Another strong plant which Gargilius included is the cultivated opium poppy (*papaveris*= *Papaver somniferum* L., (Rose, [no. 19] *Medicina*, p. 152), however Gargilius did not recommend opium. His source, Pliny (*N.H.* XX. 76. 202), said: "When the heads themselves and the leaves are boiled down, the juice is called *meconium*, and is much weaker than opium." Gargilius began the chapter with this statement from Pliny but he omitted entirely the discussion of the drug opium. Dioscorides ([n. 26] *De materia medica*. IV. 64. 7) distinguished between the latex of the *opus* or opium, and an extract of the whole plant, *mekonion*. Gargilius' usages were for simple problems, like a headache, but he did recommend another variety called a wild poppy (*Papaver rhoeas* L. or horned poppy) as effective for tumors.

84. (n. 67) *Dispensatory*, p. 1832, says that the alleged abortifacient effect is probably a product of its general toxicity.

85. Rose, (n. 19) *Medicina*, no. 46, p. 191: "Dioscorides sicca cocta aluum restringere existimat, quod Galenus non inmerito falsum esse contendit." Cf. Dioscorides, (n. 26) *De materia medica*. I. 121; Galen, (n. 26) *De simpl. med. temp. ac fac.* VII. 35.

86. Rose, (n. 19) *Medicina*, no. 56, p. 203: "adeo ut Dioscorides putet etiam cathartico dato per hanc potionem iri obviam posse, si plus quam necesse sit purget." Cf. Dioscorides, (n. 26) *De materia medica*. I. 106.

87. Rose, (n. 19) *Medicina*, no. 60, p. 207: "De hypomelidibus. Hoc pomum Dioscorides frigidissimum adfirmat atque ideo et laborem digestionis incutere." Cf. Dioscorides, (n. 26) *De materia medica*. I. 109.

On the onion, Gargilius cited Galen as stating that as an applicant it stimulates hair growth more rapidly than sea-foam.[88] The statement is found both in Galen and Dioscorides,[89] thus raising the question as to why Gargilius chose to attribute the statement to Galen and not to both. Gargilius attributed to Galen a statement of a constraining effect of green pears on the stomach but a statement to this effect is not found in those Galenic texts published by Kühn.

Such instances as these led Innocenzo Mazzini to conclude that Gargilius did not employ Dioscorides and Galen directly.[90] This postulate represents a full turn from the assertions of earlier scholars who, noting that Gargilius was the first Latin writer to cite Dioscorides and knowing that Dioscorides was translated into Latin by the sixth century, proposed that Gargilius had himself translated the full text of Dioscorides.[91] The evidence, as I see it, points to a middle position: Gargilius employed Greek sources and he made his own translations for quotation in his work. In so doing, he made errors which mean that his knowledge of Greek was poor. He often referred to "Greek writers," thus he was aware that they wrote in Greek. Had he only used Latin sources, such as Pliny, he might not have been aware of this fact. Since there is no evidence that Galen's tract on simple medicines was translated into Latin before the twelfth century, likely Gargilius read Galen in Greek. There was no intermediate source for these citations. Furthermore, there is no evidence that Diocles of Carystos, Praxagoras, and Chrysippus were ever available in Latin, but Gargilius cited them.[92] This leads me to believe that Gargilius conducted his own research by reading Latin and Greek sources as best he could and supplemented it with his experiences. Most of his citations of Latin and Greek authors are accurate. Sometimes he misunderstood his source and at other times, he summarized so severely as to misrepresent. Occasionally as on prunes, he made corrections. Finally, he either confused some other source for Dioscorides and Galen or else he had

88. Rose, (n. 19) *Medicina*, no. 27, pp. 161–2.

89. Galen, (n. 26) *De simpl. med. temp. ac fac.* VII. 58; cf. Discorides, (n. 26) *De materia medica*. II. 151.

90. Mazzini, (n. 6) *De hortis*, pp. 42–4.

91. John Riddle, (n. 4); Lynn Thorndike, *History of Magic and Experimental Science*, 8 vols., New York, Columbia University Press, 1923–58, I, 608.

92. In n. 60 above, there are Greek authors whom Gargilius cited but he took the quotations from Pliny. It remains possible that those citations to the authors not found in Pliny were also indirectly derived from some other Latin source no longer extant.

texts of Dioscorides and Galen which are different from the extant copies. Some of his citations were of such a nature that they could have been simple translation errors.

Gargilius related his own experiences with drugs. One of those experiences was unhappy. He testified to the anodyne effect of a celery (sometimes, parsley[93]) seed recipe with anise, henbane, celery seed and sprouts, formed into pills and taken with wine when one wished to sleep. "Would," Gargilius wrote, "that disaster had not forced me to learn from personal experience how much power this drink has."[94] He personally testified as to the effectiveness of horseradish boiled in barley water for chest problems.[95] A recipe of almonds (*amygdala*), gentian (*gentiana*), and wormwood (*absinthium Ponticum* = *Artemsia absinthium* L.) for the liver and spleen is strong "as I have proven by testing it in my own home [*domestica*] for by it my wife was saved."[96] Besides being our only evidence that he was married, this statement is the only indication that he may have practiced medicine. It's isolation, however, suggests that, even if he had practiced medicine, he did not necessarily do so as a physician. More likely he was a farm manager who had to treat illness and injury. The work entitled *Medicines* appears unencumbered by the preoccupations of medicine as a profession; it merely suggests the utility of simple, household remedies in the running of a farm. Some medical knowledge seems appropriate to a retired veteran of bloody military encounters.

Any judgment of Gargilius' work should be based on an understanding of the kind of book he wrote. He wrote on horticulture. For this reason he discussed those common cultivated plants and wild field plants that would be found useful and growing on and around the farm. He followed in the tradition of Cato, Varro, and Columella, authors frequently employed in the extant portions of *De hortis*. "While a garden feeds people, it also heals them," Cato said.[97] The legacy of

93. André, (n. 63) *Lexique*, p. 35.

94. Rose, (n. 19) *Medicina*, no. 2, p. 136; trans. by Tapper, (n. 7) "Materia Medica", p. 25: "quantum haec potio valeat utinam nulla calamitas coegisset ut experimento meo nossem." Cf. Pliny, (n. 23) *N.H.* XX. 441. 112–5 (*et passim.*); Dioscorides, (n. 26) *De materia medica*. III. 64; Galen, (n. 26) *De simpl. med. temp. ac fac.* VI. 51.

95. Rose, (n. 19) *Medicina*, no. 32, p. 171.

96. Ibid., no. 53, p. 200: "vehemens hoc esse etiam domesticis in uxore servata experimentis probavi." Cf. Pliny, (n. 23) *N.H.* XXIII. 75. 144–5; Dioscorides, (n. 26) *De materia medica*. I. 123; Galen, (n. 26) *De simpl. med. temp. ac fac.* VI. 36.

97. Cato. *On Farming* 8. 2, trans. Ernest Brehaut, New York, Columbia University Press, 1933.

Roman medicine had many roots on the Roman farm, as John Scarborough has shown.[98] Because it was useful information, Gargilius Martialis included a section on the medicinal uses of the plants on and around the farm. In doing this, he knew enough to go to good Greek medical authorities rather than to restrict his literary research to those who had written on horticulture. He consistently limited his selections to easily diagnosed and treated afflictions. Although some of the authorities dealt with rather complex medical issues, he selected from his sources and described medicines in what the Greek would call *euporista* or "household remedies." For an example, he did not use Book Four of Dioscorides' *De materia medica*, where there are strong medicines such as atropine alkaloids.

Even though he made errors, especially when dealing with Greek authors, he exhibited critical judgment in what he chose to include and exclude. In the words of K. D. White, he did it in a style that "is clear, simple and unaffected."[99] For these reasons, people from Cassiodorus' time regarded Gargilius as a medical authority. Undoubtedly his simple remedies using common, seemingly pharmaceutically simple plants spoke to the needs of the farm, manor and monastery in the early Middle Ages. If one today were writing a history of medicine during Antiquity, one could very well omit Gargilius Martialis and still be complete. If one were writing the same about the Middle Ages, Gargilius would have to be included although he did not live in the age.

Today we are aware of prejudices whose presence distorts values and judgments about individual people because of their race, religion, ethnicity, sex, or sexual affection. Perhaps Gargilius Martialis and other late Roman writers are victims of another kind of prejudice, when they are labelled as decadent epitomizers in the late autumn of classical civilization. Certainly in the case of Gargilius, he should not be criticized for writing a medical book because it was not such a book he wrote. He wrote on *Vegetables and Fruit Trees* and in so doing he told us fairly well what he thought useful and that included medicine. The medicines were those from mild herbal plants and how they were useful for easily treated afflictions. Martialis' contributions should be judged on the basis of what he wrote, for the purposes for which he

98. John Scarborough, *Roman Medicine*, Ithaca, Cornell University Press, 1969.
99. K. D. White, *Roman Farming*, Ithaca, Cornell University Press, 1970, p. 30.

intended, and not the purposes another age had him to serve. In the re-evaluation process, perhaps we can examine just how decadent or creative, how much of an epitomizer or how original, each of the late Roman writers was on topics judged as medicine.

XI

The Pseudo-Hippocratic Dynamidia

Recently, French. German, and Italian scholars, especially Pierre Riché, Pierre Courcelle. Robert Joly, Gerhard Baader, Augusto Beccaria and Innocenzo Mazzini, studied and observed various aspects of medicine in the late fifth and sixth century West.[1] The results show a remarkable period of acitivity probably in those areas where Byzantine. Old Roman. and Germanic cultures blended. A declaration of a Sixth Century Renaissance in Medicine is not yet justified and may never be. Nevertheless. the number of medical works, which can now be traced to the period and probably to the Ravenna region of northern Italy, are sufficient to stimulate studies of the medical and scientific originality of the period.

Part of the reason for the obscurity of time and place is the welcome of obscurity on the part of the actors who preferred to be anonymous and to present their contribution under pseudonyms of famous classical authors.[2]

One of those works is the Pseudo-Hippocratic Dynamidia[3] (or De victus ratione[4] or De virtute[s] herbarum et de cibis[5] or Liber peri diaetis ipsius Ypocratis[6]) which later was variously ascribed also to Galen[7], Pliny[8], Theodorus[9], and Oribasius[10].

1 P. Riché, Education et culture dans l'occident barbare, VIe–VIIe siècles (Paris, Editions du Seuil, 1962): P. Courcelle, Les lettres grécques en Occident. De Macrobe à Cassiodore, Paris, E. de Boccard, 1948; Robert Joly, Les versions latines du Régime Pseudo-Hippocratique. Scriptorium, 29 (1975), 3–22; Gerhard Baader, Die Anfänge der medizinischen Ausbildung im Abendland bis 1100, in: La scuola nell' occidente latine dell'alto medioevo, (Spoleto, 1972), 669–772; Augusto Beccaria, Sulle tracce di un antico canone latino di Ippocrate e di Galeno, Italia medioevale e umanistica 2 (1959) 1–56; 4 (1961) 1–75; 14 (1971) 1–23; Innocenzo Mazzini, Il latino medico in Italia nei secoli V e VI. La cultura in Italia fra tardo antico e alto medioevo 1 (1981) 433–441.

2 L. E. Voigts, The Significance of the Names Apuleius to the Herbarium Apulei. Bulletin of the History of Medicine, 52 (1978) 214–227.

3 Palatinus Ms Lat. 1088, late s. ix, fols. 91–115v; London British Library, Sloane Ms 84, s. xi, fols. 34–40. For a listing, discussion, and references to these and other Dynamidia manuscripts, see Pearl Kibre, Hippocrates Latinus. Traditio 34 (1978) 216–218.

4 Cheltenham, Phillips Ms 386, s. early ix, fols. 1–22v.

5 St. Gallen, Stiftsbibliothek Ms 762, s. ix, pp. 25–72. There is a variation, called De cibis et potibus preparandis infirmis videamus, of this text in Florence Laurentiana Ms 73. 23, s. xiii, fol. 92–95.

6 B. N. Ms lat. 7027, s. ix–x, fols. 55–66.

7 B. L. Ms Harley 5792, s. vi, fol. 273; Paris, B. N. Ms lat. 11218, s. viii-ix, fols. 42v–48v, 65–98v; Kibre, Hipp. Lat. (n. 3), 216–217.

8 Rose, Anecdota Graeca et Graecolatina, 2 pts. (Berlin 1864–1870 ; repr. Amsterdam, Hakkert, 1963), II 105–128.

9 Beccaria, I codici di medicina del periodo presalernitano (secoli IX, X e XI) (Rome, Edizioni di storia e Letterature, 1956), p. 253 for London, B. L. Harvey Ms 4986; cf. Kibre, Hipp. Lat. (n. 3), p. 218.

Most manuscripts and later citations attribute the work to Hippocrates with the title, Dynamidia. A good definition of this term is difficult, having been attempted only by Isidore in the extant documents of the early Middle Ages[11] and more recently by John Scarborough and Vivian Nutton.[12] Isidore's definition of the "power of herbs" suggests the pharmacy of all plants. By Isidore's meaning, dynamidia comes under the therapeutics subdivision of medicine in contrast to the other subdivision, dietetics. While it is true that the term dynamidia has various and evolving meanings, the term as used by the author of this tract straddles both divisions, therapeutics and dietetics.

In fact, the treatise is based on the Greek Hippocratic work, Regimen or Dietetics (*περὶ διαίτης*) and is concerned only with the plant food stuffs, most of which were discussed in the Greek work. But the information is about the *δύναμις* (pl. *δυνάμιδες*) or *medicinal properties* of these foods. If one were translating the term into modern science idiom there is no good word but there are several which convey the meaning: "the pharmacognosy of plant foods" or, in popular idiom, "the medicinal properties of plant foods." By "property," as we shall see, the meaning is not so much the pharmaceutical property in both ours and the classical senses but the qualitative effect of the food on the body. A problem for us is that we have difficulty at present in making sharp distinctions between a "food" and a "drug." When one takes, for instance, chicken soup for a cold, the distinction between food and drug becomes a matter of intention. Also foods contain organic compounds, most of which are metabolized in the body as energy, but some of which we loosely term "vitamins." And also there are minerals, some only in trace amounts. A person with deprivations of specific vitamins and minerals has a number of physiological symptoms. Ordinarily a lemon is considered food, but, when taken for scurvy, it is a drug. Although we do not conceptualize "foods" the way antiquity did, we recognize that foods have medicinal uses. Since we today cannot make sharp distinctions, all the more we cannot impose them on another era.

The treatise examines the medicinal properties and pharmaceutical usages of some seventy-seven items (counting "plums" and "prunes" as only one item despite separate chapters devoted to each). The first part is a lifting of the Latin version of Book Two of the Hippocratic Regimen, translated as De observenti ciborum in the late fifth or sixth century.[13] Dynamidia and De observantia ciborum begin with the

10 Anecd. Graec. (n. 8), II 110–114; Richard Durling, A Catalogue of the Sixteenth Century Printed Books in the National Library of Medicine (Bethesda, Md., Nat. Library of Medicine, 1967), 172.

11 Origines 4,10. Dinamidia, potestas herbarum, id est vis et possibilitas. Nam in herbarum cura vis ipso dynamis dicitur; unde et dinamidia nuncupatur, ubi eorum medicinae scribuntur. For a full discussion; see Loren C. MacKinney, Dynamidia' in Medieval Medical Literature. Isis 24 (1936), 400–414.

12 John Scarborough and Vivian Nutton, The Preface of Dioscorides' Materia Medica: Introduction, Translation, Commentary. Transactions and Studies of the College of Physicians of Philadelphia 4 (1982), 199–202 [187–227].

13 Text and discussion by Innocenzo Mazzini, De observantia ciborum. Università di Macerata. Pubblicazioni della Facoltà di Lettere e Filosofia, Instituto di Filologia Classica. No. 18

same discussion of climatic influences on human kind and plants and this is followed by a discussion on the properties of plant foods. Dynamidia omits animal foods. The text appearead inadequate to the author of Dynamidia for what he wished to convey. But the thirteenth plant, lupin, he abandoned the Hippocratic work by supplying information either from another source which is unknown to us or from information based on his own experiences.

As the tract progresses, its author relied increasingly on the treatise Medicines from Vegetables and Fruits by Gargilius Martialis (fl. 220–260 A.D.)[14] and much less on the Hippocratic work. At times Dynamidia's author copied directly from Gargilius. When Valentin Rose prepared the text of Gargilius' work, published in 1870, he included as version "b" Dynamidia's text which was printed as authored by Medicina Plinii by Stephanus Guilliretus in Rome, 1509 (and again Basel, A. Torini, 1528). Where Dynamidia had plants not in Gargilius' authentic text, Rose interpolated Dynamidia's text for those plants in version "a", which is Gargilius' authentic text minus Rose's interpolations.[15] In 1835, A. Mai published a text for Dynamidia primarily Vatican Palatinus lat. 1088 (late 9th c.) with supplementation from Vatican Reginensis 1004 (12th c.).[16] Mai's Dynamidia text is in two books, the second one of which should not be considered as part of the original.[17] Even the first book, which has fewer interpolations, contains – in the words of Robert Joly – "suppressions, additions, et déplacements."[18] Earlier in 1870, Rose published a text which is better than Mai's edition because it is based on reading from St. Gallen, Stiftsbibliothek Ms 762 and Cheltenham, Phillipps Ms 386, both of the ninth century.[19] Rose keyed the text of these manuscripts to what he considered to be a Latin Oribasius text published by J. Schottus in Strasborough, 1544, but the so-called Oribasius is actually derived from Dynamidia.[20]

(Rome, Giorgio Bretschneider, 1984), 31–34 (for dating); and earlier edition by Mazzini, De observantia ciborum. Un' antica traduzione latina del περὶ διαίτης pseudoippocratico (I, II) (edition princeps). Romanobarbarica 2 (1977), 287–357.

14 Text by Valentin Rose, ed., in: Plinii Secundi quae fertur una cum Gargilii Martialis Medicina (Leipzig, Teubner, 1863–1870), (129)–208; also see, John M. Riddle, Gargilius Martialis as a Medical Writer. Journal of the History of Medicine and Allied Sciences 39 (1984), 408–429.

15 V. Rose, Plinii (n. 14), published the readings of version "b" below the text of "a" except for the chapters on sisymbrium, portulaca, escaria, abrotanum, panagorace, and ulpicum, which he added after chapter 39 on serpyllum (p. 177) as part of the text for version "a", but Rose did not renumber the chapters. In addition version "b" contained the following chapters which had no corresponding part in version "a"; una (p. 195), mori (p. 196), tuber (p. 199), balanum (p. 204), and palmarum thebaicarum (p. 205).

16 Angelo Mai, Classicorum auctorum e vaticanis codicibus urbani. 7 (Rome, typis vaticanis, 18 –1838) 7 (1835), 399–419 (liber 1), 419–463 (liber 2).

17 Robert Joly, Versions Latines (n. 1), 11–13; V. Rose, Anecdota Graec. (n. 8), II 110 n.; L. MacKinney, Dynamidia (n. 11), 407.

18 Joly, Versions Latines (n. 1), 14.

19 Rose, Anecdota Graec. (n. 8), II 131–150.

20 The text for dynamidia is in Book 1, which is ascribed in this edition to Oribasius, fol. 143, chapter 98, beginning: "Apium mingitur magis quam egeritur . . .", and ending, fol. 149, chapter 128, "[satureia] . . . cum aceto fronti illinito, lethargum suscitat."

Professor Innocenzo Mazzini gave a welcomed notice that he and Vanda Fraticelli were working on a new critical edition for the Dynamidia.[21] Until then the work on my paper rests on a delicate foundation. I wish to approach the subject of how the Dynamidia treatise informs us about the medicine of the period of its composition. For this purpose I have relied on Rose's text based on the ninth century manuscript readings and I have employed British Library Ms Sloane 84 (670), 11th c., as a supplement and occasionally a corrective. This later manuscript for the most part drops the earlier Hippocratic text about locations and, after a short preamble, it begins – as any herbal would – with the listing of the plants, their properties and medicinal usages. The Dynamidia lacks most herbals' botanical descriptions but their inclusion would hardly be merited because these were common garden and yard plants.

With some justification Dynamidia is called a pseudo-Hippocratic work because its first part is taken almost verbatim from the Latin translation of the second book of the Regimen. Out of seventy-eight plant entries[22] (called chapters), only the text for fifteen, however, derive entirely from the Hippocratic work, thirteen of those chapters are in the first fifteen chapters, the sections on cereals and beans.[23] Around twenty-eight of the plants come directly from Gargilius Martialis' work. Of these twenty-eight, four plants – dock (lapacius, no. 25), pear (pira, 53), plum (pruna, 58), and pistachio (pistacium, 71) – are entirely derived from Gargilius without additional material.[24]

The comparison of texts for plums (no. 58) illustrates the similarity:

Dynamidia, no. 58	Gargilius, no. 46
Pruna pomum recens ventrem solvit. Stomacho contrarium iudicatur. Sicca non tantum molesta sunt. In mulsa cocta alvum commovet.[25]	Pruna recens pomum ventrem resolvit; stomacho contrarium iudicatur, sed omne hoc incommodum celeri digestione finitur. Sicca non tantum molestiae praebent. Dioscorides sicca cocta alvum restringere existimat, quod Galenus non immerito falsum esse contendit. Quis enim nesciat ex passo discocta vel mulso ad solutionem ventris operari, maximeque proficere si decoctum ipsum cui sucus admixtus est sorbetur?[26]

21 I. Mazzini, De observ. cib. (n. 13), p. 294n.

22 The numbering for the chapters is my own but it is based on Rose's text.

23 Chapters: barley (1), polenta (2), wheat (3), horse bean (4), pea (5), hyacinth bean (6), chick pea (7), millet (9), vetch (10), linseed (12), lupin (13), hedge mustard (14), sesame (15), and grape vines (63).

24 Gargilius, Medicina. No.'s 8, 40, 46 and 55 on pp. 142–143, 178–179, 191–92, and 202–203 Rose (n. 14).

25 Dynamidia, no. 58, 2 p. 145 Rose (n. 8).

26 Gargilius, Medicina, no. 46, p. 191 Rose (n. 14).

Whereas Gargilius often named his sources, Dynamidia never did. To be observed here is that Dynamidia's author saved his reader from the problem of dealing with the contradiction between Dioscorides and Galen regarding whether cooked plums had a binding or loosening effect on the bowels. Dynamidia simply stated that plums have a laxative result, as, in fact, they do.

Dynamidia's other sources are less clear. Frequently Dynamidia's text is based on Gargilius, always with editing and reduction but augmented as well with supplementary material. Dynamidia's author employed Gargilius on chichory (intibus, no. 28) – there being no discussion of it in the Hippocratic text – and he left out some medical uses, such as an applicant for gout, but he added to Gargilius that there are two kinds of intibus, a bitter kind and sweet kind.[27] Some classical writers, such as Pliny and Dioscorides, make no such distinctions.[28] Probably Dynamidia's author is distinguishing chicory (Chicorum intybus L.), the sweet kind, from endive (Chicorum endiva L.).[29]

Dynamidia's other source or sources, if any, are less clear. Possibly the Old Latin Translation of Dioscorides' De materia medica was employed as a resource but never is the wording similar enough for certainty. For example, there is the entry on the gourd:

Dynamidia, no. 22[30]	Hipp., De observ. cib., 67[31]
Cucurbita calida est et humida. Ventrem mollit in cibo sum(p)ta. Rasuram earum oculorum tumores tollit. Trita cum polenta podagricorum tumoribus medetur. Sucus earum cum rosaceo mixtum aurium dolorem tollit et humores quia humectat et deducit.	Cucurbita frigida[32] est et humectat et deducit [Old Latin Transl. 2 PIH:][33] Rasura eius cerebro inposita estigatione infantum mitigit, tumoribus oculorum opitulatur, podagricis iuvat. Sucus rasure eius dolores aurium tollit cum oleo roseo mixtus. [Gargilius, no. 6:][34] Galenus[35] umidae putat virtutis et frigidae, idque ex eo probat quod in cibo sumpta stomachum relaxat, bibendi desideria non excitat.... Crudae et tritae leniunt omnem tumorem, in cibo sumptae molliunt ventrem. Sucus earum, ut Galenus sit, ad compescendum veloriter auriculae dolorem tepefactus infunditur.

27 Dioscorides, De materia medica 1, 121 Wellmann; Galen, De simplicium medicamentorum temperamentis ac facultatibus 35. XII 32–33 Kühn

28 Dynamidia, no. 28, p. 139 Rose (n. 8); Gargilius, Medicina, no. 12, p 145–146 Rose (n. 14).

29 Jacques André, Lexique des termes de botanique en Latin (Paris, Klincksieck, 1956), 170.

30 Dynamidia, no. 22, p. 138 Rose (n. 8).

31 De observ. cib., no. 67, p. 65 Mazzini (n. 13).

32 However, the Greek was *warming* (θερμαίνει) (Regimen II 54, 46. IV 330 Jones [ed.,[Cambridge, Harvard University Press, and London Heinemann, The Loeb Classical Library, 1931]).

33 Hermann Stadler, ed., Dioscorides Longobardus. Forschungen 10 (1897) 225.

34 Medicina, no. 6, p. 140–141 Rose (n. 14).

35 Galen, De simpl. med. 7, 37. XII 33–34 Kühn.

Here with gourd as with several other plant entries, the evidence is not clear whether or not the Old Latin Translation of Dioscorides was used as a direct source. From linguistic analysis, we believe that the translation was done probably in the sixth century in or near Lombardy.[36] Throughout, Dynamidia's author modified his material to the extent that it is sometimes unclear whether he was directly employing source. The example of orache, no. 23, reveals his creative editorial propensities:

Dynamidia, no. 23	Gargilius, no. 7
Atriplices frigidam et humidem naturam habent. In cibo sumpta ventrem solvit.[37] Trita folia eius forunculos [BLs] Ms: furunculos] curat. Semen eius tritum cum vino ictericos curat. Folia eius tritia cum melle et nitro podagrae fervorem tollit.[38]	Atriplex umidae atque fridigae substantiae holus est amplius tamen ex umido possidet, et est illi sicut malvae facilis sucus ad lapsum. Inde in cibo sumptus indubitate ventrem resolvit. Crudus sive coctus inpositus duritas omnes ac furunculos sanat. Pernionibus qui ad huc aestuant, antequam invulnus erumpant utiliter inponitur. Scabros ungenes sine iniuria ulceris detrahit. Inges sacros sedat; podagrae fervorem cum nitro et aceto cum melle restingent. Galenus ad aurugenes expellendas vino tritum et in potione perductum efficacius putat semen eius.[39]

Gargilius' text is larger and he named his source, Galen.[40] Where Gargilius said that raw or cooked radishes are applied for all hardnesses (indurations) and it heals boils (or supporating tumors or furuncle), Dynamidia condensed the meaning to: *Its leaves perforated cure boils.* Gargilius: *It mitigates* (sedat) *jaundice* (ignes sacros); Dynamidia: *Its seeds pulverized with wine cure* (curat) *jaundice* (ictericos). Gargilius: [*Orache leaves?*] *with nitrum and vinegar with honey restrain the fever of gout,* Dynamadia: *Its leaves perforated with honey and nitrum get rid of fever from gout.* Do the changes indicate medical experience with such things as the force of the verbal actions (e.g., curat for sedat) or substitution of what is presumed to be a synonym for jaundice (e.g, ictericos for ignis sacer)[41], and the dropping of vinegar in the gout fever formula?

In the chapter on garlic (no. 44), Dynamidia employed almost literally the Latin translation of the Hippocratic Regimen and Gargilius' text but there is added new

36 John M. Riddle, Dioscorides, in: Catalogus Translationum et commentariorum, IV (Washington, Catholic University Press, 1981), 20–23.

37 De observ. cib., no. 63, p. 64 Mazzini (n. 13): Atriplices fridam et humidam virtutem habet, in cibo sumpta ventrem [non] solvit. (in its entirety).

38 Dynamidia, no. 23, p. 138 Rose (n. 8).

39 Gargilius, Medicina, no. 7. 142 (n. 14).

40 cf. Galen, De simpl med. 6, 74. XI 843–844 Kühn.

41 In the classical sense as used by Pliny (W. H. S. Jones, Pliny, 6, pp. x–xi, ignis sacer is a skin disease, probably shingles or lupus.

medicinal usages.[42] Some of the additional material is found in the Old Latin Translation of Dioscorides and some in Pliny, whom we can be reasonably sure was not a direct source for Dynamidia.[43]

Dynamidia's author wrote for medical purposes. His interest was the dietetical and medicinal uses of foods. While inspired by De observantia ciborum – the Latin translation of the Hippocratic Regimen, he was dissatisfied with its meager pharmacognostic content. After he dealt with the cereals, he expanded his resources by no longer relying exclusively on the Hippocratic work.

Aptly the title, Dynamidia, conveys the treatise's subject, the property of foods. It is misleading only insofar as it does not deal with drugs, pharmaca. As observed above, the Greek term dynamis has a complex and evolving concept. Its definitions in various classical Hippocratic works appear somewhat different from the understanding by the sixth century author.[44] Let me make a few general observations about the classical term which served as a foundation on which later interpretations were based. Each food, each drug, has its dynamis, its property, with an implication of potential and power. Also each body has its own dynamis so that a foreign substance, be it food or drug, introduced to it has an effect which is the combination of both the two dynamides, the body's and the object's, food or drug.[45] Therefore an effect may not merely be that of the property of, say, wine, but wine in a particular body at a particular time. One person may have a reaction different from another person with the same property in the wine.[46] Thus, a property conveys a potential but its exact activity is determined by a combination of factors.

By properties, Dynamidia's author did not distinguish primary and secondary qualities, the primary being cooling or warming and moistening or drying. He used terms with equal value, such as evacuating, restraining, tart, and irritating. Nor did the author seek to quantify the properties by the Galenic four degrees of intensity. For instance, Galen said that orache is moistening to the second degree, cooling

42 Dynamidia, no. 44, p. 142 Rose (n. 8); cf. Hippocratic. Regimen II 54, 6 Jones (n. 32) De observ. cib., no. 46, p. 62 Mazzini (n. 13); and cf. Gargilius, Medicina, no. 18, 150–151 Rose (n. 14). The text does not appear to come directly from Oribasius Euporistes (Latin), in: Ch. Daremberg and C. Bussemaker, Œuvres, 6 vols. (Paris, Imprimerie nationale, 1851–1876), 6, 403–626; cf. Henning Mørland, Die lateinischen Oribasiusübersetzungen (Symbolae Osloenses, Fasc. Suppl. 5) (Oslo, Brogger, 1932) and H. Mørland, Oribasius Latinus (S.O. Fasc. Suppl. 10) (Oslo, Brøgger, 1940); Pseudo-Theodorus, De simplici medicina, in: Theodori Prisciani Euporiston, V. Rose, ed. (Leipzig, Teubner, 1894), 401–423; Pseudo-Theodorus: Karl Sudhoff (ed.), "Diaeta Theodori". Archiv für Geschichte der Medizin 8 (1915) 377–403.

43 Latin Dioscorides 10, 230 Stadler (n. 33); Pliny, N. H. 20, 50–57.

44 Gert Plamböck, Dynamis in Corpus Hippocraticum (Akademie der Wissenschaften und der Literatur, Abh. geistes- und sozialwissenschaftl. Kl. 1964 no. 2). (Wiesbaden, Steiner, 1964); J. Soulhé, Étude sur le terme Dynamis (Paris, 1916), 32–36; Harold W. Miller, Dynamis and Physis in On Ancient Medicine. Trans. and Proceed. of the Amer. Philol. Assoc. 83 (1952) 184–197; H. Miller, The Concept of Dynamis in De victu. Trans. and Proceed. of the Amer. Philol. Assoc. 90 (1959) 147–164.

45 On ancient medicine (Περὶ ἀρχαίης ἰητρικῆς) 3, 43–44, I 18 Jones (n. 32).

46 Ibid., 5–8, 14–20 (example of wine in 20); cf. H. Miller, Concept (n. 43), 153–161.

to the first degree whereas Dynamidia said simply moistening and cooling.[47] Occasionally Dynamidia's author gave comparative values, such as a watermelon (no. 41) is *less cooling* than a canteloupe (no. 40) and a turnip (no. 31) is *most warming.*[48]

Dynamidia's theoretical basis was to administer by opposites.[49] A body in an unhealthy excessive dry condition might profit by a food or drug which moistens. Only through experience could one determine the property. Even here one had to be careful. Although Dynamidia did not copy the text of De observantia ciborum for the chapter on pomegranate (no. 79)[50], he was aware that the Hippocratic text said that acid pomegranates are cooling because Dynamidia gave pomegranate's property as warming and, uncharacteristically and unprecendentedly, Dynamidia borrowed from Gargilius' text but he omitted entirely Gargilius' assertion. *Almost all physicians agree in the opinion that the pomegranate has styptic power.*[51]

On properties Dynamidia's author seemingly had a mind of his own. Whereas De observantia ciborum said that radishes (no. 49) were moistening and Gargilius said *warming*, Dynamidia stated that they were *most warming* and he added to Gargilius' medicinal usages that they were a good emetic when taken with vinegar and honey.[52] Gargilius said that a medlar (no. 59) fruit is *most acid* (austerissimum); Dynamidia said *most sharp* (asperrimus) and added, *Before it matures, it is sticky and constrictive.*[53] Today we consider the medlar fruit as edible only when it is overripe.

In theory there is a correlation between the property (*δύναμις*) and the physical or medicinal effect on the body. The author of Regimen rejected the assertion that the same dynamis belonged to the same qualities in things: it does not follow therefore that all sweet things are laxative because some are binding, some drying, others moistening. *It is impossible to set forth these things in general,* he stated, therefore, they can be known *according to the particular* (*καθ' ἕκαστα*).[54] Without explicit acknowledgement, the author of Dynamidia accepted this. As an example among the few "cooling" remedies in this Latin treatise are orache (false spinach, no. 23), blite (no. 24), lettuce (no. 27), cantaloupe (no. 40), and prunes (no. 65), the latter called *most cooling.*[55] Nonetheless, the medicinal uses vary widely:

47 Galen, De simpl. med. 6, 73. XI 843 Kühn; Dynamidia, no. 32, p. 138 Rose (n. 8); on Galenic pharmacy theory, see Georg Harig, Bestimmung der Intensität im medizinischen System Galens (Berlin, Akademie Verlag, 1974).

48 Dynamidia, p. 141, 139 Rose (n. 8).

49 One of Dynamidia's direct sources, Gargilius, was explicit in this statement (Medicina, pp. 134–135 Rose [n. 14]).

50 De observ. cib., no. 49, p. 67 Mazzini (n. 13).

51 Medicina, pp. 179–180 Rose (n. 14). De punici arbore quod vim stypticam obtinet omnes fere medici una opinione consentiunt.

52 De observ. cib., no. 49, p. 62; Mazzini (n. 13); Gargilius, Medicina, no. 1, p. 193 Rose (n. 14); Dynamidia, no. 59, pp. 138, 141 Rose (n. 8).

53 Gargilius, Medicina, no. 47, p. 193 Rose (n. 14); Dynamidia, no. 59, p. 145 Rose (n. 8), 145.

54 Regimen II 39. IV 306 Jones (n. 32); H. Miller, Dynamis (n. 44), 155.

55 Dynamidia, pp. 138, 141 Rose (n. 8).

23. Orache: (cooling and moistening) loosens the bowels; cures furuncles (boils), jaundice and gout tumors.

24. Blite: (cooling and glueing) upsets the stomach, moves cholera, (given for) scorpion bites.

27. Lettuce: (cooling) pleasing to the appetite, causes sluggishness, makes the body weak, increases blood and lactation, and heals burns.

40. Canteloupe: (cooling) disagreeable to the stomach; alopecia; diuretic; treats stones.

As both the Greek Regimen and the Latin Dynamidia asserted, barley is cooling and moistening, but it is purging, deriving this property from the quality of the juice in the husks.[56] In classical medicine, heat was necessary for the body to cook food internally. Theoretically a cooling food would impede this process but moistening is also important to digestion. In the case of the barley, the moistening quality overcame the cooling, thus making barley laxative in its physiological effect.[57] Dynamidia's author did not have to reject a strict theoretical assertion that cold medicines are binding.

The case of lettuce serves to illustrate a point. Especially in the seeds, lettuce contains lactucarin which consists of lactucin, hyoscyamine, and mannite. Lactucarin is a narcotic and an opium substitute because of its similar but milder effects.[58] Classical medicine classified it as cooling because of its narcotic (deadening, therefore losening of innate heat).[59] Dynamidia classified it as cooling and, although employing Gargilius as its primary source[60], he contributed a revealing observation. Following the statement that lettuce causes sluggishness, Dynamidia's author added: *primarily rather it acts by its juice; the body is made weak from this part.*[61] Garden lettuce has far less lactucarin in it in comparison with wild lettuce; moreover, its leaves have but a trace. Dynamidia's concern was with its physiological reaction as food, not a pharmacon or drug. Nevertheless he seems aware of its dynamis, especially when he said: *lettuce in its different kinds has a cooling quality, not however uniformly harmful.*[62]

According to Dynamidia, some generalizations about properties were possible. In summarizing the wild vegetables, Dynamidia repeated the Latin translation of the Regimen, as follows:

56 Regimen II 40. IV 306 Jones (n. 32) (adding "drying"); De observ. cib., no. 4, p. 50 Mazzini (n. 13).

57 Regimen II 40. IV 306–310 Jones (n. 32).

58 Merck Index, 8th ed. (Rahway, N. J., Merck, 1968), 606; Dispensatory of the United States of America, 25th ed. (Philadelphia, Lippincott, 1955), 1732–1733.

59 Dioscorides, De materia medica 2, 136. I 208 Wellmann; Galen, In Hippocratis Librum de alimento commentarius eum commentarius 3, 7. XV 281 Kühn and De temperamentis 3, 4. I 677 Kühn.

60 Gargilius, Medicina, p. 144 Rose (n. 14).

61 Dynamidia, No. 27, p. 138 Rose (n. 8).

62 Ibid.

All wild vegetables are warming and they warm by the sweet smell and move the urine and pass through it. Those having a wet and cold nature have less strength and give a most harsh odor and evacuate [more easily through the bowels]. Those which are viscus and pungent will be more binding. Those that are sharp and cooling their juice moves the urine.[63]

Of all the questions yet to be addressed by historians of early medicine and pharmacy, an area of great promise for its potential insight is to evaluate the correlation between the way classical and medieval physicians matched properties and medicinal usages. To do this evaluation we must avail ourselves of the information that can only be supplied by modern science – botany, phytochemistry, pharmacognosy, medicine, to name a few. To accomplish this understanding, we need to evaluate the medicinal uses of the plants. Clearly Dynamidia is a medical work. In the sixth century, Dynamidia's author reached a decision after the data in his classical source, De observantia ciborum, proved insufficient – concerned as it was about dietetics. What were the medicinal usages which the Hippocratic writer omitted but still could usefully be employed? By the eighth plant, lentils, he supplemented the information in the Hippocratic work.

The entry on mint (no. 17) shows the concern of medicinal usages, apparently extending many beyond those in the written sources:

Mint has the property of cooling [later mss change to *warming*].[64] *With vinegar and sulphur, its juice helps jaundice* (ignos sacros); *with Attic honey and the milk of the perdicius plant, its juice wipes out darkness of the eyes* (caligo). *It checks vomiting. Its juice drunk with vinegar is good for those spitting up blood. With mastice its juice, made into a pill, glued together, settles boils/abscesses* (vocima).[65]

From Gargilius came the part about spitting blood.[66] De observantia ciborum had different properties, including calling mint a diuretic.[67] Dynamidia said (at least in the earliest extant manuscripts) that mint was cooling when both the direct Latin source, De observantia ciborum, and the Greek Regimen said *warming.*[68] Later manuscripts of Dynamdia change the property back to warming.[69] Later medieval medical works place mint as being warm and dry in the second degree of intensity.[70] Therefore, the uses for jaundice, tumors, head wounds, darkness of the

63 Ibid., pp. 141–142; cf. De observ. cib., no. 72, Mazzini ed. (n. 13), pp. 65–66.

64 St. Gallen Ms 762 has "calefacit et refrigerat"; Vatican Pal. lat. 1088 has "calidam" and both Vatican Regin. 1004 and London B. L. Ms Sloane 84 have "refrigeratoriam." De observ. cib. (n. 67 below) has "calefacit."

65 Dynamidia, no. 17, p. 136 Rose (n. 8), 136.

66 Gargilius, Medicina, no. 24, p. 158 Rose (n. 14), 158.

67 De observ. cib. no. 61, p. 64 Mazzini (n. 13).

68 Ibid.; Regimen II 54. IV 328 Jones (n. 32).

69 See note 64.

70 Constantine the African, De gradibus, in: Opera (Basel, Henricus Petrus, 1536), 359. Rufinus, Herbal, fol. 68va–b, L. Thorndike and F. Benjamin eds. (Chicago, Univ. of Chicago Press, 1946), 186–187, citing M. Platearius' Circa instans, Macer's Herbarius and Isaac's Particular Diet, as all agreeing.

eyes are either newly recorded uses or else in sources not extant or identified.[71] For sisymbrium (no. 18), which is probably a type of mint or nasturtium, Dynamidia gave a number of medicinal usages including one as an applicant on the forehead for headaches, and a treatment for eye and ear tumors, and he ended with an uncharacteristically imprecise comment: *Perforated its leaves [are put] in warm water and, if a fever is not present, in wine, and you will marvel.*[72]

Dynamidia's author and added to his source a statement that the juice of beet roots (no. 19) mixed with honey and put in the nasal passages purge the head.[73] Dynamidia said that dill (no. 29) causes sleep, an assertion that Galen had made.[74] Dynamidia added that basel (no. 32) is diuretic, good for headaches with rose oil and spitting of blood with mulsa, but he omitted its use as an ophthalmological agent, this despite the recommendation for this use by Gargilius, Pliny, Dioscorides, Aetius of Amida, and Pseudo-Apuleius.[75] Interestingly basel is not recommended for the eyes in modern herbals.[76] Cherry juice is good for coughs, Dynamidia asserted even though his working source, Gargilius, inexplicably omitted this usage.[77] Today cherry juice is frequently the base of cough syrups.[78]

Dynamidia's author directly contradicted his source. On peaches (no. 55), Gargilius wrote:

> *As a food peaches are indeed useless for the stomach because their juice quickly turns sour and their flesh likewise sours in the stomach... Galen advises us absolutely never to take them after a meal, asserting that they spoil if they float on other foods.*[79]

71 Some of the same sources checked are as in n. 42 above: see also Johann Heinrich Dierbach, Die Arzneimittel des Hippocrates (Heidelberg 1824; repr. Hildesheim, G. Olms, 1969), 168, as well as such standard authorities as Celsus, Pliny, Galen, and Dioscorides.

72 Dynamidia, no. 18, pp. 136–137 Rose (n. 8). Part of the text resembles but does not appear directly copied from Pseudo-Apuleius, Herbarius, (E. Howard and H. Sigerist, eds., Leipzig and Berlin [C.M.L., IV] 1927), no. 106, p. 189: 1. Ad vesicae dolorem et stranguiriam. Herba sisimbrium contritum except suco scripulos II. febricitanti ex aqua calida, non febricitanti ex vino potui dabis, remedialis mire.

73 Dynamidia, no. 19, p. 137 Rose (n. 8); cf. Gargilius, Medicina, p. 144 Rose (n. 14); Dioscorides (Old Latin Translation), De materia medica II PZ. 10, 220 Stadler (n. 33).

74 Dynamidia, no. 29, p. 139 Rose (n. 8); Galen, De simpl. med. 6, 45. XI 832 Kühn; cf. Paul of Aegina. Epitomae medicae, 7, 3. s.v., Francis Adams transl. in 3 vols. (London, Sydenham Society, 1844–1847) 46.

75 Dynamidia, no. 32, p. 139 Rose (n. 8); cf. Gargilius, Medicina, no. 22, pp. 156–157 Rose (n. 14); Pliny. N.H. 20, 119–124; Dioscorides, De materia medica 2, 141. I Wellmann; Aetius Iatrica 1, 418. I 146 Olivieri (C.M.G. Leipzig and Berlin, Teubner, 1935), Pseudo-Apuleius, Herbarius, no. 118, p. 204 Howald-Sigerist; cf. Dierbach, Arzn. Hipp. (n. 71), 178.

76 Wolfgang Schneider, Lexikon zur Arzneimittelgeschichte, 5 pt. 2 (Frankfurt a/M., Govi-Verlag, 1974), 368–369; M. Grieve, Modern Herbal, in 2 pts. (New York, Dover, 1971), 1, 86.

77 Dynamidia, no. 66, pp. 146–147 Rose; 146–147; cf. Gargilius, Medicina, no. 52, pp. 198–199 Rose (n. 15).

78 Varro E. Tyler, Lynn R. Brady and James E. Robbers, Pharmacognosy, 8th ed. (Philadelphia, Lea & Febiger, 1981), 71–72.

79 Gargilius, Medicina, no. 44, pp. 188–189 (Rose).

Virtually verbatim Dynamidia repeated that peaches are useless as a food but then he contradicted himself, Gargilius and, indirectly, Galen by adding: *Nevertheless if a peach is given after the meal, it is useful.*[80]

There were certain medical therapies for which Dynamidia's author was more inclined to add information. For one thing, he appeared more concerned with respiratory problems. He recommended figs, cherry juice, hazelnuts, and bitter almonds for coughs.[81] Remedies for intestinal parasites (no's. 13.70)[82] and ear troubles (70.74) are notable medical additions.[83] Certain omissions are observable. There are neither contraceptives nor abortifaciants even though they were in his direct sources' accounts. Gargilius said of summer savory:

> *Pregnant women are forbidden for this reason to eat it in their food [because it produces lust]. Crushed and applied upon the abdomen, it expels even dead fetuses.*[84]

Dioscorides recommended marjoram (3,39) as a pessary[85]; the Hippocratic Regimen said that summer savory acts the same way as marjoram.[86] While omitting any use as a pessary, Dynamidia felt obliged to say that summer savory ought not be placed in the uterus even while omitting to state why one might want to do it in the first place.[87]

Tumors were another medical interest of this unknown sixth century author of Dynamidia. To his known sources he added the following anti-tumoral remedies: celery (no. 16), mint (no. 17), sisymbrium (no. 18), and gourd (no. 22).[88] These chapters on the anti-tumoral remedies form a sequence: 16, 17, 18, and 22. Number 19 is cabbage – a classical anti-tumoral remedy – but Dynamidia omitted any explicit reference to it.[89]

In the treatise Hygiene Galen listed the moistening vegetables as follows: mallow, blite, sorrel, orache, and lettuce, as substitutes for cabbage; and the moistening fruits as: almond and terebinth seeds, gourd, mature cucumbers, prunes and black mulberries.[90] The chapter sequence in Dynamidia is as follows with a comparison to the sequence in Gargilius, Dioscorides, and Pliny:

80 Dynamidia, no. 55, p. 144 Rose (n. 8); tamen post cibum si datur utilitas est nec non. ....
81 Dynamidia, no.'s 62, 66, 68, and 74, pp. 146–148 Rose (n. 8).
82 Ibid., pp. 136, 147.
83 Ibid., pp. 147–148.
84 Gargilius, Medicina, no. 20, p. 153 Rose (n. 14).
85 Dioscorides, De materia medica 3, 39. II 52 Wellmann, 52.
86 Regimen II 54, 52. IV 332 Jones (n. 32).
87 Dynamidia, no. 51, p. 143 Rose (n. 8): Ideo in utero habentibus dare proibetur.
88 Ibid., pp. 136–137.
89 Ibid., p. 137; cf. Cato, De agricultura. 156, 1, 3–4 Hooper Ash (W. D. Hooper and H. B. Ash, eds. [Cambridge, Harvard University Press, and London, Heinemann, 1934]); cf. John Riddle, Ancient and Medieval Chemotherapy for Cancer. Isis 76 (1985),319–330.
90 Galen, Hygiene 5, 8. VI 351 Kühn.

Plant	Dynamidia	Discorides	Pliny	Gargilius
cabbage	20	II. 120	20.78–96	–
mallow	21	II. 118	20.84	5
gourd	22	II. 134	20.7	6
orache	23	II. 119?	20.83	7
blite	24	II. 117	20.93	9
sorrel	25	II. 114	20.85–6	8
coriander	26	III. 63	20.82	4
lettuce	27	II. 136	20.60	11

But Dynamidia's author said that the properties of these plants are:

cabbage	none listed
marrow	purging
gourd	warming and moistening
orache	moistening and cooling
blite	cooling and glueing
sorrel	warming and pungent
coriander	warming and astringent
lettuce	cooling

In Dioscorides' work this sequence of drugs was all for sores, ulcers, and various other dermatological afflictions where, if I understand correctly, a drying action is more appropriate. Also many were for intestinal parasites. The exception to the Dioscorides' general order is with the coriander plant which is in Dioscorides' Book Three but Galen said that Dioscorides was wrong about coriander's properties.[91] Dioscorides arranged drugs by affinities, that is to say by the physiological reactions that drugs have on and in the body.[92] The order is close to Gargilius' sequencing but Dynamidia chose not follow Gargilius' order and instead he made his own sequence. On one hand, the sequence is too close to Galen's listing of moistening plant foods for there not to have been a relationship. On the other hand, the property "moistening" is clearly not the affinity relationship that Dynamidia's author saw in these plants, because he named only two of the eight as having a moistening quality.

There is, however, a method to Dynamidia's arrangements which is not entirely clear but it is clear that there is a method, as is seen by the sequencing of the antitumoral remedies. The order is neither that of Dioscorides' sequencing by pharmaceutical affinities nor, is it on the properties as Galen and later Constantine the African proposed. Dynamidia appears to have developed his own scheme or else modified Gargilius' method because Dynamidia arranged plants on the basis of a combination of pharmaceutical affinities and botanical characteristics. For an example, Dynamidia's plants 23, 24, and 25 are:

91 Galen, De simpl. med. 6, 73. XI 843 Kühn; cf. Dioscorides. De materia medica. 3, 63. II 74 Wellmann.

92 John Riddle, Dioscorides on Pharmacy and Medicine (Austin, University of Texas Press, 1985).

orache of the Goosefoot (Chenopodiaceae) family
blite of the Cockscomb (Amaranthaceae) family
sorrel/dock of the Dock (Polygonaceae) family.[93]

While each belong to the different families, the families are in almost perfect botanical relationship. Each family is kin to the other. This sequence is not likely coincidental, but, of course, the sixth century author did not discern the fine botanical distinctions made by the Linnean system. Probably what he based his order on was the dietary affinities: things having a similar taste, smell, and dietary effect he saw as properly being in association with one another. This thesis needs further study. Part of the difficulty in trying to discern the method is that in our age dietetics is not as well advanced as pharmacognosy. We have difficulty matching our understanding of the nature of food substances to what was a natural and reasonable order to someone in the sixth century.

In summary, the sixth century author of Dynamidia was not broadly interested in drugs (pharmaca) but in the medicinal and dietary effects of foods. He based the first part of his work on what was almost a straight copying from De observantia ciborum, a sixth century literal translation from Book Two of the Hippocratic work, Regimen. He began with cereals but in the part where he came to the beans, he began to add new material, much of it coming directly from Gargilius' third century work and, possibly, some from the Old Latin Translation of Dioscorides De materia medica. What the source or sources for the other material which he used is unclear, but, whether it was largely new information derived from experience or from unidentified written sources, the author employed rational judgments about what to include and exclude. The presentation method was by gross classification of food stuffs: cereals, beans, garden vegetables, wild vegetables and herbs, sharp herbs, fruits, and nuts. Within each of these categories he arranged his order by what appears to be dietary affinities, which resemble but do not match the order by Gargilius and Dioscorides. Dioscorides and possibly Gargilius arranged drugs by pharmaceutical affinities. Dynamidia's author was concerned with properties as well as the medicinal and dietary usages of food stuffs. A theoretical basis underlies the work which rests on how the Middle Ages thought that the body worked. Further study is warranted in order to perceive the quality of their observations because clearly neither the treatise's author nor those who may have used the work in medicine during the early Middle Ages had the same understanding of the body, foods and drugs as that in the Hippocratic work on which it is based nor that in other classical works nor that in late scholastic medicine.

93 Dynamidia, no.'s 23–25, p. 138 Rose (n. 8).

KEY TO LIST OF HERBS

Dynamidia:

Valentin Rose, Anecdota Graeca et Graecolatina. 2 vols. Berlin, 1864–1870; repr. Amsterdam, Hakkert 1963. 2 (1870), 105–128.

London, British Library, Ms Sloane 84 (670), s. xi, fols. 34–40.

Regimen Hippocratis

W. H. S. Jones, Hippocrates in 4 vols. Loeb Classical Library. Cambridge, Harvard University Press; London, Heinemann 1923–1931. 4 (1931), 224–447.

De observantia ciborum

Innocenzo Mazzini, De observantia ciborum, Università di Macerata. Pubblicazioni della Facoltà di Lettere e Filosofia Instituto di Filologia Classica, No. 18, Rome, Giorgio Bretschneider. 1984.

Gargilius, Medicina:

Valentin Rose. Plinii Secundi quae fertur una cum Gargilii Martialis Medicina, Leipzig, Teubner. 1870, pp. (129)–208.

Pliny, Natural History:

W. H. S. Jones, Pliny. Natural History. in 10 vols. Loeb Classical Library, 10 vols. Cambridge, Harvard University Press, and London, Heinemann, 1969–1980. 6–8.

Dioscorides, De materia medica (Greek):

Max Wellmann, Pedanii Dioscuridis Anazarbei De materia medica libri quinque. 3 vols. Berlin, 1906–1914; repr. Berlin, Weidmann, 1958.

(Latin):

K. Hoffmann, T. M. Auracher, and H. Stadler, Dioscorides Longobardus. Romanische Forschungen 1 (1822) 49–105; 10 (1897) 181–247, 369–466; 11 (1899) 1–121; 13 (1902) 161–243; 14 (1903) 601–637.

LIST OF HERBS IN:

	Herb	Modern Name	Popular English Name	Hippocratic Regimen Bk. II *line no., Jones ed.	De observantia ciborum
1.	ordei	Hordeum vulgare	Barley [Graminea]	40.1	4
2.	polenta	Hordeum vulgare	Barley meal* *(mixture with water, wine or milk, honey and other spices)	40.8	4
3.	tritici	Triticum sp.	Wheat [Graminea]	43.1	6
4.	faba	Vicia faba L.	Horse bean [Leg.]	45.1	7
5.	pisus	Pisum arvense L.	Pea [Leg.]	45.3	8
6.	fasiolum	Dolichos Lablab. Arab.	Hyacinth bean [Leg.]	45.5	9
7.	cicer	Cicer arietinum L.	Chick pea [Leg.]	45	10
8.	lenticula	Lens culinaris L.	Lentil [Leg.]	45.14*	12*
			*Gk. text says "Lentils are warming and trouble the bowels; they are neither laxative nor astringent." Latin text has: "Lentils pull down the bowels greatly and the urine."		
9.	milium	Panicum miliaceum L.	Millet	45.10	11
	farina	Setaria italica L.	Italian millet		
10.	erbum	Vicia ervilia L.	Bitter vetch	45.15	13
11.	oridia	Oryza sativa L.	Rice		15

DYNAMIDIA HIPPOCRATIS

Properties	Gargi-lius	Pliny	Dioscorides	Latin Dios.	Source	New Information or from unknown source
Cold & wet		18.13 71–14.74	2.86	ΞΘ	Hipp.	No
Wet		18.18.78f			Hipp.	No
		18.20.85f	2.85	ΞΗ	Hipp.	No
Nourishing & Astringent			2.105	ΠΗ	Hipp.	No
Evacuating & less inflative		18.31.123f			Hipp.	No
Evacuating, inflative & nourishing					Hipp.	No
Mollifying, diuretic & nourishing		18.32.124	2.104		Hipp.	No
Binding of bowels & kidneys [deducit]		18.31.123f	2.107	Q	Hipp.	No
Dry & binding		18.22.96f	2.97–8	OΘ Π	Hipp.	No
Very strong: binding, strengthening, fattening		18.37.137–8	2.108	QA	Hipp.	No
Constraining the stomach & slowing evacuation*			2.95	OZ	?	

*Latin Dios. says: [orizia] eustomaca est, ventrem abstines.

	Herb	Modern Name	Popular English Name	Hippocratic Regimen Bk. II *line no., Jones ed.	De observantia ciborum
12.	lini semen	Linum usitatissimum L.	Linseed [Linaceae]	45.17	14
13.	lupinus	Lupinus sp.	Lupin [Leg.]	45.20	16
14.	herysimum (crisimum)	Sisymbrium officinale L.	Hedge mustard [Cruciferae]	45.22	17
15.	sesamum	Sesamum indicum L.	Sesame (seeds)	45.25	19
16.	apium	Apium graveoleus L.* *Sometimes combined with parsley	Celery (Umbelliferae)	54.25	55
17.	menta	Menthe sp.	Mint (Libiatae)	54.37	61
18.	sisymbrium	Mentha genilis L. Sisymbrium sophia L. Tanacetum Balsemita L. Nasturtium officinalis L. Stachy germanica		–	–
19.	beta nigra beta alba	Beta vulgaris L.+	Beet	54.45	64
20.	caulium	Brassica sp.	Cabbage	54.43	65
21.	malva	Malva sylvestris L.	Mallow		
22.	cucurbita	Citrullus colocynthis L.	Gourd	54.46	67

DYNAMIDIA HIPPOCRATIS

Properties	Gargilius	Pliny	Dioscorides	Latin Dios.	Source	New Information or from unknown source
Nourshing, restraining & cooling		19.2.7f	2.103	ΠZ	Hipp.	No
Warming, very strong		18.36.133–136	2.109	QB	Hipp.	Yes
Moistens and evacuates		18.22.96	2.158	PMΔ	Hipp.	No
Evacuating, filling & fattening		18.22.96	2.99	ΠB	Hipp.	No
Diuretic & evacuating	2	20.44 112–5	3.64	ΞH	Hipp.	Yes
Cooling [Warmin in some later Mss]	24	20.53. 147–151	3.34	ΛZ	?	
[Later Mss add "warming"]	Interpolated	20.91.247–8	3.41	MΓ	?	
	10	20.27.69–72	2.123	PZ	Latin Diosc. +	Yes
	30	19.41.139–41 20.34.84–96	2.120	PΔ	Hipp. + (poss. four words)	Yes
Purging	5	20.84.222–30	2.118	PB	?	
Warming, moisturing & evacuating	6	20.7.13, 8.14–17	2.134 [135]	PIH	Gargilius, Latin Diosc?	Yes

LIST OF HERBS IN:

	Herb	Modern Name	Popular English Name	Hippocratic Regimen Bk. II *line no., Jones ed.	De observantia ciborum
23.	atriplex	Atriplex sp.	Orache [Chenopodiacea]	54.41	63
24.	bletus	Amaranthus blitium L.	Blite [Amaranthacese]	54.42	64
25.	lapacius	Rumex sp.	Dock or Sorrel [Polygonacese]	54.41	62
26.	coriandrum	Coriandrum sativum L.	Coriander [Umbelliferae]	54.22	52
27.	lactuca	Lactuca sp.	Lettuce	54.24	53
28.	intibu	Cichorium intybus L.*	Chicory		
		C. endiva L.	Endive		
			*Dyn. says that there are two kinds: one bitter, one sweet		
29.	anethum	Anethium graveolens L.	Dill	54.26	54
30.	pastinaca	Pastinaca sp. (incl. P. satival L.)	Wild parnip [Umb.]		
		Daucus carota L.	Wild carrot		
31.	rapus napus*	Brassica Rapa L.+?	Turnip	54.49	68
		*Dyn conflates two terms rapus and napus, for two kinds of turnips			
32.	ocymum	Ocimum basilicum L. [Libiatae]	Basil	54.27	56
33.	olisatrum	Smyrnium olusatrum L.	Alexanders		
34.	portulaca	Portulaca deraca L.	Purslane	54.33	60

DYNAMIDIA HIPPOCRATIS

Properties	Gargilius	Pliny	Dioscorides	Latin Dios.	Source	New Information or from unknown source
Cooling & moistening	7	20.83.219–21	2.119? Interpolation		Gargilius	Yes
Cooling & glueing	9	20.93.252	2.117	PA	Gargilius?	Yes
Warm, tart	8	20.85.231–3	2.114	QH	Gargilius	No
Warming & astringent	4	20.82.216	2.63	PΞ	Hipp. & Gargilius	Yes
Cooling	11	20.26.60f	2.136	PKA	Hipp. & Gargilius	Yes
	12	20.29.73, 30.74–5	2.132	PIZ	Gargilius	Yes
Warming & restraining	28	20.74.196	3.58	ΞΓ	Hipp. & (?) Gargilius	Yes
Warming & tart	33	20.14.29	3.52	NE	Gargilius	Yes
Most warming, disquieting & diuretic	34.35	20.9.18–11.21	2.110	QΓ QΔ	Hipp.	Yes
Drying & stringent	22	20.48.119–24	2.141	PKZ	Hipp. & Gargilius	Yes
Warming & tart	26	20.46.117	3.67	OB	?	
Fesh, cooling, later warming & purging	Interpolation from Dyn.		2.124	PH	Hipp.	Yes

LIST OF HERBS IN:

	Herb	Modern Name	Popular English Name	Hippocratic Regimen Bk. II *line no., Jones ed.	De observantia ciborum
35.	escaria	Isatis sp.?	Woad (possibly)		
36.	abortanum	Artemisia arb-orescema L.	Southern wormwood		
37.	ruta	Ruta graveo-lens L. +	Rue	54.30	57
38.	feniculus	Foeniculum vulgare Gaert.	Fennel	54.64	73
39.	panagorace	?			
40.	cucumeris	Cucumis melo L.	Cantaloupe	55.24(?)	18(?)
41.	pepo	Citrullus vul-garis Schradar	Watermelon		
42.	carduo	Cynara car-dunculus L.	Artichoke		
43.	papaver	Papaver sp.	Poppy	45.29	20
44.	alium	Allium sp.	Garlic	54.6	46
45 a.	cepa	Allium cepa L.	Onion	54.8	47

DYNAMIDIA HIPPOCRATIS

Properties	Gargilius	Pliny	Dioscorides	Latin Dios.	Source	New Information or from unknown source
Neutral (mediam)	Interpolation from Dyn.	20.25 59	2.184–5	,,	?	
Warming	Interpolation from Dyn.	21.34.60	3.24	KE	?	
Warming	3	20.51 131–43	3.45	MZ	?	
Warming, sharp	25	20.45. 254	3.70	OE	Gargilius	Yes
Warming	Interpolation from Dyn.				?	
Cooling	16	22.5.10	2.135	PIΘ	Gargilius	Yes
Less cooling	15	20.6.11–2			Gargilius	Yes
Caustic & less sharp (mordax et sub austera)	17	20.99. 262	3.14	IΔ	Gargilius	Yes
Restringent, replenishing, and most strong	19	20.76. 198–78. 206	4.63–4	no.59–60	Hipp.	Yes
Warming & diuretic	18	20.23. 50–7	2.152	PΛH	Hipp. Gargilius(?)	Yes
Warming & irritating	27	20.20. 39–43	2.151	PΛZ	Hipp., Gargilius?, Latin Dios.?	Yes

LIST OF HERBS IN:

	Herb	Modern Name	Popular English Name	Hippocratic Regimen Bk. II *line no., Jones ed.	De observantia ciborum
45 b.	ulpicum*	Allium ursinum L. A. vineale L. + sp. *Not in BLS/84	Wild onion		
46.	rafanus	Raphanns sativus L.	Radish	54.15	49
47.	porros	Alium porrum L.	Leek	54.12	48
48.	sinapus	Sinapis alba L.	White mustard	54.19	51
49.	nasturcium [cardamonum-BLs] ms]	Lepidium sativum L.	Garden cress	54.18	50
50.	eruca	Eruca sp.	Rocket	54.12	51* *with sinapus
51.	satureia	Satueria hortensis L.	Summer savory	54.52	70
52.	malus	Malus domestica L.	Apple	55.8	76–77
53.	pira	Pyrus communis L.	Pear	55.3	74
54.	cidonie	Cydonia oblonga L.	Quince	55.9	
55.	persica	Prunus persica L.	Peach		

DYNAMIDIA HIPPOCRATIS

Properties	Gargilius Interpolation	Pliny	Dioscorides	Latin Dios.	Source	New Information or from unknown source
Most warming	1	20.13. 23–8	2.112	PZ	Hipp., Gargilius	Yes
Less warming, diuretic & evacuating	21	20.21. 42–22. 49	2.149	PΛE	Hipp., Gargilius(?) Latin Dios. (?)	Yes
Warming & evacuating	29	20.87. 236–240	2.154	PM	Hipp, Gargilius(?)	Yes
Warming	13	20.50. 127–30	2.155	PMA	Hipp., Latin Dios(?)	Yes
Warming & caustic	14	20.49. 125–6	2.140	PKE PKZ	Gargilius	Yes
Warming, almost fiery	20	19.50. 165	3.37	ΛΘ	Gargilius	Yes
Moistening & cooling; wild apples [crab apples?] are astringent	42	23.54. 100f.	1.159	PKB	Gargilius	Yes
Styptic	40	23.62. 115–6	1.116	PKZ	Gargilius	No
Styptic, sharp	43	23.54. 101f	2.115	PKΓ	Gargilius	Yes
	44	23.67. 132	1.129	PKE	Gargilius	Yes

	Herb	Modern Name	Popular English Name	Hippocratic Regimen Bk. II *line no., Jones ed.	De observantia ciborum
56.	armoniaci	Prunus armeniaca L.	Apricot		
57.	citrus	Citrus medica L.	Citron		
58.	pruna	Prunus domestica L.	Plum		
59.	mespela	Mespilus germanica L.	Medler	55.10	75
60.	zyzavarum	Ziziphus jujuba Miller	Jujube		
61.	sorba et precordia	Sorbus domestica L. poss. S. torminglis L. or Prunus ameniaci L.	Service tree (sometimes used for apricots)	55.15	78
62.	ficas	Ficus sp.	Figs	55.26	82
63.	uva uva passa	Vitis sp.	Grape vines Grapes	55.22	81
64.	pomum mori (mora)	Morus nigra L.	Mulberries	55.72	74
65.	Nixum	from Prunus domestica L.	Prune (cf. n. 58)		
66.	cerasi	Prunus cerasus L. + sp.	Cherry		
67.	tuberus	Crataegus azarolus L.			

DYNAMIDIA HIPPOCRATIS

Properties	Gargilius	Pliny	Dioscorides	Latin Dios.	Source	New Information or from unknown source
Warming, styptic	Interpolation	16.42.103	1.115		?	
Center is warming; seeds, acid & styptic	45	23.56.105	1.115	PKE(?)	Gargilius	Yes
Drying	46	23.66 132	1.121	PΛB	Gargilius	No
Most sharp	47	23.73.141	1.118	PKΘ	Gargilius	Yes
Warming	48				Gargilius	Yes
Sticky & constrictive, most warming	50		1.120	PΛ	Hipp.	Yes
Moistening, evacuating & warming	49	23.63.117–64.130	1.28	PM	?	
Warming, moistening & evacuating	49b		5.1f	A	Hipp.	No
Cooling		23.70.134–71.140	1.126	PΛH	?	
Most cooling	46	23.66.132	1.121	PΛB	?	
Moistening	52	23.72.141	1.113	PKA	Gargilius, Latin Dios.?	Yes
Styptic		23.73.141	1.118	PKΘ	?	

	Herb	Modern Name	Popular English Name	Hippocratic Regimen Bk. II *line no., Jones ed.	De observantia ciborum
68.	abellana	Corylus avellana L.	Hazel nut		
69.	castania	Castanea sativa Miller	Chestnut	55.37	85
70.	balamus	from Quercus sp.	Acorn	55.37	85
71.	pistacium	Pistachia lentiscus L.	Pistachio		
72.	iugulandis	Juglans regia L.	Walnut	55.36	84
73.	amigdala dulcia	Amygdalus communis var. Sativa Ludw.	Sweet almond	55.32	83
74.	amigdala amara	A. communis var. Amara D.C.	Bitter almond	55.12	83
75.	puncia	Puncia granatum L.	Pomegranate	55.16	79
76.	pinorum nucleos	from Pinus sp.	Pine cones		
77.	palmarum tebaicarum	Hyphaena thebaica Mart.	Doum palm		
78.	pira matura	? [Test not found in BLs/ms]			

DYNAMIDIA HIPPOCRATIS

Properties	Gargi-lius	Pliny	Diosc-orides	Latin Dios.	Source	New Infor-mation or from un-known source
Styptic	54	23.78. 150	1.125	PΛZ	Gargilius	Yes
Very strong ("fortissimum")	56		1.106		Gargilius	Yes
Stringent			1.106		?	
Sharp, styp-tic	55		1.177	PΛϛ	Gargilius	No
Styptic, cool-ing	47	23.77. 147–9	1.125	PΛZ	Hipp., Gargilius	Yes
Most warming, nutricious	53		1.123	PΛE	Hipp., Gargilius	Yes
Stronger than sweet almond	53	23.75. 144.5	1.123	PΛE	?	
Warming-sweet kind Cooling-bitter kind	41		1.110	PIΘ	Gargilius	No
Most warming	58	23.74. 142–3	1.69	OZ	?	
Nutritious & soporific			1.109	PIH	?	
Warming						

XII

Ancient and Medieval Chemotherapy for Cancer

IN 1916 DR. WILLIAM S. STONE, who became the director for cancer research at New York Memorial Hospital, addressed his colleagues about cancer. Both his own and his father's generation, he explained, treated cancer mostly by surgery; chemical treatments had been virtually abandoned long before. His argument calling for reexamination of the issue was largely historical, based on the observation that classical and early medieval "treatment of the disease . . . almost invariably consist[ed] of arsenic, zinc, or the alkaline caustics." The historical testimony ought to be presumption, he implied, that chemical agents had some beneficial results, even though in his age there had been, in his words, "unqualified condemnation" of them.[1]

Stone's exhortation did not usher in a "second age of chemotherapy" for cancer, however. That age can perhaps be dated to 1938, when A. P. Dustin published his report about the antimitotic properties of colchicine, found in *Colchicum autumnale* L. C. Gordon Zubrod would date modern cancer chemotherapy to about 1935, with the investigation of the effect of bacterial toxins on human sarcomas. Others argue that the true beginning of modern cancer chemotherapy was in World War II, with the research on nitrogen mustards, but, because of security, the results were not published until after the war. Finally, a few note that the experiments by Paul Ehrlich in 1908 on transplantable tumors in rodents anticipated modern chemotherapy.[2] No one, however, disputes that

I express my appreciation to Allen Vegotsky and Samuel Tove for their expert suggestions and to the Division of Cancer Treatment (National Cancer Institute, National Institutes of Health) for helpful information.

[1] W. S. Stone, "A Review of the History of Chemical Therapy in Cancer," *Medical Review*, 7 Oct. 1916, *90*:628–634, quoting pp. 628, 633.

[2] See A. P. Dustin, "Nouvelles applications des poisons caryoclassiques à la cancerologie," *Sang*, 1938, *12*:677–697, based on his earlier study on the mitotic changes induced by colchicine in a rat's Crocker sarcoma: Dustin, "Contribution à l'étude des poisons caryoclassiques sur les tumeurs animales . . . ," *Bulletin de l'Academie Royale de Médecine de Belgique*, 1934, *14*:487–502; on bacterial toxins, see C. Gordon Zubrod, "Origins and Development of Chemotherapy Research at the National Cancer Institute," *Cancer Treatment Reports*, 1984, *68*:9–19, on p. 9; on mustard gas, see Forest Ray Moulton, ed., *Approaches to Tumor Chemotherapy* (Washington, American Association for the Advancement of Science, 1947); and for Ehrlich see Paul Ehrlich, *Experimental Researches on Specific Therapeutics*. (Harben Lectures for 1907) (London: H. K. Lewis, 1908); and Vincent T. DeVita, Jr., "Principles of Chemotherapy," in *Cancer: Principles and Practice of Oncology*, ed. DeVita, Samuel Hellman, and Steven A. Rosenberg, (Philadelphia: Lippincott, 1982), pp. 132–155, on pp. 132–133. A few oncologists look to an earlier remedy as a stimulant to chemical therapy. In 1865 Lissauer ("Zwei Falle von Leucaemie," *Berliner Klinische Wochenschrift*, 1865, *2*:403–404) reported a useful systemic agent in the treatment of neoplastic diseases. The agent was potassium arsenite, which became know as Fowler's solution, but it also produced arsenical keratosis and carcinomas, as reported by Jonathan Hutchinson, "On Some Examples of Arsenic-Keratosis of the

in recent decades complex organic compounds, often plant alkaloids, have produced increasingly successful results as one by one new agents are found and clinically tested.

In 1955 the United States Cancer Chemotherapy National Service Center (NSC) began cataloguing potential plant antitumor agents.[3] Many plants were nominated as candidates for listing by "both the technical literature and folklore." Although historical sources were included under the rubric "folklore," no qualitative historical research was employed to identify potential agents. Many major medical writings were not systematically searched and, for the most part, they were read in translations. The resultant NSC catalogue was impressive in size, but because a single suggestion of a plant in any type of source qualified the plant for the list, so many were listed—over 3,000 species—that using the guide for laboratory testing is difficult.

A more historically oriented approach could well constitute such a guide. A search through the leading pharmaceutical and medical authorities of the Greco-Roman, classical Islamic, and medieval periods reveals that they recommended many of the same natural sources as those for the compounds discovered in the 1960s and 1970s and currently utilized in cancer treatments. For example, in the first century Dioscorides (fl. ca. A.D. 50–79) employed a drug made from autumn crocus (*Colchicum autumnale* L.), the very plant investigated by A. P. Dustin in 1938, as an antitumor agent. Dioscorides recommended that the plant (*kolchikon*) be "soaked in wine and administered to dissolve tumors (*oidêmata*) and growths (*phumata*) not yet making pus."[4] Compounds from this and other plants were neither historically nor are they now the "magic bullet," but they are helpful, sometimes very helpful, in cancer therapy.

"CANCER" IN ANTIQUITY AND THE MIDDLE AGES

Several questions must be answered before recommendations like Dioscorides' can be evaluated, whether historically, for the light they shed on the medicine of the time—especially its probable efficacy—or scientifically, for the direction they might give to current research. First, we need to know whether the ancients had cancers and whether their medicine was capable of distinquishing between benign and malignant neoplasms. The answer to the first question is assuredly affirmative. There is persuasive paleopathological evidence, and such authorities

Skin and of Arsenic-Cancer," *Transactions of the Pathological Society of London*, 1888, *39*:352–363. For a review of systemic therapy of cancer, see Michael B. Shimkin, *Some Classics of Experimental Oncology: 50 Selections, 1775–1965* (NIH Publication No. 80-2150) (Washington, Department of Health and Human Services, 1980), pp. 651–704.

[3] J. L. Hartwell, "Plants Used Against Cancer," *Lloydia*, 1967, *30*:379–436; 1968, *31*:71–170; 1969, *32*:79–107, 153–205, 247–296; 1970, *33*:97–194, 288–392; 1971, *34*:103–160, 204–255, 310–361, 386–438; reprinted in Hartwell, *Plants Used Against Cancer: A Survey* (Lawrence, Mass.: Quarterman Publications, 1982). For an excellent discussion of advantages and disadvantages of "folklore" nomination of plants for screening, see Matthew Suffness and John Douros, "Drugs of Plant Origin," *Methods in Cancer Research*, 1979, *16*:76–126, on pp. 76–77.

[4] Dioscorides, *De materia medica*, 4.84, ed. Max Wellmann, 3 vols. (Berlin: Weidmann, 1906–1914; rpt. 1958). This and other translations, unless otherwise noted, are my own. For what can be deduced about Dioscorides' life and career, see John Scarborough and Vivian Nutton, "The Preface of Dioscorides' *Materia Medica*: Introduction, Translation, Commentary," *Transactions and Studies of the College of Physicians of Philadelphia*, 1982, N.S. *4*:187–227, on pp. 192–194; and John Riddle, *Dioscorides in Medicine and Pharmacy*, (Austin: Univ. Texas Press, 1985).

as Galen (A.D. 129–post 210) and Avicenna (ca. 980–1037), gave good descriptions of neoplastic tumors.[5] Galen and the Byzantines used the term *onkos* to cover swellings, all types of tumors, and lesions. Ancient and medieval writers employed a variety of terms to describe tumors and other lesions, many of which will be discussed in this article.

From the Hippocratic period, the belief in the etiology of cancer was fairly constant. It was an inflammation (Greek *phlegmonê, phlogôsis*; Latin *inflammatio*) derived from an excess of black bile. Avicenna describes a "malignant" tumor as follows:

> Cancer [*cancer* in Gerard of Cremona's Latin translation] is an atrabilious [black bile] swelling (tumor); its development is from combustible (metabolized) atrabile through a biliary substance or through a substance in which there is a biliary element combusted (metabolized) from it, not through turbid drainage. It differs from *scirrhus* [benign solid tumor which may turn malignant] by being accompanied by pain, acuteness and some degree of beating (throbbing) and rapid growth because of increase of (its) substance and swelling as a manifestation of this substance boiling at its junction with the organ. It differs also (from the scirrhus) by the vessels which formed around it to the organ in which it exists simulating the legs of cancer crab and it is not red as *cellulitis* but "with a trend" to blackness, heat and greenness. . . . And it differs from the true scirrhus by being sensitive while the former has no sensitivity. On its onset it (cancer) is concealed and when it is manifested it is problemic in most cases. Then its signs become apparent. And the initial manifestation is a small solid rounded sprout, dark in color, with some kind of warmth. And there is a kind of cancer that is very painful and there is a kind that produces little pain; silent. And there is a kind of cancer that is unchanged, does not ulcerate.[6]

Galen and Avicenna both characterized most malignant tumors as potentially suppurating, and Galen was especially careful to distinguish suppurating atrabilious metabolizations from those excretions that come from boils, carbuncles, and ulcers.[7]

Greek and Latin had a number of terms that covered malignant tumors; many that may refer to a malignant tumor will be discussed in this article, but only in specific contexts about their therapy. Dioscorides' terms *oidêmata* and *phumata* probably included malignancies, but they were not restricted to that condition. Also there is Galen's Greek term *karkinos* (sometimes *karkinôma*; Latin, *cancer*) which often meant malignant lesions, but not always. Obviously the ancients could not have had the histological diagnosis for malignant neoplasms that

[5] For paleopathological evidence, see D. Brothwell, in *Diseases in Antiquity* (Springfield: Thomas, 1967), pp. 320–345; Keith Manchester, "Secondary Cancer in an Anglo-Saxon Female," *Journal of Archaeological Science*, 1983, *10*:475–482; Aidan and Eve Cockburn, *Mummies, Disease and Ancient Cultures* (Cambridge, Cambridge Univ. Press, 1983), pp. 37–38; for descriptions, see Galen, *De tumoribus praeter naturam*, in *Opera omnia*, ed. C. G. Kühn, 20 vols. (Leipzig, 1821–1833; Hildesheim: Olms, 1965), Vol. VII, pp. 705–732; Avicenna, *Canon*, 1.2.1.5–4.3.1.15 (Venice, 1507; facs. ed. Hildesheim: Olms, 1964); Aristotelis Eftychaidis, "The Oncology of Nicolaos Myrepsus in Byzantium of the 13th Century" (in Greek), *Hellenic Oncology*, 1981, *17*:38–47, and Eftychaidis, "Oncological Opinions of Byzantine Medical Writers: Neophytus, Maximus Planudes, and John, Bishop of Prisdaunon" (in Greek), *Hell. Onc.*, 1981, *17*:109–116; for an excellent discussion of the Greek terms for cancer, see L. J. Rather, *The Genesis of Cancer: A Study in the History of Ideas* (Baltimore: Johns Hopkins Press, 1978), pp. 9–13.

[6] Avicenna, *Canon*, 4.3.1.15, trans. from Arabic in I. Eltorai, "Avicenna's View on Cancer from his Canon," *American Journal of Chinese Medicine*, 1979, *8*:276–284, quoting from pp. 277, 280.

[7] Galen, *De tumoribus*, 3, in *Opera*, ed. Kühn, Vol. VII, pp. 715–716, trans. in Jeremiah Reedy, "Galen on Cancer and Related Diseases," *Clio Medica*, 1975, *10*:227–238, on p. 232.

we have. We can only conclude that their terms had the lexical range to include malignancies in our sense of the term. In the instance above, Dioscorides probably meant his therapy to apply to malignant neoplastic lesions, for we know the ancients had cancer, that they recognized it (although not precisely), that Dioscorides was correctly pointing to it when he implied suppuration, and that this particular therapy, because of its side effects, would probably not have been resorted to for a benign tumor.

Any claim that the ancients had an effective cancer "cure" must be qualified, perhaps even denied. Since Dioscorides gives no information about the exact preparation, concentration of colchicine, dosage, frequency, or administration site, the likely efficacy of his treatment cannot be estimated. Such information, critical to modern evaluations, was not usually given by classical and medieval authorities. Any instructions given are never adequate when judging potential effects of toxic—antimitotic and cytotoxic—drugs employed in cancer therapy. Premodern authorities assumed that their work was to guide those already knowledgeable in the observation of plants (especially proper harvesting periods), drug preparation, dosage, and frequency, as well as in making good diagnoses. Without this information, we can only make informed conjectures about what they were treating and how they were doing it. Autumn crocus contains a sufficient concentration of colchicine for pharmaceutical efficacy, but on the basis of modern studies, we conclude that the drug would arrest tumor mitoses in man but would not produce a complete regression in a malignant tumor.[8] An ancient or medieval physician, treating a malignant growth topically and possibly internally, would probably observe a beneficial response but not a "cure."

Not all early authorities recommended autumn crocus as an antitumor agent. While Dioscorides reported its use, Pliny (A.D. 23–79) recommended it only as an emetic. Galen recommended the plant as a medicine against tumors (*phumata*); Oribasios (325–403) again recommended it only as an emetic. Paulos Aegineta (seventh century) wrote only of its being a "breaking up" agent. Some Latin writers, such as Constantinus Africanus (d. ca. 1087) and Hildegard of Bingen (1098–1178), did not recommend it at all against tumors, despite knowing the plant; Matthaeus Platearius (d. 1161?) and Avicenna employed the plant in ways that suggest antitumoral activity. Platearius, for example, recommends it "contra morbos ex flegmate; . . . . Carnem superfluam corrodit . . . et licinium intinctum fistule imponatur." Abū Manṣūr (fl. 968–977) said that the drug concocted from it is poisonous but dries up old sores.[9] In light of this evidence, one can conclude that prior to the thirteenth century autumn crocus was em-

[8] The antitumor agent in colchicine is demecolcine (desacetyl-N-methylcolchicine), a bona fide anticancer drug whose use the Federal Drug Administration has not approved in the United States. Because the premodern physicians were dealing with crude drugs, I shall use the broad term colchicine. On demecolcine, see Irving S. Johnson, "Plant Alkaloids," in *Cancer Medicine*, ed. James F. Holland and Emile Frei III, 2nd ed. (Philadelphia: Lea & Febiger, 1982), pp. 910–920. On colchicine, see O. J. Eigsti and Pierre Dustin, Jr., *Colchicine—in Agriculture, Medicine, Biology, and Chemistry* (Ames: Iowa State College Press, 1955), p. 264; and William A. Remers, ed., *Antineoplastic Agents* (New York: Wiley, 1984), p. 214. John Edmund Driver and George E. Trease, *The Chemistry of Crude Drugs* (London: Longmans, Green, 1938), p. 92, give the colchicine concentration in the cormseeds of autumn crocus as between 2% and 8%. Experimental dosages of the cormseeds have ranged from 130 mg to 300 mg; *Dispensatory of the United States of America*, 25th ed. (Philadelphia: Lippincott, 1955), pp. 351–357, on p. 357. Mammary tumors in dogs have been treated with colchicine: 2 dosages of 0.25 mg, 2 dosages of 0.5 mg, and 2 dosages of 1 mg over a six day course, *Merck Index*, 8th ed. (Rahway, N.J.: Merck, 1968), p. 278.

[9] Pliny, *Natural History*, 28.45.160, ed. W. H. S. Jones, 10 vols. (Loeb Classical Library)

ployed as an anticancer agent, but that its use was not widespread. The reluctance may have been due to the belief expressed by Hildegard, who said that it was more of a poison than a medicine. An interesting and possibly significant footnote: in a field study of traditional medicine in Greece conducted between 1947 and 1960, autumn crocus was reported to be taken internally against cancer.[10]

METHODOLOGY

In what follows I identify modern agents and then seek their counterpart in the historical records. Some historians may object that it would be better methodology to list all the remedies employed as cancer agents in the historical records and then evaluate them in light of modern medical studies. In general, I agree with the objection, but for the purposes of this article, the better method would produce a much longer study without appreciably different results as to the question whether the premoderns had some effective cancer drugs. A major obstacle is that the longer process would produce many plants that cannot be firmly identified. For instance, in his pharmaceutical treatises, Galen employed only three herbs in the treatment of *oidêmata* (whose meaning we established includes malignant tumors): *akantha(-os) leukê, damasônion,* and *orchis.*[11] The identification of all three is uncertain. *Akantha leukê*—"white thorn"—may be *Acacia albida* Delile, *Euphorbia antiquorum* L., or *Cnicus arvensis* Hoffm., or possibly something else. Each of these is reported in modern studies as being used in various East Asian cultures for cancer therapies. Galen's *damasônion* may be our *Alisma plantago* L., and *orchis* may be either *Ophrys apifera* Huds. or *Orchis* sp. Alisma is reported in modern Chinese medicine as treating leukemia patients effectively, and various species of orchis have been employed for a long period in Western European medicine as an anticancer drug.[12] Beyond problems of plant identification, other uncertainties involved in evaluating Galen's drugs for *oidêmata*, such as uncertain diagnosis and a lack of corresponding modern clinical studies, make difficult even tentative conclusions about these remedies'

(London: Heinemann; Cambridge, Mass.: Harvard Univ. Press, 1938–1962), Vol. VII, p. 110; Galen, *De simplicium medicamentorum temperamentis ac facultatibus,* 6.25, s.v. *ephêmeron* (= *kolchikon*), in *Opera,* ed. Kühn, Vol. XI, pp. 879–880; Paulos Aegineta, *Epitomae medicae,.* 7.3., s.v. *ephêmeron,* trans. Francis Adams, 3 vols. (London: Sydenham Society, 1847), Vol. III, pp. 119–120; Oribasios, *Collectiones medicae reliquae,* 11.29, s.v. *ephêmeron,* ed. Johannes Raeder, 4 vols. (Corpus Medicorum Graecorum, 6.1, 2) (Leipzig: Teubner, 1928–1933), Vol. II, p. 111; Constantinus Africanus, *Liber de gradibus,* in *Opera* (Basel, 1536), p. 379, s.v. *hermodactilus* (= *colchicum*); Hildegard von Bingen, *Physicas,* 2.91, s.v. *hermodactylus* (Strassbourg, 1533); ed. and trans. I. Muller (Salzburg: Muller, 1982), p. 99; Matthaeus Platearius, *Circa instans,* s.v. *hermodactilis,* ed. H. Wölfel (Berlin: Preilipper, 1939), p. 61; Avicenna, *Canon,* 2.2.354, fols. 122v–123r; and Abū Manṣūr Muwaffaq ibn Ali Harāwī, *Die pharmakologischen Grundsätze (Liber fundamentorum pharmacologiae),* trans. Abdul-Chalis Achundow, *Koberts historischen Studien aus dem Pharmakologischen Institute der kaiserlichen Universität Dorpat,* 1893, *3*:137–481, on p. 222, no. 330. Kurt Ruegg, *Beiträge zur Geschichte der officizinellen Drogen: Crocus, Acorus calamus und Colchicum* (Basel: Schahl, 1936), pp. 231–232, believes that Pliny and Galen may have intended *Iris agrestis* rather than *Colchicum autumnale*; however, in my opinion the traditional identification of autumn crocus is correct.

[10] G. Lawrendiadis, "Contribution to the Knowledge of the Medicinal Plants of Greece," *Planta Medica,* 1961, 9:164–169.

[11] Galen, *De simplicium facultatibus* 6.1, 6.4, 7.15, in *Opera,* ed. Kühn, Vol. XI, pp. 819, 861; Vol. XII, p. 93.

[12] Hartwell, "Plants," *Lloydia,* 1970, *33*:98–99 (*Acacia* sp.); 1969, *32*:159 (*Euphorbia antiquorium*); 1968, *31*: 134, 137, 138, 146 (*Orchis* sp.); 1967, *30*:389 (*Alisma plantago*); 1970, *33*:309 (*Orchis* sp.).

relation to modern scientific studies. A comprehensive approach examining all ancient and medieval anticancer drugs would, I suspect, run into the same problems as those attendant on Galen's *oidêmata* remedies, and the main point would be obscured. If, however, it can be shown that modern chemotherapy agents for cancer were employed in much the same way by ancient and medieval peoples, the case can be made that other drugs which they used and we have not evaluated would be a rational place to begin screening tests.

For example, one ancient and medieval remedy not employed in modern scientific medicine is nightshade (Greek *strychnos*; Latin *solanum* = *Solanum* sp. in Linnean classification). It is a poisonous, alkaloid plant, and Galen thought it especially helpful as an applicant for "ulcerated cancers" (*hêlkêka karkinos*). Dioscorides applied nightshade externally for *erysipelas* and *herpês*. While Pliny gave no specific medicinal uses for it, Celsus applied it on *erysipelas*. Later writers continue the prescription. Today in traditional medicine around the world, nightshade is used to treat cancers, but modern Western medicine does not employ the plant.[13]

Although making an exact count of remedies such as nightshade is impossible, for it would depend on the criteria followed, the number of drugs used in cancer therapy both in modern Western medicine and in ancient and medieval Western medicine is small. One study in 1977 showed only ten plant species employed or being tested in actual clinical studies.[14] While the number of plants used by ancient and medieval authorities is larger, it is not so large that statistical probability alone would account for several drugs used in modern chemotherapy appearing among them, rather than the early authorities' recognition of antitumoral properties. For instance, in the first two books of his work, Dioscorides prescribes only two drugs for *oidêmata,* both in contexts that do not suggest anticancer activity. One, kermes oak, "helps" the tumor, which suggests symptomatic relief; the other, myrrh, is used against tumors caused by poisonous snake bites.[15] He gave only three treatments for *karkinas* (*karkinôma*): frankincense, nettle (*Urtica pilulifera* L. and *U. urens* L.), and figwort (*Scrophularia peregrina* L.).[16] In his entire work, Dioscorides discussed only about seven hundred plants.

ANCIENT AND MEDIEVAL CANCER DRUGS

Of all the classical authorities, only Dioscorides appears to have recognized the actions of plant alkaloids. First he grouped them together by drug affinities: for

[13] Galen, *Ad Glauconem de medendi methodo*, 2.12, in *Opera*, ed. Kühn, Vol. XI, p. 143; cf. Galen, *De simplicium facultatibus*, 8.19., s.v. *truchnon ê strychnos*: "*ἕλκη κακοήθη καὶ νομώδη θεραπεύει,*" *Opera*, ed. Kühn, Vol. XII, p. 146; Dioscorides, *De materia medica*, 4.70, ed. Wellmann, probably for *Solanum nigrum* L.; Pliny, *Natural History*, 27.107.132; Celsus, *De medicina*, 5.26, 33a–b, ed. W. G. Spencer, 2 vols. (Loeb Classical Library) (London: Heinemann; Cambridge: Harvard Univ. Press, 1935–1938), Vol. II, p. 102; Paulos Aegineta, *Epitomae mediciae*, 7.3., s.v. *strychnos*; Platearius, *Circa instans*, 718, ed. Wölfel (cit. n. 13): "contra apostemata in stomacho et intestinis"; Rufinus, *Herbarius*, fol. 104rb–104va, in *The Herbal of Rufinus*, ed. Lynn Thorndike with Francis S. Benjamin, Jr. (Chicago: Univ. Chicago Press, 1945). On modern use for *Solanum dulcamara* L., see George Edward Trease and William C. Evans, *Pharmacognosy*, 11th ed. (London: Tindall, 1978), p. 621.

[14] Walter H. Lewis and M. P. Elvin-Lewis, *Medical Botany* (New York: Wiley, 1977), p. 133.

[15] Dioscorides, *De materia medica*, 1.87, 106, ed. Wellmann.

[16] *Ibid.*, 1.68, 4.93–94.

example, he put plants containing the papaverine alkaloids in one group and those containing tropane alkaloids in another.[17] Second, he employed many of the same plants that we have rediscovered and currently employ. Many of those alkaloids he said were good as antitumor agents. One such plant is the squirting cucumber (*Ecballium elaterium* L.). In 1958 a chemical compound from this plant was found to have "strong antitumor activity against sarcoma."[18] Almost alone among the classical writers, Dioscorides recommended squirting cucumber to "dissolve old, soft tumors (*oidêmata*)." Pliny recommended this same plant as a remedy for a variety of skin conditions, including *psora, lichen,* and *parotis.*[19] These terms may have had the lexical range to encompass malignancies, but Latin and Greek dermatological afflictions are notoriously difficult to translate into modern terminology. For example, Galen said that *psora* was called cancer (*karkinos*), if it "occurred in the veins and flesh."[20] Scribonius Largus (fl. reign of Claudius, A.D. 41–54) prescribed squirting cucumber for *condylomata,* or lumps associated with the anus. These could be malignant anal lesions, but one has no justification to conclude that they were—merely that they could be. Galen, Paulos Aegineta, Cassius Felix (fl. 447), Constantinus Africanus, and Rufinus (fl. 1287) gave no clear recommendations for the plant in conjunction with tumors and neither did such Islamic authorities as Avicenna, Ibn Sarābī (or Serapion, d. ca. 1074), and Māsawaih (or Mesue, 925–1015).[21] This evidence suggests that although the plant was not widely employed against tumors (many of which were malignant lesions), the continuous reliance on the authority of Dioscorides makes it nonetheless likely that there was occasional use of the plant for cancer treatments. This remedy has persisted in folk medicine, so that modern investigators learned in 1952–1953 that the squirting cucumber was taken orally for cancer.[22]

In the same section of his treatise Dioscorides recommended the bulb of *Narcissus* sp. for a variety of skin afflictions (*epsêlis, alphos, helkos,* and *apostêma*). Narcissus contains colchicine, and an extract from the bulb is employed in modern chemotherapy for cancer. But the plant also contains calcium oxalate, and because some of these afflictions were sores and wounds, the action may have been cleansing owing to the calcium oxalate rather than to antitumoral activity.[23] Also in the same sequence Dioscorides prescribed the castor bean (*Ricinus communis* L.) for *oidêmata* and *erysipelata,* the latter being, according

[17] *Ibid.*, 4.63–67 (for papaverine-yielding plants); 4.70–75 (for tropane-yielding plants), ed. Wellmann.

[18] D. Lavie and D. Willner, "The Constituents of *Ecballium elaterium* L. III. Elatericin a and B[1, 2]," *Journal of the American Chemical Society*, 1958, *80*:710–714.

[19] Dioscorides, *De materia medica*, 4.150, ed. Wellmann; Pliny, *Natural History*, 20.2.4, ed. Jones.

[20] Galen, *De tumoribus*, 13, in *Opera*, ed. Kühn, Vol. VII, p. 727; trans. Reedy in "Galen on Cancer" (cit. n. 7), p. 236.

[21] Scribonius Largus, *Compositiones*, 224, ed. Sergio Sconocchia (Leipzig: Teubner, 1983); Galen, *De simplicum facultatibus*, 8.15, s.v. *sikuos* in *Opera*, ed. Kühn, Vol. XII, p. 122; cf. Galen, *Hippocratis Epidemiorum libri II*, 5.7, in *Opera*, Vol. XVIIA, p. 472; Paulos Aegineta, *Epitomae medicae*, 7.3., s.v. *elatêrion*; Cassius Felix, *De medicina*, 8, ed. Valentin Rose (Leipzig: Teubner, 1879), p. 15; Constantinus, *De gradibus* (no entry); Rufinus, *Herbarius* (cit. n. 13), fol. 49vb; Avicenna, *Canon*, 2.2.181, s.v. *cucumer asininus*; Ibn Sarābī, *Simplicibus medicinis*, 196, ed. Otto Brunsfels (Strassbourg, 1531), p. 133; and Māsawaih al-Mārdīnī, *De simplicibus*, 2.7 (Venice, 1558), fol. 64.

[22] Hartwell, "Plants against Cancer," *Lloydia*, 1969, *32*:96, citing the National Cancer Institute's central file.

[23] Dioscorides, *De materia medica*, 4.158, ed. Wellmann; for the narcissus as containing colchicine and calcium oxalate, see Lewis and Elvin-Lewis, *Medical Botany* (cit. n. 14), pp. 135, 78, 80.

to Galen, a protocancerous condition.[24] The castor bean contains ricin, currently recognized for its antitumorous qualities and employed in cancer chemotherapy research, although because of its high cytotoxicity, present attention is directed towards binding monoclonal antibodies to it to impart tumor specificity.[25] Following his discussion of the castor bean plant, Dioscorides gave a number of recommendations for spurge (*Euphorbia* sp.)—which is in the same family, Euphorbiaceae, as castor bean—as a remedy for afflictions suggestive of cancer. He added that spurge causes loss of hair, weight, and color, and that it even causes death.[26]

Some later writers recommended narcissus, castor bean, and spurge as antitumoral drugs, but many were silent.[27] In one of his pharmaceutical treatises, Galen clearly used narcissus for cleaning wounds (*traumata*) and not as an antitumor agent, but he recommended spurge for a number of types of tumors (*helkos, lichên, psôra, phagedaina, anthrax,* and *gangrainôde*), which in his treatise on tumors he said were often malignant. A preparation of spurge, called *elatêrion,* is given for an incipient cancer (*karkinos genomenos*), according to Galen.[28] Galen described castor bean as good for its dispersing and discutient property (*diaphorêtikos dynamis*), which could very well apply pharmaceutically to antitumoral action, although he did not specify that action, merely the property. Similarly Constantinus Africanus said that spurge was warming and drying to the fourth degree of intensity, thereby making it an extremely dangerous drug, and that it acted to purge black bile and viscous humors.[29] In the context of medieval science, these properties would be sought in a drug against cancer because that disease was in theory an excess of black bile, and any drug having the property of purging black bile would be suitable for testing as an antitumor agent. Drugs so strong in intensity as the fourth degree were considered drastic, life-threatening poisons, to be administered only in extremely severe conditions.[30]

Avicenna recommended narcissus for a variety of dermatological afflictions, none suggestive of cancer, but Rufinus clearly stated that a drug from the plant

[24] Dioscorides, *De materia medica,* 4.161, ed. Wellmann; Galen, *De tumoribus,* 9, in *Opera,* ed. Kühn, Vol. VII, pp. 723–724; trans. Reedy in "Galen on Cancer" (cit. n. 7), p. 235.

[25] Emil Frei, "Pharmacology," in *Cancer: Achievements, Challenges, and Prospects for the 1980's,* ed. Joseph H. Burchenal and Herbert F. Oettgen, 2 vols. (New York: Grune & Stratton, 1981), Vol. I, pp. 108–122, on p. 113; Lewis and Elvin-Lewis, *Medical Botany* (cit. n. 14), p. 135.

[26] Dioscorides, *De materia medica,* 4.164–169, s.v. *sikuos agrios,* ed. Wellmann.

[27] Hartwell, "Plants against Cancer," *Lloydia,* 1967, *30*:391, citing a quotation in Aetios of Amida, alleges that Soranus recommended narcissus for scirrhous tumors of the uterus. My reading of Soranus's statement was that narcissus was employed as a uterine injection to treat an atonic womb. See Soranus, *Gynecology,* 3.13, trans. Owsei Tempkin (Baltimore: Johns Hopkins Univ. Press, 1956), p. 172; Aetios of Amida recommended narcissus as a cleansing agent in *Libri medicinales,* 1.293, ed. A. Oliveri, 2 vols. (Corpus Medicorum Graecorum, 8) (Leipzig: Teubner), Vol. I (1935), p. 114.

[28] Galen, *De simplicium facultatibus,* 8.13., s.v. *narkissos,* in *Opera,* ed. Kühn, Vol. XII, pp. 85–86; *ibid.,* 8.19., s.v. *tithymalli* (=spurge), in *Opera,* Vol. XII, p. 142; Galen, *Hippocratis Epidemiorum libri II,* 5.8, in *Opera,* Vol. XVIIA, p. 477 (*elatêrion* = a preparation from spurge); on relating terms to cancer, cf. Galen, *De tumoribus,* 6–9, in *Opera,* Vol. IX, pp. 719–724, and trans. Reedy in "Galen on Cancer," pp. 234–235; Galen, *De simplicium facultatibus,* 7.10, s.v. *kikeôs,* in *Opera,* Vol. XII, p. 26.

[29] Galen, *De simplicium facultatibus,* 7.10.24, in *Opera,* ed. Kühn, Vol. XII, p. 26; Constantinus, *De gradibus,* p. 387.

[30] Georg Harig, *Bestimmung der Intensität im medizinischen Systems Galens* (Berlin: Akademie Verlag, 1974); Jerry Stannard, "The Theoretical Bases of Medieval Herbalism," *Medical Heritage,* 1985, *1*:186–198, on 189.

was applied topically on tumors (*super tumores*). Henri de Mondeville (ca. 1260–1320) prescribed narcissus for indurations and making various tumors soft. On the other hand, Matthaeus Platearius omitted all these poisonous plants, that is narcissus, castor bean, and spurge, from his popular herbal pharmacy. Abū Manṣūr prescribed the castor bean as an antitumor remedy.[31] Some of these drugs, however, are found in folk usages against cancer. The castor bean is or was employed for cancers and tumors in traditional Chinese medicine, Ayurvedic, South American, Indian, San Dominican, and modern Californian folk medicine. Various species of spurge are employed against cancer among the Bantu tribes of South Africa, India, and Finland, among other traditional medicine systems.[32]

Dioscorides placed yet another plant, *Vinca major* L., in the same sequence with plants containing alkaloids having antitumor activities, but he did not list the plant as specifically active against tumors. Pliny, however, said that *vicapervica* (= *Vinca*) "dried tumors."[33] A genus closely related to *Vinca* is *Catharanthus*. From one of its species, *C. roseus* G. Don, comes the present source for vinblastine and vincristine, which are remarkably effective against acute lymphocytic leukemia, Hodgkin's disease, carcinoma, and lymphosarcoma. Until 1948, *C. roseus* was classified as *Vinca rosa* L.[34] *Vinca major* has no active antitumor compounds, just as Dioscorides observed by omitting this use in discussing the plant. *Vinca* plants were found in the various regions of the eastern Mediterranean where Dioscorides traveled, but *C. roseus* is found in tropical settings, such as Madagascar and India. Many drugs, however, came to the Greeks and Romans from these regions, for example, cassia, cinnamon, and pepper; it is possible that Pliny was referring to a drug taken from the *Catharanthus*, inasmuch as the two genera are so similar that, despite the plant's importance, botanists did not reclassify *Vinca rosa* L. as *Catharanthus roseus* G. Don until recently. Even if Pliny (or his sources) intended the plant that is the source for our cancer therapy, we can be certain that the classical therapeutic use of the catharanthic alkaloids did not have the success that the present therapy has, with its isolation and concentration of active compounds and well-regulated administration. Nonetheless we can hypothesize that some ancient physicians may have observed some beneficial actions as a result of their treating cancers with *Catharanthus*. Possibly their inability to distinguish *Vinca* sp. and *C. roseus* hindered their confidence in the drug derived from the correct species.

Other plants, non-alkaloid-producing but nonetheless toxic, were used against cancers. One, a legume, provides an interesting insight. The plant is one or two species of *Vicia*, *V. ervilla* L., bitter vetch, or *V. fava* L., horse bean. Its seeds are poisonous but edible if properly prepared and cooked. Dioscorides

[31] Avicenna, *Canon*, 2.2.514; Rufinus, *Herbarius* (cit. n. 13), fol. 73rb; *Chirurgie de Henri de Mondeville*, 3. Chir. sp. Apostemes. Doct. 2.7.2, 18.2; 4. Doct. 2; Antidotaire. 3.B.2, 5.1, 8.2, 11. 118, ed. A. Bos (Paris, F. Didot, 1897–1898); Abū Manṣūr, *Liber fundamentorum pharmacologiae*, 174, in "Die pharmakologischen Grundsätze," trans. Achundow (cit. n. 9), p. 195.

[32] Hartwell, "Plants against Cancer," *Lloydia*, 1970, *33*:120–122 (castor bean); 158–167 (spurge).

[33] Dioscorides, *De materia medica*, 4.147, s.v. *chamaidaphnê*; and Pliny, *Natural History*, 21.99.172: "vicapervica sive chamaedaphne . . . tumores siccat."

[34] R. L. Noble and Cutts Beer, "Role of Chance Observation in Chemotherapy, *V. rosea*," *Annals of the New York Academy of Science*, 1958, *76*:882; cf. B. Oliver-Bever, "Vegetable Drugs for Cancer Therapy," *Quarterly Journal of Crude Drug Research*, 1971, *11*:1661–1671, on pp. 1665–1671.

recommended *Vicia* for "cleaning ulcers with honey, moles (*phakoi*), skin spots (*spiloi*), freckles or rough spots (*ephêles*). . ;. [and] it stops boils/ulcers (*nomai*), gangrene or running sore (*gangraina*); it softens hardness (*sklêriai*) in the breast, malignant ulcers (*thêriôdai*), malignant pustules (*anthrakai*), and *kêria* [= yellow and bad skin swelling or ulcer]."[35] The range of contexts suggests that some of the terms would include cancers, especially deep-seated, papillary, and superficial epithelioma and nonspecific, metastatic inflammatory lesions associated with cancer in the stage of ulceration. The vetch plant (*Vicia* sp.) contains vicianin, a cyanogenic glycoside, and was given for cancer into the nineteenth century.[36] Dioscorides did not recommend apricot pits, the source of amygdalin or laetrile, for cancer. Amygdalin, like vicianin, allegedly is effective because it causes cyanide production upon ingestion. Modern science has not found laetrile an effective antitumor agent despite its popularity in underground medical practices.

Certainly not all antitumor discoveries were classical. There is at least one fascinating Byzantine modification. An anonymous herbalist called Pseudo-Apuleius, who lived in the fourth century A.D., wrote in Latin that birthwort (*Aristolochia clematitis* L.), commonly recommended for parturition, was good for nasal carcinoma. Although the Greek term *karkinôma* primarily meant malignant tumors, in this case the context suggests a polyp of the nares, usually a benign tumor in the nasal passage, displaying a pedicle, especially on the mucous membrane. Other surviving classical authorities do not ascribe antitumoral qualities to birthwort. But in or before the fourteenth century, a Byzantine commentator added to a text of Dioscorides a statement that birthwort "helps nose [or, skin?] carcinomas (*ἐν ῥινὶ καρκινώμασι βοηθεῖ*)." The Greek word *ῥίς, ῥινός*, means nostril and *ῥινός, ῥινοῦ* means skin. Whether the commentator meant birthwort to be applied to benign nasal tumor or skin cancer is unclear. Whatever the interpretation, another Byzantine scholium sought to strengthen the claim by changing the verb from "it helps" to "it cures (*ἰᾶται*)."[37] In 1969 aristolochic acid from birthwort was found to have antitumoral qualities, and it is now used in cancer chemotherapy.[38]

In 1971 and in 1972, Lee Wattenberg published studies on the effects of cab-

[35] Dioscorides, *De materia medica*, 2.108, ed. Wellmann.

[36] R. J. McIllroy, *The Plant Glycosides* (London: E. Arnold, 1951), pp. 22–23; *Merck Index* (cit. n. 8), 8th ed., p. 1107; cf. 9th ed., pp. 9624–9625; and Hartwell, "Plants against Cancer," *Lloydia*, 1970, *33*:120–122.

[37] Pseudo-Apuleius, *Herbarius*, 19.7, ed. Ernst Howald and Henry Sigerist (Leipzig: Teubner, 1927): "Ad carcinomata, quae in naribus nascuntur. Herba aristolochia cum cipero et draconteae semen cum melle inpositum emendat." The first scholium is found in Paris, BN MS Gr. 2183, (15th c); Venice, San Marco MS Gr. Z 271 (15th c.); and Salamanca MS 2659 (15th c.); the second in Vienna ON MS Gr. 16 (15th c.); and Vatican MS Palatinus Gr. 77 (15th c.). See John M. Riddle, "Byzantine Commentaries on Dioscorides," in *Byzantine Medicine*, ed. John Scarborough (Washington, D.C.: Dumbarton Oaks, 1984), pp. 95–102; see also Schol. Dioscorides, *De materia medica*, 3.4(5), ed. Wellmann, Vol. II, p. 8n (*apparatus criticus* to line 10). On Pseudo-Apuleius, see Linda E. Voigts, "The Significance of the Name *Apuleius* to the *Herbarium Apulei*," *Bulletin of the History of Medicine*, 1972, *52*:214–227. Pseudo-Apuleius is a highly unlikely source for the Byzantine commentator's scholium because the Latin herbal ascribed to Apuleius had no Greek counterpart or Greek translation.

[38] S. Munavalli and C. Viel, "Etude chimique, taxinomique et pharmacologique des aristolochiacées," *Annales pharmaceutiques français*, 1969, *27*:449–464, on p. 463; Trease and Evans, *Pharmacogonosy* (cit. n. 13), pp. 98, 577; and *Chemical Abstracts*, 1974, *80*:24780g for (*A. baetica*), 1974, *81*:111458z (for *A. clematitis*.)

bage on drug and carcinogen metabolism, and in 1978 he reported that the compounds in cabbage inhibit chemically induced carcinogenesis in rats. In the same year Japanese researchers found antimutagenic action by cabbage juice.[39] While the research on cabbage and other *Brassica* species is promising, the candidacy of drugs from the genus, most especially cabbage, developed late in modern cancer research. But Cato the Elder (234–149 B.C.) spoke of cabbage around 2,200 years ago: "Of the medicinal value of cabbage: It is cabbage which surpasses all other vegetables. . . . It can be used as a poultice on all kinds of wounds and swelling; . . . it will cleanse suppurating wounds and tumors (*vulnera putida canceresque*), and heal them, a thing which no other medicine can do. . . . An ulcer on the breast and a cancer (*in mammis ulceris natum et carcinoma*) can be healed by the application of macerated cabbage." Similarly Dioscorides prescribed that cabbage be applied directly on tumors (*oidêmata*) to cause them to shrink.[40] The therapeutic use of cabbage by the Greek, Roman, and medieval peoples was chiefly as a drug. Modern research investigates it for desmutagenic activity chiefly in diet;[41] this action, prevention of carcinogenesis, is different from the antitumor activity attested by Cato and Dioscorides. Possibly it is only coincidence that ancient and modern attention focused on cabbage. Possibly also the ancients observed that those whose diet was heavy in cabbage were less susceptible to cancers. Possibly cabbage contains an antitumorial compound. The point is that modern attention to it was not, as best as I can determine, first directed by the history of the substance. Most chemotherapeutical agents of today were rediscovered without benefit of history.

There are animal sources for drugs as well as plant sources, although many fewer. Traditional Chinese medicine employed a drug made from the blister beetle (*Mylabris phalerata* Pall.) for the treatment of malignant diseases. Dioscorides also said that the drug from the beetle was effective against a malignancy (*karkinôdê*), as well as *lepra* and *leichênê*. Pursuing suggestions from a study of the historical traditions, modern Chinese investigators isolated from the crude drug a compound, cantharidin, that is therapeutic for primary heptocarcinoma, intestinal carcinoma, and other cancerous neoplasms.[42]

[39] L. Wattenberg, "Studies of Polycyclic Hydroxylases of the Intestine Possibly Related to Cancer," *Cancer,* 1972, *28*:99–102; Wattenberg, "Enzymatic reactions and carcinogenesis," in *Enviroment and Cancer* (Baltimore: Williams & Wilkins, 1972), pp. 241–255; Wattenberg and W. D. Loub, "Inhibition of Polycyclic Aromatic Hydrocarbon-induced Neoplasia by Naturally Occurring Indoles," *Cancer Research,* 1978, *38*:1410–1411; T. Kada, K. Morita, and T. Inoue, "Anti-mutagenic Action of Vegetable Factor(s) on the Mutagenic Principle of Tryptophas Pyrolysate," *Mutation Research,* 1978, *53*:351– 353; and K. Morita, M. Hara, and T. Kada, "Studies on Natural Desmutagens," *Agricultural Biological Chemistry,* 1978, *42*(6):1235–1238.

[40] Cato, *On Agriculture,* 156.1.–157.4, ed. and trans. W. D. Hooper and H. B. Ash (Loeb Classical Library) (London: Heinemann; Cambridge, Mass.: Harvard Univ. Press, 1934); and Dioscorides, *De materia medica,* 2.121, ed. Wellmann.

[41] Michael Albert-Puleo, "Physiological Effects of Cabbage with Reference to its Potential as a Dietary Cancer-Inhibitor and its Use in Ancient Medicine," *Journal of Ethnopharmacology,* 1983, 9:261–272.

[42] Bin Hsu, "The Use of Herbs as Anticancer Agents," *Amer. J. Chin. Med.,* 1980, *8*:304–305; Dioscorides, *De materia medica,* 2.61, ed. Wellmann. On the widespread knowledge and use of cantharidin in Greek and Roman pharmacy, see John Scarborough, "Some Beetles in Pliny's *Natural History,*" *Colepterists Bulletin,* 1977, *31*:293–296, and Scarborough,"Nicander's Toxicology, II: Spiders, Scorpions, Insects and Myriapods," *Pharmacy in History,* 1979, *21*:73–92, on pp. 73–80. Cantharidin is used in the United States pharmacopeia to remove warts, molluscum, and other benign epithelial growths; see *Physicians' Desk Reference,* 37th ed. (Oradell, N.J.: Medical Economics Company, 1983), pp. 827–828, 1882.

In this study I have developed essentially two lines, one modern and the other ancient and medieval, without showing a definite relationship (except in the case of cantharidin). If extreme care is used, the historian can find it useful to evaluate pharmaceutical records in the light of scientific studies, in order to learn whether early practitioners were, in our judgment, "rational" users of medicines. Medical anthropologists have taught us to be cautious because there are many factors that may determine whether a person finds a drug effective. Nonetheless, the historian wishes to know as a matter of curiosity what the physical effects of given drug therapies might have been. Since most of the plants discussed in this paper are sources of alkaloids, which have a toxic effect (cabbage excepted), it is difficult to believe that they could qualify as placebos, at least in the traditional sense. A drug user would seek positive effects to outweigh the deleterious side effects of these toxins. On the other hand, it is probable that premodern users saw some beneficial responses to these drugs when treating tumorous growths, but, since they lacked the ability to control concentration, dosages, and frequencies, the drugs were probably only marginally efficacious.

In contrast, the modern scientist might employ the history of a drug, especially in the works of the leading medical authorities, as a starting point for conducting animal and clinical tests. Important clues exist in the historical records about which drugs might be worth testing. While colchicine is not a drug of choice for cancer therapy, its chemical analogues are employed, and colchicine proved an important first step in modern chemotherapy.[43] William Stone's speech in 1916 was prophetic. For too long we have believed that the past was filled more with superstition and stupidities than with experienced judgments about medicine.

[43] Remers, *Antineoplastic Agents* (cit. n. 8), p. 214.

XIII

BYZANTINE COMMENTARIES ON DIOSCORIDES

In the mid-first century, Dioscorides had written "And some have recorded that if someone were to bury rams' horns broken into small pieces, asparagus grows,"[1] but a Byzantine scribe, living no later than the fourteenth century, simply could not accept this assertion. Reacting strongly, he wrote, "it seems incredible to me" (ἐμοὶ δὲ ἀπίθανον).[2] Thereafter the texts of at least ten Dioscorides Greek manuscripts incorporated the phrase into the chapter on this common vegetable.[3] This added comment must have appeared strange to later readers, confronted by "Dioscorides" expressing skepticism about what he had just written, and doing so in the first person.

Having interrupted Dioscorides with his own doubt, the scholiast decided to add new material to Dioscorides' pharmaceutical descriptions of asparagus. Dioscorides had set down the following about the plant:

> Growing in rocky soil, asparagus or "spiky-mushroom,"[4] which some term a sage,[5] has a stalk which boiled and eaten softens the bowels and is also a diuretic. When drunk, the decoction of its roots is helpful for those having difficulty micturating, and for those afflicted by jaundice or sciatica; when decocted with wine, the roots are helpful for those bitten by a poisonous spider (φαλάγγιον),[6] and those suffering from toothache are benefited when the decoction is applied to the painful tooth. Also asparagus seeds made into a drink provide the same effects [as the root decoction]. And also they say that dogs die after they have drunk the decoction of asparagus.[7] And some have recorded that if someone were to bury rams' horns broken into small pieces, asparagus grows.[8]

The commentator added, "it seems incredible to me," even though the tenth-century Byzantine compilation of agricultural lore, the *Geoponica*, had honored the same tradition as follows:

> If one wants to produce an abundance of asparagus, chop up (κόψας) wild rams' horns into small pieces, throw them onto the [asparagus] beds, and water. Some say even more incredibly (παραδοξότερον) that if whole rams' horns are bored and laid down, they will bear asparagus.[9]

[The reader is referred to the list of abbreviations at the end of the volume.]

[1] Dioscorides II, 125 (ed. Wellmann, Vol. I, p. 198).

[2] *Ibid.*, *apparatus criticus* to line 2.

[3] I have noted the commentary in the following manuscripts (an asterisk indicates the manuscripts used by Wellmann): Leiden, Bibl. Univ., MS Voss Gr. F. 58, 14th cent.; *Vatican, MS Palatinus gr. 77, 14th cent.; Paris, B.N., MS gr. 2182, anno 1481; *Paris, B.N., MS gr. 2183, 15th cent.; Salamanca, Bibl. univ. MS 2659 (formerly *Madrid, MS palat. Reg. 44), 15th cent.; *Venice, San Marco, MS Gr. Z 271, 15th cent.; Venice, San Marco, MS Gr. Z. 272, 15th cent.—Michael Apostoles, scribe; Venice, San Marco, MS Gr. Z. 597, 15th cent.; El Escorial, MS T-II-12, 16th cent. Generally throughout I shall not give foliation. While I have seen all these manuscripts, I normally follow Wellmann's critical apparatus and list the manuscripts which have the commentary and were not included by Wellmann. My expanded list includes those I studied and in which I observed the particular scholium; therefore, the actual number of texts with the scholium under discussion will probably be larger than what is recorded in this article. Still, the number of manuscripts will be greater than known by Wellmann.

[4] This translation of μυάκανθος is offered as an approximation of what appears to be the meaning suggested by Dioscorides' sources. The literal roots of the term suggest both a "mouse" and a "mushroom." R. Strömberg, *Griechische Pflanzennamen* (Göteborg, 1940), 28; Alexander of Tralles IX, 1 (ed. Puschmann, Vol. II, p. 395), and Dioscorides III, 151, and IV, 143.2 (ed. Wellmann, Vol. II, pp. 159 and 287), show that this name (μυάκανθος) was given to the shoots of butcher's broom (*Ruscus aculeatus* L.), which explains why Dioscorides would say some call it a "sage"—even though ὅρμινον is definitely another plant.

[5] Ὅρμινον is probably red-topped sage (*Salvia horminum* L.), considered separately by Dioscorides (III, 129). The plant certainly does not resemble asparagus.

[6] For a discussion of the identities of this venomous spider, see Scarborough, "Nicander II," 7–14.

[7] According to Pliny, *Natural History* XX, 43.111, the assertion that asparagus will kill dogs was made by Chrysippus (4th cent. B.C.). See *RE*, Vol. III, pt. 2 (Stuttgart, 1899), cols. 2509–10.

[8] Dioscorides II, 125 (ed. Wellmann, Vol. I, pp. 197–98).

[9] *Geoponica* XII, 18.2–3 (ed. Beckh, p. 365).

It is quite probable that the Byzantine scholiast was well aware of this venerable "rams' horns" custom for cultivators of asparagus—quite similar to modern gardeners in their adding bone meal to certain vegetable plots—but the commentator has chosen to supplement Dioscorides with a botanical morphology very much in keeping with the pattern of description laid down by Theophrastus,[10] and then to add further pharmacological details about asparagus:

> Be that as it may (μέντοι), this asparagus shrub is multibranched, has many leaves, and is large, and is similar to fennel.[11] The roots are rounded off, are large, and have a knob, and their stalks, made soft with white wine, abate phrenitis.[12] Taken either boiled or baked, they slake strangury, difficulty in micturation, and dysentery. Boiled down in vinegar or wine, the roots alleviate sprains; taken boiled with figs and chickpea,[13] they cure jaundice and alleviate sciatica and strangury. Hung as an amulet and drunk as a decoction, the root causes barrenness (ἀτοκία) and sterility (ἄγονος).[14]

The Byzantine commentator has added a botanical description, frequently omitted by Dioscorides, especially for common plants. Unlike the scribe's classical model Theophrastus, Dioscorides normally provided topical habitats, information probably helpful for finding it in the wild. The commentator properly terms asparagus a "shrub" because it grows to a height of one and one-half meters. He says that it is multibranched, and calls the leaves "large," somewhat inaccurate by modern botanical morphology: technically, according to modern botany, asparagus has no leaves, simply modified branchlets which serve that morphological function. The scribe, however, likens asparagus leaves to fennel leaves. The modern botanist would state that fennel (*Foeniculum vulgare* Miller) has true leaves, much divided and feathery, but the casual observer could easily compare fennel leaves with those of asparagus.

The commentator's purpose in supplementing Dioscorides' text was therapeutic, not botanical, and one may assume that he was attempting to explicate the medical and pharmacological properties of asparagus, as contrasted to their fusion with farm lore, seen both in Dioscorides and the abridgment of Didymus in the *Geoponica*. The scholiast adds medicinal employment for phrenitis, dysentery, and sprains, and the use of asparagus as an antifertility agent. There is repetition: he repeats Dioscorides and he repeats himself. Dioscorides had said that the root was good for those with difficulty in micturation, and the Byzantine commentator repeats this twice and adds the affliction called strangury, a painful and interrupted urination in drops, produced by spasmodic muscular contraction of the ureter and bladder. Asparagus remains a strongly recommended diuretic in folkmedicine.[15] Dioscorides had prescribed a boiling of the root, and the scholiast has added "or baking." Lest one conclude too quickly from the skepticism about ram's horn growing into asparagus that the Byzantine scribe was more "rational" than Dioscorides, one should note his statement of asparagus' use as an amulet: the scholiast has included the amuletic asparagus without Dioscorides' manner of disclaiming folklore with such phrases as "they say" and "it is reported."

The final aspect of the scribe's additions is the use of asparagus as an antifertility agent. Curiously, a Hippocratic work suggests that asparagus seeds are to be used in a pessary to promote conception, not contraception.[16] In 1952, Russian investigators reported that a decoction of asparagus (*A. acutifolius officinalis*) was used in folkmedicine for its contraceptive effect.[17] While asparagus has asparagin, an amino acid, its use for the regulation of fertility cannot be verified.[18] In 1975, however, the *Journal of Pharmaceutical Sciences* published an article which suggested asparagus as a future can-

[10] Schol. Dioscorides II, 125 (ed. Wellmann, Vol. I, p. 198: *app. crit.* to line 2, lines 1–2). Cf. Theophrastus, *HP* I, 3.1.

[11] *Foeniculum vulgare* Miller. Cf. Theophrastus, *HP* I, 11.2.

[12] φρενῖτις. LSJ, *s.v.* wrongly defines this as "inflammation of the brain," whereas the cited texts show an inflammation of the diaphragm. Berendes, in translating Dioscorides (p. 222), included the commentary as part of Dioscorides' text, and interpreted the meaning as an affliction of the bladder or spleen. A long discussion of phrenitis is given by Caelius Aurelianus, *On Acute Diseases* Bk. I (ed. and trans. Drabkin), who certainly included febrile delirium and several psychotic states within the meaning of phrenitis. One of the better discussions on the φρένες among the Greeks is R. B. Onians, *The Origins of European Thought* (Cambridge, 1951), esp. 13–15, 23–28, 29–32, 37–40, and 116–17.

[13] *Cicer arietinum* L.

[14] Schol. Dioscorides II, 125 (ed. Wellmann, Vol. I, p. 198: *app. crit.* to line 2, lines 1–8).

[15] W. Schneider, *Lexikon zur Arzneimittelgeschichte* (Frankfurt, 1974; 7 vols.), Vol. V, pt. 1, 147–49.

[16] The Hippocratic *Diseases of Women* I, 75 (ed. Littré, Vol. VIII, p. 166). Cf. J. H. Dierbach, *Die Arzneimittel des Hippokrates* (Heidelberg, 1824; rptd. Hildesheim, 1969), 20.

[17] V. J. Brondegaard, "Contraceptive Plant Drugs," *Planta Medica*, 23, 2 (1973), 169.

[18] P. G. Stecher, *et al.*, eds., *The Merck Index*, 8th ed. (Rahway, New Jersey, 1968), 106–7; J. E. Driver and G. E. Trease, *The Chemistry of Crude Drugs* (London, 1928), 8.

didate for the testing of antifertility agents in natural products.[19] Aside from the possible effectiveness of asparagus as a contraceptive, it is important to note that the Byzantine commentator has recorded data otherwise unknown to us, either from earlier authorities now lost, or as testimony of contemporary late Byzantine medical pharmacognosy.

Commentaries and scholia on Dioscorides are rather common in the manuscript traditions. The famous alphabetical Greek codex of c. A.D. 512, the so-called Anicia Juliana, contains numerous scholia and commentaries, but the Anicia Juliana is excluded from consideration in this study because there exists a good scholarly literature on the commentaries to the Vienna codex.[20] The concentration in this study is on later manuscripts, since many preserve Dioscorides' original (non-alphabetical) order and have fewer alterations than found in the Anicia Juliana and the later Greek texts which descend from it. Wellmann, in the critical apparatus to his edition of the Greek text of Dioscorides' *Materia medica*, faithfully recorded most of the scholia and commentaries in the manuscripts he employed to establish his text, but Wellmann used less than half of the Greek manuscripts of Dioscorides now known to be extant. For example, the earliest manuscript employed by Wellmann for the asparagus scholium is Vatican Palatinus MS graec. 77 (fourteenth century). One other manuscript is at least as early as the Palatine, and it was not known to Wellmann: the marvellously illustrated manuscript at Padua's seminary library (MS 194).[21] The scribe or scribes of the Padua manuscript use the text and iconographical tradition of the Anicia Juliana, but when the plants beginning with the letter *Omega* are reached, the scribes show awareness of another Dioscorides text with its own set of illuminations. Thus, the scribes start over with *Alpha* and go again through *Omega*. In this second text, the copyists include plants omitted in the initial manuscript, and the second text contains substantially different readings in many instances. It is in the second copying that the scribes of the Paduan manuscript include the additional material on asparagus, significantly by using a Greek text far less corrupted than that represented by the Anicia Juliana and its descendants. Since the Paduan manuscript did not employ the non-illustrated Palatine text, it is clear that both of these fourteenth-century manuscripts had a common source for the scholia on asparagus.

Wellmann's stemma stands in need of revision, but until this arduous task is performed, one may make general assumptions concerning the commentaries and scholia to Dioscorides by observing when they appear in the manuscripts. Since there are a variety of styles, forms, and quality of comments in the scholia, and since the commentaries are in various combinations of manuscript families, one may assume that there were certain scribes who hoped to supply addenda or corrections to the Greek texts of Dioscorides. Both the Byzantine Greek vocabulary and the dates of the manuscripts which contain commentaries show that most scholia were appended after the tenth century but not later than the fourteenth. Consequently, these Byzantine commentaries and scholia indicate numerous facets about the nature and quality of Byzantine medicine.

Generally, the commentaries were attached at the conclusions of Dioscorides' chapters, and most of them consider therapeutics. In one instance, Dioscorides had written about a plant called γιγγίδιον, probably a species of wild carrot, *Daucus gingidium* L.,[22] as follows:

> It grows plentifully in both Cilicia and Syria, a little herb like the wild carrot (σταφυλῖνος = *Daucus carota* L. [*D. guttatus* Sibthorp])[23] but thinner and more bitter; its root is somewhat white, pungent. It is grown as a pot herb, eaten raw, and boiled and pickled. It is good for the upper digestive tract, and is diuretic.[24]

To which a copyist adds:

> boiled down and drunk with wine, it is useful for the bladder.[25]

At least eight manuscripts subsequently integrated

[19] N. R. Farnsworth, *et al.*, "Potential Value of Plants as Sources of New Antifertility Agents. I," *Journal of Pharmaceutical Sciences*, 64, 4 (1975), 544.

[20] There are two facsimile printings, each with lengthy commentaries: J. de Karabacek, ed., *De codicis Dioscuridei Aniciae Iulianae, nunc Vindobonensis Med. Gr. I* (Leiden, 1906; 4 vols.); and H. Gerstinger [Kommentarband zur Faksimileausgabe (1970)], *Dioscurides Codex Vindobonensis med gr. 1 der Österreichischen Nationalbibliothek* (Graz, 1965–1970; 5 vols.). See also O. Mazal, *Pflanzen, Wurzeln, Säfte, Samen: Antike Heilkunst in Miniaturen des Wiener Dioskurides* (Graz, 1981). For a partial bibliography, see J. Riddle, "Dioscorides," in *Catalogus*, 14–15.

[21] See E. Mioni, "Un novo erbario greco di Dioscoride," *Rassegna Medica. Convivium Sanitatis* [Milan], 36 (1959), 169–84.

[22] Berendes, trans., *Dioskurides*, p. 228; Carnoy, 130; LSJ, *s.v.*

[23] Berendes, trans., *Dioskurides*, p. 299; Carnoy, 252.

[24] Dioscorides II, 137 (ed. Wellmann, Vol. 1, pp. 208–9).

[25] Schol. Dioscorides II, 137 (ed. Wellmann, Vol. 1, p. 209; *app. crit.* to line 3).

the new line into Dioscorides' chapter.[26] From the view of pharmacological chemistry, the carrot is not known to have an effect on the bladder,[27] except as a diuretic through the kidneys. Possibly the scholiast intended his addition as an elaboration, but this seems implausible, since the appended data is superfluous. Another reason is more likely. In a chapter on the plant called λεπίδιον, Dioscorides gives γιγγίδιον as its synonymn.[28] Identified either as dittander (*Lepidium latifolium* L.) or broad-leaved pepperwort (*L. sativum* L.) in the family Cruciferae, these pepperworts are in distinct contrast to a carrot in the Diapensiaceae family.[29] It is likely that the Byzantine scholiast thought that γιγγίδιον was pepperwort, and added the line to correct Dioscorides' omission. In the Latin West during the Middle Ages, *lepidium* and *gingidion* were often presumed to be the same plant, a pepperwort,[30] and through the nineteenth century folkmedicine used pepperwort in the treatment of bladder ailments.[31]

In almost half of the manuscripts that contain the scholium on pepperwort,[32] there is an interesting commentary added to Dioscorides' chapter on plantain (*Plantago* spp.):

> The Syrians say that the broth [of plantain], and of the catmint (χαλαμίνθη: prob. *Nepeta cataria* L.), with honey, cures the fevers; the broth is given for a quotidian, a quartan, just in a preparation; accept this as some secret talisman (μυστήριον).[33] For this is very true, even through experiences.[34]

These comments are quite distinct from other scholia, since they may be connected with Hermetic literature or other magical texts.[35]

In other instances, Byzantine scholiasts give a classical source as the authority. In his original, Dioscorides had referred to at least two species of plants—by our system of taxonomy—with a single Greek name, ἀσφόδελος, which would include both *Asphodelus ramosus* L., and *A. albus* Miller (a St. Bernard's lily, and white asphodel) in Liliaceae. The following appears in a number of manuscripts:[36]

> Another kind flowers at harvest time. It is necessary to cut the white asphodel during the spring equinox before its fruit increases. It is said that its root taken in a drink creates an appetite for sexual activity.[37] And Crateuas the Rhizotomist said the same thing, and also that the root drunk with wine successfully treats the pain in those who suffer from gout.[38]

These comments are important because if we knew their origin we then would know when a "true" cure for gout was first discovered. Our natural product drug of choice for gout is colchicine, which breaks the chemical chain of excessive uric acid deposits on joint tissue and tophoi.[39] Colchicine is present in asphodel.[40] One needs more data than what ancient, medieval, and Byzantine sources tell us, before there is assurance that this is a cure for gout, and such information would include the concentration of colchicine, particular species, preparation method, and dosages and frequency of administration. Lacking these details, one suspects that pre-modern use of the drug would have been less spectacular than the modern synthesized drug, which gives a clinical response within twenty-four hours. Nevertheless, in all probability, the ancient and Byzantine asphodel preparation for gout would have been effective.

The earliest test of this scholium ends with "an appetite for sexual activity."[41] Later manuscripts add the fragment attributed to Crateuas, who had written a medical tract on root medicine in the second

[26] Leiden, Bibl. Univ. MS Voss G. F. 58, 14th cent.; *Vatican, MS Pal. gr. 77, 14th cent.; *Venice, San Marco, MS Gr. Z. 271, 15th cent.; Salamanca, Bibl. univ. MS 2659, 15th cent.; *Paris, B.N., MS gr. 2183, 15th cent.; Paris, B.N., MS gr. 2182, anno 1481, fol. 62; El Escorial, MS T-II-12, 16th cent.; Paris, B.N., MS gr. 2185, 16th cent., fol. 64.

[27] Carrot juice, however, is sometimes substituted for coffee as a stimulating beverage. Lewis and Elvin-Lewis, 387.

[28] Dioscorides II, 174 (ed. Wellmann, Vol. I, pp. 241–42).

[29] Schneider, *Lexikon* (n. 15 above), Vol. V, pt. 2, 17–19 and 246–48.

[30] H. Fischer, *Mittelalterliche Pflanzenkunde* (Munich, 1929), 273; Schneider, *Lexikon* (n. 15 above), Vol. V, pt. 2, 246–47.

[31] Schneider, *Lexikon* (n. 15 above), Vol. II, 73.

[32] To the three manuscripts identified by Wellmann (Paris 2183, Salamanca 2659, and Venice Z. 272), one adds another in which the scholium also appears (Paris, B.N., MS gr. 2182, fol. 50), but it is not in other codices in which there are scholia already mentioned, e.g. Leiden, MS Voss. Fr. F. 58 (fols. 266ᵛ–67 have plantain), El Escorial MS T-II-12, and Venice, San Marco MS Gr. Z. 597.

[33] *PGM*, XII, 331–34 [talisman]. This is also the name of a particular drug, "The Secret," or "The Talisman," as recorded by Galen (ed. Kühn), XIII, 96, quoting Niceratus; cf. Alexander of Tralles V, 4 (ed. Puschmann, Vol. II, p. 161), and Oribasius, *For Eunapius* IV, 135 (ed. Raeder, p. 496).

[34] Schol. Dioscorides II, 126.4 (ed. Wellmann, Vol. I, p. 200: *app. crit.* to line 15).

[35] J. M. Riddle, *Marbode of Rennes' De lapidibus* (Wiesbaden, 1977 [*SA* Beiheft 20]), 3–5, 10, and 28–30.

[36] Leiden, Bibl. univ., MS Voss. Gr. F. 58; *Vatican, MS Pal. gr. 77; Paris, B.N., MS gr. 2182; *Paris, B.N., MS gr. 2183; Paris, B.N., MS gr. 2185; El Escorial, MS T-II-12.

[37] Vatican, MS Pal. gr. 77 ends here.

[38] Schol. Dioscorides II, 169.3 (ed. Wellmann, Vol. I, p. 236: *app. crit.* to line 8).

[39] A. Goth, *Medical Pharmacology*, 9th ed. (St. Louis, 1978), 533–34. Lewis and Elvin-Lewis, 199 and 219.

[40] J. A. Duke, "Phytotoxin Tables," *Critical Reviews in Toxicology* (Nov. 1977), 215.

[41] Schol. Dioscorides II, 169.3 (ed. Wellmann, Vol. I, p. 236: *app. crit.* to line 8 [line 4]).

century B.C.[42] An extensive fragment on asphodel from Crateuas' treatise is preserved in the Anicia Juliana, and the text is separate from that of Dioscorides; the use of asphodel for gout appears in this fragment.[43] The extant texts suggest the following: Crateuas was the first known writer on herbal medicine to recommend an effective remedy for gout, but the drug was not employed by his successors, including Dioscorides.[44] The copyist of the Anicia Juliana manuscript in the early sixth century recognized that Dioscorides' account could be augmented, and so he added the quotation from Crateuas, but in a separate section, clearly identified as a different source. After the citation of the Anicia manuscript, there is no evidence before the fourteenth century that asphodel was used against gout, even by the Byzantine commentator who provides information about its collection and employment as an aphrodisiac. The old Latin translation of Dioscorides (c. sixth century) does not include asphodel as a remedy for gout.[45] It first reappears in extant texts of the late fourteenth century by a Byzantine scholiast who again recognized asphodel as a treatment for gout, and he appended it to a previous commentary on this section of Dioscorides' text. Credit for this rediscovery should be given to this unknown Byzantine scribe, who perceived important data inexplicably lost for 800 years, and added the information to the text of Dioscorides.

In a similar manner, new information is appended to the description of another plant, emerging partially from Crateuas and Galen, but with a possible major innovation. In the chapter on the birthwort (ἀριστολοχεία), Dioscorides had written that there was a third kind (κληματῖτις) with the same pharmaceutical properties as the other two (probably *Aristolochia pallida* Willd., and *A. sempervirens* L.), but this third kind was not as strong.[46] Some Byzantine scholiasts were not satisfied by this terse description, and chose to elaborate on what is probably our *Aristolochia clematitis* L.:

> [The *klēmatitis*] is called by some *araniza*, as well as *melekaproum*, *erestios*, *lestitis*, *pyxionyx*, *dardanon*, and *iontitis*; the Gauls call it *theximon*, the Egyptians *sophoeph*, the Sicilians *chamaimēlon*, the Italians *terra mala*, the Dacians *apsinthion chōrikon*. It grows in mountainous country, in warm and flat places or rough and rocky areas. It "works" in the treatment of an oppressive fever in this way: [have the patient] with fever [breathe the odors] from a charcoal fumigator with birthwort [on it], and the fever will subside. And applied as a plaster, birthwort cures wounds. With nut grass (*Cyperus rotundus* L., possibly a galingale, *C. longus* L.) and the tuber of the dragon arum (*Dracunculus vulgaris* Schott)[47] and honey, it helps [Paris, Venice, and Salamanca MSS: "cures" Vienna 16 MS and Vatican MS] those with carcinomas of the skin. Boiled in oil, or pig's fat, and rubbed on, it is a treatment for periodic shivering fevers [Paris, Venice, and Salamanca MSS end here]. And Crateuas the Rhizotomist and Galen [or Galos] have said the same things [El Escorial MS ends], and it also helps those with gout.[48]

This commentary is more complete than many others on Dioscorides: it has synonyms, plant habitat, and medicinal usages. Wellmann thought that this scholium had come from the Pseudo-Apuleius *Herbarius*.[49] While there are similarities, the Byzantine commentator's source is not the *Herbarius*, a work in Latin composed perhaps in the fourth century, and not, as previously believed, based on an original Greek work.[50] The list of synonyms resembles that in the *Herbarius*, but there are notable differences.[51] Pseudo-Apuleius has no recommendation for gout, and prescribes *clematitis*-birthwort for nasal carcinoma[52]—probably a polyp of the

[42] M. Wellmann, *Krateuas* (Berlin, 1897 [AbhGöttingen, Phil.-hist.Kl., n.f. 2, no. 1]).

[43] Vienna, Nationalbibliothek MS med. gr. 1 (= Anicia Juliana MS), fol. 27ʳ, published as Crateuas fragment No. 5 in Wellmann, ed., Dioscorides, Vol. III, p. 145.

[44] E.g., the discussion of asphodel in Galen, *Properties of Foods* II, 55, and *Mixtures and Properties of Simples* VI, 77 (ed. Kühn, VI, 651–52, and XI, 842), and the fragment of Galen in the Vienna Anicia Juliana MS, fol. 27. Cf. Paul of Aegina VII, 3 (ed. Heiberg, Vol. II, p. 198). For Hippocratic works, see Dierbach (n. 16 above), 99–100.

[45] Munich, MS lat. 337, fol. 66ᵛ–7, published by H. Stadler, "Dioscorides Langobardus," *Romanische Forschungen*, 10 (1897), 238–39.

[46] Dioscorides III, 4.5 (ed. Wellmann, Vol. II, p. 8).

[47] The scholiast's δρακοντίου σπέρματος is probably to be rendered "tuber," given the manner of reproduction of the dragon arum.

[48] Schol. Dioscorides III, 4.5 (ed. Wellmann, Vol. II, p. 8: *app. crit.* to line 10). This is appended in at least the following MSS: •Vatican MS Pal. gr. 77; Vienna, N.B., MS gr. 16, 15th cent.; •Paris, B.N., MS gr. 2183; •Salamanca, MS 2659; •Venice, San Marco, MS Gr. Z 271; El Escorial, MS T–II–12.

[49] Ed. Wellmann, Vol. II, p. 8: *app. crit.* to line 10 init.

[50] H. E. Sigerist, "Zum Herbarius Pseudo-Apulei," *SA*, 23 (1930), 197–204, esp. 200.

[51] Pseudo-Apuleius, *Herbarius* 19 (ed. Sigerist, p. 57, lines 24–27), has the following synonyms not found in the Greek scholium: *feuxicterus*, *erectitis*, *Itali opetes*. The Greek scholium has ἰοντῖτις and θέξιμον, not found in the Latin *Herbarius*. Also variant is *Dardani sopitis*, cf. χαμαίμηλον. Both the Byzantine scribe and the author of the *Herbarius* apparently employed the same source. For an early study of plant synonyms, especially those appearing in the Anicia Dioscorides manuscript, see M. Wellmann, "Die Pflanzennamen des Dioskurides," *Hermes*, 33 (1898), 360–422.

[52] *Herbarius* 19.7 (ed. Sigerist, p. 57, lines 20–22): *Ad carcinomata, quae in naribus nascuntur. Herba aristolochia cum cipero et draconteae semen cum melle inpositum emendat.*

nares, usually a benign tumor in the nasal passage, displaying a pedicle, especially on the mucous membrane. Most of the medicinal suggestions in the commentary originated in the Crateuas fragment found in the Anicia Juliana on two separate folios,[53] and from Galen who clearly borrowed from Crateuas for the description of birthwort.[54] The major difference in the Byzantine scholium is the use of the herb for skin carcinomas (ἐν ῥινὶ καρκινώμασι). Byzantine diagnostics certainly did not include malignant neoplastic lesions as in modern oncology, but there is little doubt that they suffered from various kinds of malignant cancers,[55] and one of several terms to describe them was καρκίνωμα.[56] Recently, aristolochic acid, found in *Aristolochia baetica* and *A. clematitis*, was discovered to have antitumor properties,[57] and currently it is employed in chemotherapy for cancer.[58] It seems that a Byzantine physician, in or before the fourteenth century, had discovered *clematitis*-birthwort's pharmaceutical properties in use against skin cancers, and the scribe thereby modified the Greek text derived from Crateuas and added the scholium to Dioscorides' account, writing that *klēmatitis* "helps" skin cancer. Significantly, another copyist strengthens the claim by changing the verb from "helps" to "cures." This last alteration is correct, as judged in 1983, a fact we have had to rediscover. In early modern employment of the plant in Europe, it was apparently not used against cancer, but its history requires further research.[59]

There is a similar scholium attached to Dioscorides' account of βολβὸς ἐδώδιμος, one of the grape hyacinths, and most likely tassel hyacinth (*Muscari comosum* [L] Miller).[60] At the end of *Materia medica* II, 170.2, the scribes of three manuscripts have appended:

> [tassel hyacinth] boiled with barley meal[61] and pig's fat causes οἰδήματα and φύματα quickly to suppurate and break up.[62]

Oidēmata and *phymata* are two other Greek terms for tumorous growths or lumps, the lexical range of which include our "malignancies," "carcinoma," and "sarcoma."[63] An extract from the bulb of tassel hyacinth is currently used in chemotherapy for cancer.[64]

Not all commentaries and scholia attached to Dioscorides are rational or even empirical. Appended to the same group of manuscripts which include the tassel hyacinth scholium is a short text at the end of Dioscorides' clipped description of the herb called *mōly* (prob. *Allium* spp.):[65]

> The roots being cut and gathered up and carried next to the body, *mōly* helps against drugs [or poisons: φάρμακα] and frees one from his enemies.[66]

In this case, the Byzantine scholiast may have borrowed from the anonymous first- or second-century work called *Carminis de viribus herbarum*,[67] a collection of poems retailing quasi-magical properties of certain herbs. Even if the scholium can be traced to an ultimate source in Greek from the early Roman Empire, the data has been filtered and changed through centuries of transmission.

In other instances, the contents of the commentaries are apparently new, and one may also judge them rational. The same manuscripts that have the scholium on *mōly*, as well as the Anicia Juliana, also

[53] Vienna, Nationalbibliothek, MS med. gr. 1, fols. 18 and 19ᵛ; printed as Crateuas, Frgs. Nos. 1 and 2 in Wellmann, ed., Dioscorides, Vol. III, p. 144. A Galen fragment on *klēmatitis* is in fol. 19ᵛ of the Vienna MS, but it also does not include the statement on *karkinōma*.

[54] Galen, *Simples* VI, 56 (ed. Kühn, XI, 835–36).

[55] D. Brothwell, "The Evidence for Neoplasms," in D. Brothwell and A. T. Sandison, eds., *Diseases in Antiquity* (Springfield, Illinois, 1967), 320–45, using the findings of paleopathology. See also J. Reedy, "Galen on Cancer and Related Diseases," *Clio Medica*, 10 (1975), 227–38.

[56] L. J. Rather, *The Genesis of Cancer* (Baltimore, 1978), 9.

[57] G. E. Trease and W. C. Evans, *Pharmacognosy*, 11th ed. (London, 1978), 98 and 577; S. Munavalli and C. Viel, "Etude chimique, taxonomique et pharmacologique des Aristolochiacées," *Annales pharmaceutiques français*, 27 (1969), 449–64 [463]; *Chemical Abstracts*, 80 (1974), 24780g for *A. baetica*, and 81 (1974), 111458z for *A. clematitis*. Cf. earlier uses as listed in *Dispensatory of the United States*, 25th ed. (Philadelphia, 1955), 1841.

[58] Lewis and Elvin-Lewis, 134.

[59] Schneider, *Lexikon* (n. 25 above), Vol. V, pt. 1, 124–29.

[60] Dioscorides II, 170 (ed. Wellmann, Vol. I, pp. 236–37); Berendes, trans., *Dioskurides*, p. 247; Carnoy, 51.

[61] ἄλφιτον.

[62] Schol. Dioscorides II, 170.2 (ed. Wellmann, Vol. I, p. 237: *app. crit.* to line 14).

[63] Rather, *Genesis of Cancer* (n. 56 above), 9–13.

[64] Lewis and Elvin-Lewis, 135.

[65] J. Stannard, "The Plant Called Moly," *Osiris*, 14 (1962), 254–307, traces the remarkable history of plants called by this name in Greek. Cf. Schneider, *Lexikon* (n. 15 above), Vol. V, pt. 1, 65, and B. Langkavel, *Botanik der spaeteren Griechen* (Berlin, 1866; rptd. Amsterdam, 1964), 12.

[66] Schol. Dioscorides III, 47 (ed. Wellmann, Vol. II, p. 61: *app. crit.* to line 2).

[67] E. Heitsch, ed., *Carminis de viribus herbarum fragmentum*, 179–91 (esp. 190–91) in *Die griechischen Dichterfragmente der römischen Kaiserzeit*, Vol. II (Göttingen, 1964), pp. 35–36; Stannard, "Moly" (n. 65 above), 286; Wellmann, ed., Dioscorides, Vol. II, p. 61: *app. crit.* to line 2 (accepting the *Carminis de viribus*—known in Wellmann's day as *Carmen de herbis*—as the source).

have added details on κρόμυον) or onion (prob. *Allium cepa* L.).

> Thus boiled and laid on in a plaster with stavesacre (*Delphinium staphisagria* L.) or fig, onion softens and breaks up tumors (φύματα) very quickly.[68]

Modern Chinese medicine employs the onion for its anti-tumor properties,[69] and western folkmedicine uses it as a stimulant for the nervous system.[70] The scholium also suggests stavesacre, which contains a strong alkaloid which may have anti-tumor properties as do many alkaloids, but no ancient author on pharmacy recommends the onion for treatment of tumors.[71] Therefore, this discovery can be assumed to be early Byzantine, since the addendum on onion for tumors is first found in the Anicia Juliana manuscript.[72]

Some of the scholia are botanical, but clearly with a medicinal purpose. Dioscorides had written that the stem of the reedmace, a kind of cattail (prob. *Typha latifolia* L., possibly *T. angustifolia* L.) was smooth and uniform;[73] a Byzantine scribe added "the stem white, uniform."[74] Modern botanical manuals describe two types of spikes for *T. latifolia*, a female which turns brown, and a male which forms a yellow spike but which later falls off to leave a slender, colorless terminal axis,[75] so that the Byzantine addition of "white" probably aided identification.

Some of these manuscripts[76] have added a habitat description to Dioscorides' ἄκανθα 'Αραβική, with "It grows in rugged places." Sprengel believed that Dioscorides' "Arabian acanthus" was *Onopordon arabicum* [= *acanthium* L.], but Berendes thought it was no particular species, simply "acanthus" from Arabia.[77] Dioscorides says only that "Arabian acanthus" is similar to "white acanthus," identified as a thistle,[78] and several other plants.[79] A larger number of species passed under the name of "acanthus," as recorded in Theophrastus.[80] The illumination of the "Arabian acanthus" in the Anicia family of Dioscorides manuscripts, as well as the textual description are, however, more appropriate for *Onopordon acanthium*, Scotch thistle, sometimes also called cotton thistle from its fluffy purple flowers.[81] Scotch thistle grows on waste ground, which is in keeping with the "rugged places" in the scholium. Whatever might have been Dioscorides' intent regarding the plant, the Byzantine commentator most likely understood the description as that of Scotch thistle, and so described its habitat, since this was omitted in Dioscorides' text. In a modern herbal, Scotch thistle is recommended as an astringent,[82] the same use as given by Dioscorides, which makes the identification of Scotch thistle appropriate in its pharmacognosy. Not surprisingly, the Byzantine scribe is seeking clarity in the confusing nomenclature of plants called "acanthus," and his appended remark would be helpful.

In correcting Dioscorides' description of "wild isatis," a Byzantine scholiast shows remarkable botanical observation, surpassing by far Dioscorides. In this instance, moreover, the scribe says that Dioscorides is wrong. From a modern perspective, Dioscorides is not incorrect as the Byzantine scho-

[68] Schol. Dioscorides II, 151.2 (ed. Wellmann, Vol. I, p. 217: *app. crit.* to line 7).

[69] Bin Hsu, "Use of Herbs as Anti-Cancer Agents," *American Journal of Chinese Medicine*, 8 (1980), 305.

[70] *Dispensatory* (n. 57 above), 1538. Cf. V. E. Tyler, Lynn R. Brady, and J. E. Robbers, *Pharmacognosy*, 8th ed. (Philadelphia, 1981), 482, who write: "Further chemical and pharmacologic research is needed to determine the real value of garlic and onion for the many conditions in which they are reputed to be effective."

[71] No such recommendation appears in the Hippocratic corpus, Galen, Aetius of Amida, and Theophrastus, among the Greek sources, and none appears in Latin in the tracts by Pliny, Gargilius Martialis, Pseudo-Apuleius, and Scribonius Largus.

[72] The copyists of the early sixth-century Anicia Juliana MS, or an earlier prototype (the text is also in Naples, N.B., MS suppl. gr. 28, 7th cent.), were apparently of the opinion that Dioscorides had not given enough attention to plants of the genus *delphinium*, of which stavesacre is one species. After δαῦκος (Dioscorides III, 72) in the original order, the Anicia Juliana and the Naples MSS add two more plants, called δελφίνιον and δελφίνιον ἕτερον, along with descriptions. Venice, San Marco, MS Gr. Z 273 (12th cent.) is a fragmentary Dioscorides in the regular order, and this allowed Wellmann to discern the chapter's proper position in Dioscorides' work. Book III in the Venice MS begins on folio 21.

[73] Dioscorides III, 118 (ed. Wellmann, Vol. II, p. 129); Berendes, trans., *Dioskurides*, p. 342; Carnoy, 271.

[74] Schol. Dioscorides III, 118 (ed. Wellmann, Vol. II, p. 129: *app. crit.* to line 3).

[75] Polunin, *Flowers of Europe*, nos. 1827–28.

[76] Schol. Dioscorides III, 13 (ed. Wellmann, Vol. II, p. 20: *app. crit.* to line 11). *Vatican, MS Pal. gr. 77; *Paris, B.N., MS gr. 2183; *Venice, San Marco, MS gr. Z 271; Vienna, Nationalbibliothek, MS gr. 16; and El Escorial, MS III–R–3. The first three MSS also have the scholium to Dioscorides III, 118.

[77] Berendes, trans., *Dioskurides*, 271.

[78] *Ibid*. *Cnicius ferox* L; Langkavel, *Botanik* (n. 65 above), 74.

[79] E.g. *Acacia albida* Delile; *Cnicius arvensis* Hoffm. = *Cirsium arvense* (L.) Scop.; Carnoy, 3.

[80] Theophrastus, *HP* IV, 2.8 (tree); IV, 10.6 (creeping thistle, prob. *Carduus* [= *Cirsium*] *arvense* [L.] Scop.); IX, 12.1 (pine thistle, *Atractylis gummifera* L.), *etc*.

[81] Polunin, *Flowers of Europe*, no. 1494.

[82] M. Grieve, *A Modern Herbal* (New York, 1931; 2 vols.; rptd. 1971), Vol. II, 798.

liast alleges, but the scribe apparently believes that Dioscorides was describing a plant other than the one we now think he intended. Knowing it to be wrong, the Byzantine commentator hoped to correct the description with details so exact that we can be virtually certain which plant he intended.

Dioscorides devotes one chapter to woad (ἰσάτις [*Isatis tinctoria* L.]) and another to "wild woad" (ἰσάτις ἀγρία),[83] which modern authorities agree is another species of woad, while disagreeing on the exact nomenclature.[84] He writes that the plant is similar to ordinary woad except that it has larger leaves, like lettuce, but with slender stems which are reddish and multi-branched, on the end of which hang many tongue-like pods containing the seeds, the flowers being yellowish and small.[85] Modern descriptions add only that woad has petals up to twice as long as the sepals.[86] The Byzantine scribe believes he is correcting Dioscorides as he writes:

> One must consider faulty the information on woads. The cultivar (ἡ ἥμερος) bears a quince-yellow flower, thinner and greatly subdivided branches, and little pods from the top which are like tongues, in which are the seeds; but there is enclosed in these a black seed like black cummin (μελάνθιον, *Nigella sativa* L.),[87] and its stalk grows to a height of over two πήχεις (c. 3 ft./95 cm.), not to a height of a πῆχυς (c. 1½ ft./47 cm.). The wild kind, however, bears blacker leaves than the cultivar, and the wild kind has a shorter and thicker stalk, a purple or blue flower, and a prickly fruit shaped like a cross, in which the seed is as if divided into five equal small leaflets.[88]

The scholiast's description compares well with technical, modern depictions of cow basil (*Vaccaria pyramidata* Medicus) and its flowers, stalk, ovary, and seeds.[89] The Byzantine commentator observes that the seed pod has five small equal leaflets, and the *Hortus Third*, a modern botanical reference, says "epicalyx absent, calyx 5-lobed, 5-winged, inflated petals 5 . . . seeds nearly globose."[90] By contrast, woad's seed is black, but flat and pendulous, and does not compare to the seed of black cummin in the manner of cow basil's seed. In summary, this scholium reveals excellent attention to botanical detail rarely equaled in ancient or medieval herbals. Although the scholiast probably has mistaken Dioscorides' intended plant, he has boldly and explicitly written that Dioscorides was wrong and proceeded with his corrections. The unknown Byzantine commentator has trusted his observation of the plant in nature in a way that his western counterpart would not have done.

Byzantine commentaries on Dioscorides are apparently carefully pondered, and their contents are rationally constructed corrections and supplements to the text. A certain number of them are clearly derived from classical authorities, but most seem to be the results of Byzantine medicine's experience with the drugs mentioned in Dioscorides' *Materia medica*. By comparison, the manuscripts of the Old Latin Translation of Dioscorides reveal clumsy copyist errors by scribes who knew little about the material they were handling. It was not until the late eleventh century, when Constantine the African (or someone from his school) rearranged the Old Latin Translation in alphabetical order, that a large scale,[91] rationally designed set of commentaries were attached to Dioscorides' Latin text. By contrast, the Byzantine commentaries were more modest, but generally of a high medical and botanical quality. These Byzantine scholia show the purpose toward which Dioscorides' works were directed: medicine. The texts were not exclusively warehoused in isolated monastic libraries awaiting a Renaissance dusting. They must have been used by physicians.

[83] Dioscorides II, 184 and 185 (ed. Wellmann, Vol. I, pp. 253–54).

[84] Berendes, trans., *Dioskurides*, 258, with list of suggested spp.

[85] Dioscorides II, 185 (ed. Wellmann, Vol. I, p. 254).

[86] Polunin, *Flowers of Europe*, no. 292. *Hortus Third*, 606.

[87] Cf. Dioscorides III, 79 (ed. Wellmann, Vol. II, pp. 92–93).

[88] Schol. Dioscorides II, 185 (ed. Wellmann, Vol. I, p. 254: *app. crit.* to line 11). *Vatican, MS Pal. gr. 77, and Paris, B.N., MS gr. 2182 end with οἱονεὶ διειλημμένον (line 8 of scholium); but three earlier MSS add five further lines (as printed by Wellmann).

[89] Polunin, *Flowers of Europe*, no. 182; *Hortus Third*, 1142.

[90] *Hortus Third*, 1142.

[91] J. M. Riddle, "The Latin Alphabetical Dioscorides," *Proceedings of XIIIth International Congress of the History of Science, Moscow, August 18–24, 1971* Sections III & IV (Moscow, 1974), 204–9, and Riddle, "Dioscorides," *Catalogus*, 23–27.

XIV

Folk Tradition and Folk Medicine: Recognition of Drugs in Classical Antiquity

IN the late nineteenth century the History of Medicine and Pharmacy came to be studied for what was learned about history rather than about lost secrets in medicine. Although the romance of lost medical secrets attracted increased scorn from professional historians, many of the same historians harbored a romantic infatuation with Hippocrates, as the ancient founder of medicine. As early as Hellenistic Alexandria, he was venerated and regarded as the founder of scientific medicine for allegedly separating it from empirical practices, magic, superstition, and priestly rituals. All diseases are equally divine and equally natural.[1] This expression, found in the Hippocratic treatise *Sacred Disease*, came to embrace the philosophy of science on which the foundation of modern science and medicine rested. In the last twenty years, however, Hippocrates is regarded more as a legend, than as a founder. There are more than sixty treatises ascribed to Hippocrates but mostly written between 430 and 330 B.C. Now we place all of these works under the generic rubric "Hippocratic Corpus" (*HC*).[2] Regardless of authorship, they all seemed to share some common sentiments, preeminently among them, a prejudice in favor of rationality. In the hundreds of years of scholarship on the *HC*, there is no serious challenge to the assertion that the writers of these nascently scientific works founded a rational medicine different from folkish ways, summarized in a phrase often quoted from the Hippocratic Corpus: "witch-doctors [or 'magicians'], faith healers [or 'purifiers'], charlatans and quacks."[3]

In the history of pharmacy, the fact that there was little therapeutic intervention found in the Hippocratic Corpus was seen positively in contrast to the primitive, empirical medicine in what was known of Egyptian and Mesopotamian medicine. When we had the contexts to identify the plant, mineral, and, above all, animal substances in the ancient tablets, stones, and papyri, we saw a legacy of the doctrine of signatures and, less often, of opposite qualities as a means of explaining active pharmacy. All too often in Near Eastern medicine, magic appeared lurking near the front, enough so that we distrusted the medical rationality of the document's worth. Instead, modern historians agreed with the Alexandrians and some Romans that the Hippocratic physician was the founder of scientific medicine. Moderns regarded the Hippocratic physician as one who knew that he knew little about disease, made his patient comfortable, removed by regime all that might hinder nature, and finally and above all, described with a keen eye and precise language the course of disease and recovery from injury.

In his herculean *Introduction to the History of Science* (1927–1948) George Sarton declared that he would not include magic because its study would be about unreason while science was the study of reason, that is to say, progress. W.H.S. Jones declared, "if we take the Hippocratic collection we find that in no treatise is there any superstition."[4] The *HC* author of *Ancient Medicine* captured the eternal aspiration of medicine when he wrote: "Medicine has for long possessed the qualities necessary to make a science."[5]

In pharmacy these extremely postivistic assertions are troublesome. On one hand, there are modern scientists and scholars who believe as does Arthur K. Shapiro that the only linkage between modern and ancient medicine is the placebo effect, and Henry F. Dowling, who simply says, "Less than two dozen effective drugs were known before the year 1700."[6] In 1927, the same year as Sarton's first volume appeared, W.H.R. Rivers wrote the classic *Medicine, Magic, and Religion,* which defined medicine as part of a cultural system. Historians of pharmacy were faced with a problem either to accept the whig school of progress in the separation of the rational from the irrational, science from magic, or to view ancient pharmacy on the same grounds as the medical anthropologists, that is to say, engage in descriptive analysis in much the same way as the Hippocratic physician apparently treated his patients.

In contrast, Erwin H. Ackerknecht estimated that medical people in some traditional medicine groups employ a pharmacopoeia that consists of twenty-five to fifty per cent "objectively active" drugs.[7] What ever the drugs our ancestors had, whether effective or not in our sense, is beside the point as to when scientific medicine came to view folk drugs usages as beneath the dignity of a learned physician. When we study the early drugs that the early Greeks used, a different picture about early medicine emerges. Enough information recently has come to light so that we can reexamine the interrelation between science and folklore in classical culture. The ghosts, goblins, and malignant spirits were not driven from medicine by the Hippocratic rationalists, nor did these low level elements have an entirely inhibiting effect to "progressive developments" in medical history.

Edith K. Ritter's study of Assyrian tablets makes clear that the ancient Babylonians distinguished two types of medical practitioners: the *āšipu* or magical-expert and the *asû*, physician.[8] The *āšipu* viewed disease in a broad context of natural and supernatural powers. Treatment consisted of incantations, rituals, and various regimens designed to drive away the malignant influences on the sick person. In contrast, the *asû*, physician in a broad interpretation, did not affix supernatural causes to disease. Indeed, normally he did not inquire into the etiology or make a prognosis. He treated specific symptoms by empirical therapies. Both the *āšipu* and the *asû* employed drug therapy, but the *āšipu's* cupboard was relatively bare, showing a preference for stones, wool, and aromatic drugs. On the other hand, the *asû* prepared drugs and treated patients on an empirical basis. Prescription tablets sometimes begin: "A proved prescription of the hands of the master"; and "A proved/tested [tried and true] prescription. . . ." More detail is given concerning preparation and administration (*e.g.*, bandages, massages, lavages, salves, potions, pills, suppositories, tampons, and enemas). Even though many of the plant names especially are difficult to translate and place in modern terminology, there are familiarities with such drugs as colocynth seeds, chaste tree, garlic, cress, onions, thyme, and juniper.[9]

Texts for the *asû* and *āšipu* are prevalently separate and distinct, but occasionally there are texts which show that the patient tried one type of practitioner unsuccessfully and went to the other type for a different treatment. The inference is made in a few instances that there was some cooperation between the two types of practitioners.[10] This should not be surprising to us in the modern world because medical anthropologists describe communities that have both native medicine practitioners and modern, Western ones. People seem to know generally what types of problems to take to what kind of healer. If one type does not give successful treatment, the patient takes his or her problem elsewhere.[11] The point is not to reaffirm historically what we moderns already know from evidence much more direct than the ancient Greeks. Instead we observe that Ancient Near Eastern cultures may have evolved the distinction between spiritual healers and empirical healers long before any famous man by the name of Hippocrates was on Cos or anyone wrote a word in Greek attributed to the Ancient Founder.

An apparently distinguishing characteristic of the Hippocratic writings, however, is a contentiousness against faith healers, magic, and superstition. Beginning in the late fifth century B.C. there appeared a new type of practitioner, a person of learning and philosophy, whom we have come to name as the true physician (*iatros*). As one Hippocratic writer expressed it, "Each [disease] has its own nature [*physis*] and property [*dynamis*] and there is nothing in any disease which is unintelligible or which is insusceptible to treat. . . . He [i.e., a person of the art of medicine] would not need to resort to purifications and magic and all kind of charlatanism."[12] In medical therapy, a chief distinguishing feature of the new medicine is the emphasis on diet as the principal means of health maintenance and restoration.[13] Drug therapy, while not prohibited, appeared too close to purifications, magic, and charlatanism for too cozy an embrace.

In the *HC* there is not a kind word said for the older practitioners despite the voluminous discussion of diseases, injuries, health, water, airs, foods, anatomy—to a lesser extent—and other health issues. Occasionally the writings contradict one another, but never on the issue of unlearned medical practitioners. Although to some degree the Hippocratic physicians were like-minded,[14] because they were trained by the apprenticeship mode, there was no Hippocratic doctrine, indeed no oath, but there was an attitude. In the entire *HC* there is no work devoted to pharmacy *per se* and, for medical works, precious few concerns with therapy, except for diet. Dietlinde Goltz names only six works as therapeutically centered, two being on women's diseases:[15]

Diseases: **Peri nousōn** Bks. II & III: De morbis.[16]

Internal affections: **Peri tōn entos pathōn;** De affectionibus interioribus.[17]

Affections: **Peri pathōn:** De affectionibus.[18]

Places in Man: **Peri topōn tōn kata anthrōpon:** De locis in homine.[19]

Women's Disorders: **Gynaikeia**: De mulierum affectionibus.[20]

The Nature of Women: **Peri gynaikeiēs physios:** De natura muliebri.[21]

Argumentatively, the list could be expanded by: **On visions, Fistulas, Purgatives, Ulcers, Diseases V,** and **Machinery for reducing dislocations.**[22]

Drug Nomenclatures

I took the drug list compiled and published in 1824 by Johann Heinrich Dierbach, *Die Arzneimittel des Hippokrates* (Heidelberg), and compared its natural product drugs with modern pharmacy and pharmacognosy guides. My identifications were guided by Dierbach but in many cases I have made corrections of obvious errors. There are many plants imperfectly identified because the species are often uncertain. Treatises in the *HC* treatises give neither descriptive detail about the drugs nor detail about preparation, as this example from *Internal Affections* illustrates: "If that be the case [it is necessary] to purge the bowels with spiny spurge (*hippophaes*), then afterwards with hellebore, and to purge the head with antimony. . . ."[23]

I selected the modern guides because each one had a different purpose. The eighth edition (1981) of *Pharmacognosy* by Varro E. Tyler, Lynn R. Brady, and James E. Robbers is a hardline science of pharmacy approach to natural products. The twenty-fifth edition of the *United States Dispensatory*, Arthur Osol, George Farrar Jr., *et al.* (Philadelphia, 1955) contains more than 500 non-official drugs according to the United States Pharmacopoeia and other official guides. Walter Lewis and Memory Elvin-Lewis's *Medical Botany* is a guide to plants affecting health and it includes information derived from both anthropology and science studies. Trease-Evan's *Pharmacognosy* is more of a research reference to the scientific study of natural product drugs. Given these disparate guides, it is not surprising to find uneven results in the listings, but, although uneven, the data are revealing.

The comparison of the Hippocratic drugs with the modern guides unveils a surprising correspondence. Of the 257 drugs in the *HC* only twenty-seven or 10.5% are not listed in at least one of the modern guides. Of the twenty-seven, six to eight are more often classed as foods rather than drugs: blite, cucumber, turnip, lentil, medlar, cress, and, possibly, black cumin and asphodel. The twenty-seven have three animal products: eggs, castoreum (from beaver), and horn. Water and horn are two which one would not expect to find in a pharmacognosy guide, although most recipes contain water and calcium in the horn may have some physiological effects. The remainder are: cotyledon (50), hares tailgrass (56), ceterach (78), thorny bunet (81), lepidium (112), shepherd's purse (113), rocket salad (115), hartwort (196), alexanders (200), samphire (201), horse fennel (202), caucalis (205), daucos (206), and potter's earth (255).

The identification of eleven of the 257 is so uncertain that a tentative suggestion was not made. The reason for difficulty in identifying these plants is because they are not common, and this probably means that any use of them as a drug was slight. Sporadically, the only reference for an unidentifiable term in Greek is here in the *HC*. The plants contributing the greatest usages in pharmacy tend to be extensively used throughout the years from the time of *HC* to the time of Linnaeus, such as drugs from almonds, lettuce, fenugreek, mistletoe, licorice, willow, poppy, white hellebore, black hellebore, stavesacre, colocynth, cassia, scammony, spurge, rue, calamus, cinnamon, horehound, thyme, cat mint, wormwood, anise, coriander, juniper, storax, myrrh, henbane, and hemlock. Some plants are included in the *HC* list that clearly were little used as drugs. House leek or hen-and-chickens, for example, is mentioned only once and that comes in the treatise *On the Nature of Women* where it is described as a good additive in drink for nursing women. Willow leaves are used solely as a fumigant to promote menstruation.[24] This observation about willow leaves points out a weakness of these data: they identify the medicinal plants and other drugs but do not evaluate their usages.

Another approach to these data adds insight. Tyler-Brady-Robbers's *Pharmacognosy* has a chapter on resins and resin combinations in which some eighteen natural product medicinal plants are discussed. Eight of the eighteen are plants indigenous to North and South America. Of the remainder, eight are found in the *HC*, leaving only two: cannabis and storax. The medicinal use of cannabis was known later in antiquity to Dioscorides (fl. 40–80 A.D.)[25] and storax from liquid amber is a medieval substitute discovered when the old source of a similar resin was harvested almost to extinction.[26] The correlation between the Hippocratic drugs (*HC*) and modern ones available in Europe then is quite close; this phenomenon could not be due to random selection of drugs by classical peoples employing only placebos with their magic and superstition. Something more, something much more, is happening here, as evident from this historical data.

Even more startling is the correlation with the alkaloidal plant drugs. Of the thirty-four alkaloids listed in the modern sources, eighteen are New World, East African, Australian or Oceania—in other words, not indigenous to Europe, the Mediterranean or its immediate trading areas. Two, ergot and tryptophan, are derived from microorganisms which we do not expect to find in pre-modern sources. In one case, hydrastis, the source, *Hydrastis canadensis* L., is not found in the *HC* but the crude source, berberine, is found in rue which was employed by the Hippocratic authors.[27] Three which were not, withania from *Withania somnifera* Dunal, nux vomica from *Strychnos nux-vomica* L., and, possibly, stramonius from *Datura stramonium* L., are found in Dioscorides' *De materia medica*.[28] Regarding the last one, catharanthus alkaloids, I am uncertain whether the plant was known in antiquity because of the confusion between the Catharanthus and Vinca species.[29] These data demonstrate decisively that what there was to be discovered was discovered by the time that these medicinal substances were recorded in the first so-called scientific writings.

Empirical Tradition

The question now comes down to how did the *HC* writers learn which plants, which animal products, and which minerals were useful? On the basis of all evidence, explicitly and implicitly derived, there is no serious claim that the Hippocratic physicians had research laboratories where substances were tested. By elimination of alternative hypotheses, this leaves folklore, or—searching for words—folk usage, or empirics who practiced medicine much as the *asû*, and probably the *āšipu*, did in Babylonia. A number of terms are available, such as ethnopharmacy, ethnomedicine, folk medicine, popular medicine, popular health culture, ethnoiatry, and ethnoiatrics to describe this but, in keeping with this Symposium title, I shall use 'folk medicine' to denote medical practice before the *HC* and the traditional medicine that competes with scientific medicine after the fifth century B.C.

Many of the drugs found in the *HC* are found in earlier Near Eastern works. More research is needed to confirm more certainly the early evidence. There is little evidence that native Greek medical practitioners earlier than the *HC* writers employed written Near Eastern sources, and no Hippocratic works could be called pharmaceutical, not even the short work on laxatives, which is a medical discussion about their administration and not about specific drugs.[30] Dietlinde Goltz believes that references in *Affections* to a source called *pharmakitis* means that there is a lost work on Hippocratic drugs, but her suggestion is emphatically rejected by Georg Harig.[31] An interesting corollary is why many, if not most, of the drug references in the *HC* derive from two treatises on women's disorders?[32]

In stark contrast to the disdain of folk medicine shown by the Hippocratic writers, Theophrastus (*d. ca.* 287 B.C.) readily accepted information from common people and ordinary folk medicine practitioners, herbalists, or druggists called *pharmakopōloi* and *rhizotomoi* in his work called *Inquiry into Plants.*[33] Not only did he accept their information but he valued their knowledge. In relating that wolf's bane supposedly kills scorpions, Theophrastus wrote, "Now if what has been told already about the scorpion be true, then other similar tales are not incredible. And in relation to our own persons, apart from their effects in regard to health, disease, and death, it is said that herbs have also other properties affecting not only the bodily but also the mental powers."[34] Certain areas were noted for their drug knowledge especially about plants which are either indigenous to their region or grow there more abundantly. Aconite grew at Akonai "from whence it gets its name," he wrote about this Bithynian village. Anticyra was associated with hellebore, Chaeronea with spurge, Tyrrhenia with meadow saffron, and Mount Deta with black hellebore, while the more distant Libyians were known for silphium, the Scythians for licorice, and the Sabateans for myrrh.[35] Particular physicians (*iatroi*) were associated with specific drugs. Thrasyas of Mantineia and his pupil Alexias were known for a prescription for a deadly poison that had hemlock as a base. Drug vendors called *pharmakopōloi* and herbalists called *rhizotomoi* supplied information about the medicinal usages of plants, which Theophrastus readily accepted, in one case giving the name of the vendor, Eudemus the Chian. In relating information about the emetic and purgative qualities of wild carrot (*thapsia*), Theophrastus gave information helpful to our understanding how folk learned of the medicinal qualities in the first place. He observed that, "The cattle of the country [Attica] do not touch it, but imported cattle feed on it and perish of diarrhea."[37] Medical anthropologists raise the question about how the plants with beneficial medicinal properties are first separated from the half million or so species which are inert or harmful, but provide no conclusive or hard answers. The medical historian, Erwin Ackerknecht suggested that the separation came the same way that ill animals seem to know by instinct which plants to eat. But anthropologist Francis J. Clune, Jr., says that this is too big a burden to place on instinct alone. Ackerknecht rejected primitive experimentation on the grounds that there is no historical or anthropological evidence that this occurred or occurs. Clune disagrees. He believes that he has seen primitive experimentation in Peru and among Indians in Ecuador. How else, he poses, could the pre-modern people have discovered the psychogenic property in practically every plant possessing those properties, plants such as coffee, tea, tobacco, yerba maté, peyote, marijuana, opium, alcohol, hallucinogenic mushrooms, and several other drugs? Some modern scholars believe that there is some evidence to suggest that there may be a pathological explanation whereby organoleptic hints about chemical effects may reside in plants and can be detected by peoples who learned that a plant with one taste may have the same medicinal effect as a plant with a similar taste.[38]

Modern people are not the only ones who raised the question about how medicines first were discovered. Theophrastus gives us some insight about the discovery of early medicines in his story about the discovery of the purgative properties of wild carrot learned through the observation of cattle feeding on it. A recent discovery that plants could have an effect on fertility occurred when Australians noted the miscarriages in sheep that had grazed on a type of clover.[39] The ancient author of the Hippocratic treatise, *Ancient Medicine*, said that medicines were discovered in the same way that primitive man tested potential foods to determine nutritional, beneficial, and healthy things to eat. But, he added, research by physicians takes into account the accumulative folk experiences and forms the art of medicine. "The discovery of medicine," he wrote, "came about by much investigation and art."[40] Now that the art of medicine has been established, he dismisses folk experiences as being outdated. As I stated above, a reason Hippocratic physicians took this stance may have much to do with their attempts to establish themselves as sole conveyors of medical services. Theophrastus, in contrast, was not a physician, and he both valued and acknowledged traditional folk experience with medicines. The Hippocratic physicians, lacking a comprehensive theoretical basis to apply, simply took the vast data supplied by folk medicine and contemptuously dismissed the source. Just the same, they had to rely, as Geoffrey Lloyd said, "on observation of what worked."[41]

Greco-Roman Use of Folk Medicine

The Western cultural die was cast in its attitude towards folklore. On one hand, high science rejected magic and superstition and, because of its connection with them, folklore. On the other hand, it relied on data supplied by it.[42] Two of the best of the brightest of the Hellenistic-Roman scientists and medical persons were Dioscorides and Soranus of Ephesus (second century A.D.). Both of them openly relied on folk medicine and folk lore in their medical writings but they were critical and evaluative in their approach. In the Preface to *De materia medica*, Dioscorides explained how he arrived at his *logos* of *pharmaka*, that is his science of drugs: first he made direct and personal observations of "most" drugs beginning with identifying, harvesting, and preparing them in the field; second, researching pharmacy data in the written authorities; third, clinical observation—his words, "measuring the activities of drugs experimentally"—of drugs in trials on patients; fourth, personal field inquiries of folk practices "in each botanical region;" and, finally, arranging them by affinities.[43] While my summary here may sound suspiciously modern, it is only to the degree to which I have placed the sequence of Dioscorides' method stated in his own words. His objective was to impose order on scientific and traditional folk experiences with drugs, data from both communities being the means by which full knowledge of his science would be brought to the attention of the health service people, including the common person, we presume, assisting himself with self-prescribed remedies. In short, with the use of reason, traditional or folk medicine was not only valuable but critical in obtaining data.

There is another practical use of folk medicine for the scientific physician that was elaborated on by Soranus, a second century writer on gynecology. In his description of the ideal midwife, he gave these qualities: "She must be literate in order to be able to comprehend the art through theory too; . . . she will be free from superstition so as not to overlook salutary measures on account of a dream or omen or some customary rite or vulgar superstition."[44] But he also requires her to be sympathetic with the patients. He valued the use of amulets and any number of harmless superstitions because they seem to help the patients' psychological state. Superstitions and folkish practices, however, that resulted in harm or discomfort, he rejected. Folk medicine is useful to the learned physician if its use makes the patient feel better and more receptive to take the good advice of rational therapy. In the words of Lloyd, Soranus "puts his concern for his patients' feeling and their state above his own conception of the futility of superstitious belief."[45]

In contrast to the positive benefits Dioscorides and Soranus saw in traditional folk medicine, two Roman writers espoused traditional medicine in distrust of scientific medicine of the Greeks. Cato simply was anti-Greek and pro-Roman. A Roman learned from his father what he ought to know about medicine and cures. Folk medicine was superior medicine to him, because he distrusted Hellenic ways and trusted things that sprang from the soil of the Roman farm. Magic was employed, but W.H.S. Jones believes only to supplement the feeble curative effect of most of the folk drugs. Pliny noted that for quartan fevers "ordinary medicines (*medicina clinica*) are practically useless; for which reason I shall include several of the magician's remedies." Celsus (*fl. c.* A.D. 14–37), another Roman writer on medicine, said that rustics used germander in water for pleurisy "not having the remedies prescribed by medical practitioners."[46]

Pliny (d. A.D. 79) certainly knew a lot of remedies because he describes around a thousand plants and over a hundred animal derived drugs, but his positions on folk medicine, scientific medicine, and magic are at once more complex and more important than Cato's because his large sized *Natural History* is very influential. Pliny even joked about magic as when he wrote: "The Magi add also other details [about frogs], and if there is any truth in them, frogs should be considered more beneficial than laws to the life of mankind." He quite rightly observed that the Greeks supported magic and superstition as well as scientific medicine as when he said, "Another extraordinary thing that both these arts, medicine I mean and magic, flourished together, Democritus expounding magic in the same age as Hippocrates expounded medicine, about the time of the Peloponnesian War." The art of the magi, "the most fraudulent of arts," Pliny saw as springing from *medicina* and reinforced by *religio* and *artes mathematicae*.[47] But this did not prevent him from using magicians' remedies for fevers when traditional Roman medicine proved ineffective. Just the same, he had little patience for all the shrill arguments of the high medicine Greeks (*medici*), those practicing scientific medicine, with their contradictions endlessly expounded. In the words of Vivian Nutton, Pliny delivered "the most sustained, influential and potentially devastating attack on doctors and their medicine ever mounted."[48] Pliny sought to provide the means by which the ordinary Roman could arm himself and the family with the practical knowledge to protect himself from the harm done by Greek physicians and all forms of foreign magic and superstition. Like Dioscorides and Celsus, Pliny saw experimentation as a means of proof of a medicine's effectiveness, [49] which he even did himself as when he said—strangely enough to us: "I find that a heavy cold clears up if the sufferer kisses a mule's muzzle." Folk learning with medicines provided that proof and freedom from foreign influences. The smart person, however, learns all that he can. Even though he counselled the use of amulets employed by the magi for quartan fevers because "ordinary medicines are practically useless," Pliny bemoans that the exotic remedies from abroad are preferred to those available in the local garden.[50]

The last representation of classical thinking about folk medicine comes from Marcellus (*fl* 379–395), who wrote in the late Autumn of classical thought, when the sun was setting on the Roman Empire. He began his work with the following statement: "While I follow the aspirations of learned people, who to be sure may be strangers to the practice of medicine, however, despite their objective of producing cures by rational procedures, I have written this book about empirical cures, resourcefully and diligently collected, of natural remedies, reasonable preparations and observations with resources provided me from all kinds of sources." Marcellus claims that he has assembled information not only from the learned written authorities, but "fortunate remedies and simples from rural folk and lower class people."[51] Indeed, he did and uncritically at that. His work, *On Medicines*, combines Hippocratic knowledge together with Roman and Celtic popular remedies and rank superstition. If he were placed in modern terminology, we would call him an integrationist. Information about drugs was information about drugs, regardless the source of the information.

Conclusion

There are a number of ways to view folk medicine. Many people in today's learned communities regard folk medicine as thoroughly old fashioned, at best quaint, at worst dangerous for its deceptive practices, when scientific medical procedures are available by professionally trained personnel. These people share the same view as the Hippocratic writers. Another school of thought holds that folk medicine is a form of experience, an uncontrolled laboratory, which, if examined carefully and critically, can provide helpful information for modern science. Adherents of this school share the same position as Theophrastus and Dioscorides. Some people in the modern world, frequently they are social scientists although not exclusively, regard folk medicine within a cultural frame and they see that it can be valuable to modern medical practitioners in so far as they can know the psychological state of their patients and possibly build on that knowledge empirically. These people regard folk medicine much the same as did Soranus. Another school of modern people really wish that they were not so modern, because the old fashioned ways of their fathers and mothers were better. They stand with Pliny who stood with Cato. And finally, there is a small group of people who believe that facts are only functional things that work within a context and are discarded when they do not. Procedures, methodology, and rational judgments are set aside. Best it is to integrate knowledge from science, tradition, East and West. These people share the same position as Marcellus. It would seem that the principal positions that one can take in respect to folk medicine had been taken already by classical writers. What is new? partly my appreciation of what is old.

References

1. *De morbo sacro*, 1 (ed., W. H. S. Jones [Cambridge, Mass., 1923–1931; Loeb Classical Library, 4 vols.] II, 138–83, on 138).
2. For the best overall perspective, see Wesley D. Smith, *The Hippocratic Tradition* (Ithaca, 1979), and review by John Scarborough, *American Journal of Philology*, 103 (1982):340–344.
3. *De morbo sacro* (n. 1), 2 (ed. Jones, II, 141).
4. G. Sarton, *Introduction to the History of Science*, 3 vols. in 5 pts. (Baltimore, 1927–48), I, 19; Jones (n. 1), I, xiv.
5. *De prisca medicina*, 2 (= ed., Jones [n. 1]) I, 12–64, on 14; translation by G. E. R. Lloyd, *Hippocratic Writings* (New York, 1978), 71.
6. Arthur K. Shapiro, "The Placebo Effect in the History of Medical Treatment: Implications for Psychiatry," *American Journal of Psychiatry*, 116 (1959): 298–304; Henry F. Dowling, *Medicines for Man* (New York, 1973), 14.
7. Erwin H. Ackerknecht, "Problems of Primitive Medicine," *Bulletin of the History of Medicine*, 11 (1942): 503–521 [esp. p. 512].
8. Edith K. Ritter, "Magical-Expert (=ĀŠIPU) and Physician (=ASÛ). Notes on Two Complementary Professions in Bablylonian Medicine," in *Studies in Honor of Benno Landsberger on his Seventy-fifth Birthday, April 21, 1965*. (Chicago, 1965; "Assyriological Studies," No. 16), 299–313.
9. Ritter (n. 8), pp. 308, 311, 313; Franz Köcher, *Keilschriften zur assyrisch-babylonischen Drogen- und Pflanzenkunde*. (Berlin, 1955; Deutsche Akademie der Wissen-

schaften zu Berlin. Institut für Orientsforschung. Veröffentlichung), 28; Reginald C. Thompson, *Assyrian Medical Texts From the Originals in the British Museum* (Oxford, 1923); Reginald C. Thompson, *The Assyrian Herbal* (London, 1924).

10. Ritter (n. 8), pp. 314–5.
11. Richard W. Lieban, "The Field of Medical Anthropology," in: *Culture, Disease and Healing*, David Landy, ed. (New York, 1977), 27 refs.; and David Landy, "Traditional Cures Under the Impact of Western Medicine," *ibid.*, 471 refs.
12. *De morbo sacro* (n. 1), 21 (ed. Jones, II, 182).
13. I. M. Lonie, "A Structural Pattern in Greek Dietetics and the Early History of Greek Medicine," *Medical History*, 21 (1977): 235–260.
14. Peter M. Fraser, *Ptolemaic Alexandria* (Oxford, 1972; 3 vols.), I. 353.
15. D. Goltz, *Studien zur altorientalischen und griechische Heilkunde. Therapie—Arzneibereitung—, Rezeptstruktur* (Wiesbaden, 1974; *Sudhoffs Archiv*, Beiheft 16), 102.
16. *Oeuvres complètes d'Hippocrate*, E. Littré, ed. (Paris, 1839–1861; repr. Amsterdam, 1979; 10 vols.), Vol. VII, 8–114. 118–160.
17. *Ibid.*, VII, 166–302.
18. *Ibid.*, VI, 208–270.
19. *Ibid.*, VI, 276–349.
20. *Ibid.*, VIII, 10–406.
21. *Ibid.*, VII, 312–430.
22. Georg Harig, "Anfänge der theoretischen Pharmacologie im Corpus Hippocraticum," *Hippocratica* (Paris, 1980; Colloques internationaux du Centre National de la Recherchée Scientifique, No. 583), 223–45, on 227.
23. *De affect.* (n. 18) 49 (= ed. Littré, VII, 290).
24. *De natur. mul.* (n. 21), 32 (VII, 348); 78 (VIII, 186).
25. Dioscorides, *De materia medica*, IV. 148 (= M. Wellmann, ed., *Pedanii Dioscuridis Anazarbei De materia medica* [Berlin, 1906–1914; 3 vols.] Vol. II, 157.
26. John M. Riddle, "Quid pro quo. Pharmacy in the Middle Ages," *Medical Heritage*, forthcoming.
27. *E.g., De morbis III.* 15. 9 (= ed. Paul Potter, *Hippokrates Über die Krankheiten III* [Berlin, 1980; Corpus Medicorum Graecorum, I 2, 3], 86); *De mulierum affectionibus* (n. 20), II. 206 (= ed. Littré, n. 16, VIII, 402).
28. Dioscorides (n. 25), IV, 71–74 (= ed. Wellmann, II, 229–233); Wolfgang Schneider, *Lexikon zur Arzneimittelgeschichte* (Frankfurt, 1968–1975; 7 vols.), V, pt. 3, 294–296.
29. John M. Riddle, "Ancient and Medieval Chemotherapy for Cancer," *Isis*, 76 (1985): 319-330 [esp. p. 327].
30. *De purgantibus* = *De remediis* (ed. Hermann Schöne, "Hipp. Peri pharmakon," *Rheinisches Museum für philologie.* N.F. 73 [1924]: 434–448 [text, pp. 440–443 with Latin trans]).
31. Goltz (n. 15), 139; Harig (n. 22), 225.
32. I know of no satisfactory explanation for this apparent phenomenon. For recent work on the *HC* gynecological treatises see Hermann Grensemann, ed. and trans., *Hippokratische Gynäkologie* (Wiesbaden, 1982); see also, Danielle Gourevitch, *La mal d'être femme. La femme et la médecine à Rome* (Paris, 1984).
33. Theophrastus, *Enquiry into Plants* (= Arthur Hort, ed. and trans. [Cambridge, Mass., 1916; Loeb Classical Library, 2 vols). Theophrastus' authorship of Bk. IX—where the medical and folklore material is discussed—is challenged but for the purposes of this article the real author is not important so long as the writer lived about the same time and voiced the sentiments that he did in the work. For further references, see Jerry Stannard, "The Herbal as a Medical Document," *Bulletin of the History of Medicine*, 43 (1969): 212–220, [esp. p. 213], and John Scarborough, "Theophrastus on Herbals and Herbal Remedies," *Journal of the History of Biology* (1978): 353–385.
34. *Enquiry* (n. 33), IX. 18. 2–3 (= ed. Hort, II, 308–310).
35. *Ibid.* IX. 16. 4, 9.2, 11.1, 16.7, 2.5, 7, 10. 2, 1.7, 13. 2, 4. 5, 2. 3, 5; 3. 3 (= ed. Hort, II, 298, 260, 268, 302, 226, 228, 266, 222, 282, 236, 224, 226, 232).

36. *Ibid.* IX. 17. 3 (= ed. Hort, II, 306).
37. *Ibid.* IX. 20. 3 (= ed. Hort, II, 316).
28. Ackerknecht (n. 7) [esp. 512], citing as supporters of trial and error discovery: Castiglioni, Meyer-Steineg and Sudhoff, Neuburger, Diepgen, and Pagel; Francis J. Clune, Jr., "Witchcraft, the Shaman, and Active Pharmacopoeia," in: *Medical Anthropology*, Francis X. Grollig and Harold B. Haley, eds. (The Hague, 1976), pp. 5–9, on 7; on organoleptic detection, see introduction by C. Pfaffman to *Taste, Olfaction and the Central Nervous System*, ed. D. W. Pfaff (New York, 1985); John K. Crellin, "Traditional Medicine in Southern Appalachia and Some Thoughts for the History of Medicinal Plants," in: *Botanical Drugs of the Americas in the Old and New Worlds. Invitational Symposium at the Washington-Congress 1983*, ed. Wolfgang-Hagen Hein (Stuttgart, 1984; Veröffentlichungen der Internationalen Gesellschaft für Geschichte der Pharmazie e.V., vol. 53), 65–78 [esp. p. 67]; and Philip M. Teigen, "Taste and Quality in 15th- and 16th-Century Galenic Pharmacology," *Pharmacy in History*, 29(1987): 60–68. (I am grateful to John Crellin for helpful advice about this problem.)
39. J. H. Harborne, *Introduction to Ecological Biochemistry* (London, 1977), 83–89.
40. *Ancient Medicine* (n. 1), 4 (= ed., Jones, IV, 20)
41. G. E. R. Lloyd, *Science, Folklore, and Ideology* (Cambridge, 1983), 134.
42. On the concurrence between traditional medicine and scientific medicine, see Antje Krug, *Heilkunst und Heilkult. Medizin in der Antike* (München, 1985).
43. Dioscorides. *De materia medica.* Preface. 1–2, 5 (= trans. John Scarborough and Vivian Nutton, in: "The Preface of Dioscorides' *Materia Medica*: Introduction, Translation, Commentary," *Transactions and Studies of the College of Physicians of Philadelphia* 4 [1982]: 187–227 [on pp. 195–6]; John M. Riddle, *Dioscorides On Pharmacy and Medicine* (Austin, 1986), 164.
44. Soranus, *Gynecology*. I. 2. 3–4 (= trans. Owsei Temkin, *Soranus' Gynecology* [Baltimore, 1956], pp. 5–7).
45. Lloyd (n. 41), 182.
46. Cato. *On Agriculture* (= eds. and trans. William D. Hooper and Harrison B. Ash [Cambridge, Mass., 1934; Loeb Classical Library]); Pliny, *Natural History*, XXX. 30. 98 (eds. and trans., W. H. S. Jones, H. Rackham, and D. E. Eichholz [Cambridge, Mass., 1938–1963; Loeb Classical Library, 10 vols.], Vol. VIII, 340); W. H. S. Jones, "Ancient Roman Folk Medicine," *Journal of the History of Medicine and Allied Sciences. 12* (1957): 459–472, on 462; Celsus. *On Medicine*, IV. 13. 3 (= ed. and trans. W. G. Spencer (Cambridge, Mass., 1935–1938; Loeb Classical Library; 3 vols.) I, 406.
47. *Natural History* (n. 46), quoting XXXII. 18. 49, XXX. 2. 10, 1.1 (VIII, pp. 494, 284, 278).
48. Vivian Nutton, "Murders and Miracles: Lay Attitudes Towards Medicine in Classical Antiquity," in: *Patients and Practitioners*, ed. Roy Porter (Cambridge, 1985), 23–53 [on p. 43].
49. Dioscorides (n. 43), Preface. 1–5 (= trans. Scarborough-Nutton, 195–6); Celsus (n 46), V. 28. 7B; *VI*. 9. 7 (= ed. Spencer, II, pp. 142, 250); Pliny (n. 46), XXX. 29. 95 (= eds. Jones, Rackham, Eichholz, VIII, p. 338).
50. Pliny (n. 35), *Natural History*, XXX. 11. 31 (eds. Jones, Rackham, Eichholz, VIII, p. 298); XXX. 30. 98 (= VIII, p. 340); XXIV. 1. 4–5 (= VII, pp. 4, 6).
51. Marcellus, *De medicamentis liber*, prol. 1–3 (= ed. and trans. Max Niedermann, *Marcellus Uber Heilmittel* [Berlin, 1968; Corpus Medicorum Latinorum, V; 2 vols.], I, 2 (trans. from Latin by J. Riddle).

TABLE

Drugs in the Hippocratic Corpus Compared to Pharmacognosy Guides

Guide to Table:

Dierbach, Johann Heinrich. *Die Arzneimittel des Hippokrates.* Heidelberg, 1824; rpt. Hildesheim, Olms, 1969.

Tyler = Tyler, Varro E., Lynn R. Brady, James E. Robbers. *Pharmacognosy.* Eighth Edition. Philadelphia, Lea & Febiger, 1981. (pp. 468–502 = herbs and health foods)

Dispensatory = *Dispensatory of the United States.* Twenty-Fifth Edition. Arthur Osol, George E. Farrar, Jr., *et al.* eds. Philadelphia, Lippincott, 1955. (official drugs, pp. 1–1521; unofficial drugs, pp. 1523–1933; veterinary biological products, 1935–2057)

Lewis = Lewis, Walter H., and Memory P. F. Elvin-Lewis. *Medical Botany. Plants Affecting Man's Health.* New York, Wiley, 1977.

Trease = Trease, George Edward and William Charles Evans. *Pharmacognosy.* Eleventh Edition. London, B. Tindall, 1978.

The number in the left column next to the Greek term is the author's numbering. Some drugs have more than one name in Greek that may appear in various Hippocratic works. Normally employed is the most common name. The number in the second column is Dierbach's number. Not all of Dierbach's identifications are acceptable. Occasionally I have corrected his identifications and substituted my own. The identification of the Greek terms are generally made to correspond with the modern binomial classification system—a necessary step in relating modern information about natural plant drugs. Nevertheless, this practice may convey a deceptively incorrect impression that there is more accuracy than is merited. The number under each source is pagination in the modern guide. An asterisk (*) denotes that the modern reference is not to the same species but one closely related.

	Common Name	Scientific Name	Tyler	Dispensatory	Lewis	Trease
1. *hydōr*	1. water					
	Animal drugs:					
2. *gala*	2. milk		29			
3. *ōa*	3. eggs					
	Cereals:					
4. *krithē*	1. barley	*Hordeum vulgare* L.	287	1713	190, 219	768
5. *pyros*	2. wheat	*Triticum vulgare* L.	38	1910	98	154
6. *zeia trynis*	3. spelt	*T. spelta* L.	38*	1910*		
7. *brōmos*	4. oats	*Avena sativa* L.			21ff	154
8. *elymos*	5. millet, Italian	*Panicum italicum* L.			18, 59	
9. *kenchros*	6. millet	*Panicum miliaceum* L.			18, 59	
10.*asparagos*	7. asparagus	*Asparagus officinalis* L.	293–4*	51*	259ff	272
11. *aigyptios kyamos*	8. Egyptian bean	*Nelumbium speciosum* L. (1) *Nymphaea nelumbo* L. (2)			326(2)	95–7(2)
12. *tribolos*	9. tribulus	*Tribolos terrestris* L.		1671	313	107–8
13. *phoinix*	10. date palm	*Phoenix dactylifera* L.			70	155
14. *andraphaxis*	11. orach	*Atriplex hortensis* L.			[69]	[90]
				no medicinal usages given		
15. *teuflion*	12. beet	*Beta vulgaris* L.		1344	69, 93	90
16. *bliton*	13. blite	*Amaranthus blitum* L.				[90]
		no medicinal usages given; Dioscorides (*2.* 117) explicitly says that it has no medicinal usages				

	Common Name	Scientific Name	Tyler	Dispensatory	Lewis	Trease
17. *drys*	14. oak	*Quercus* sp.		1820	245ff	367
18. *karya*	15. nut	*Juglans regia* L. + refs. to walnuts only		1725	282ff.	
19. *morea*	16. mulberry	*Morus nigra* L.			[69]	403
20. *knidē, akalyphē*	17. nettles	*Urtica* sp.			387ff	
21. *sykas, kradē*	18. fig	*Ficus* sp.		1691	253ff	332
22. *sikyos pepōn*	19. canteloupe	*Cucumis melo* L.			119	
23. *kolokyntē*	20. gourd	*Cucurbita maxima* L. + sp.				
24. *sikyos*	21. cucumber	*Cucumis sativus* L.	479	1818	291	119
25. *krambē*	22. cabbage	*Brassica oleracea* L.			218ff	
26. *gongulis*	23. turnip	*Brassica rapa* L.				
27. *rhaphanis*	24. radish	*Raphanus sativus* L.			361	
28. *thermos*	25. white bean	*Lupinus albus* L.		1744	93f	
29. *dolichos*	26. bean	1-*Vicia faba* L. 2-*Phaseolus vulgaris*			1–45f 2–99f	
30. *ōchros*	27. yellow pea	*Pisum ochres* L.? + sp.				
31. *pisos*	28. garden pea	*Pisum sativus* L.			98	
32. *orobos*	29. bitter vetch	*Vicia ervila* L.			98	
33. *phakos*	30. lentil	*Ervum lens* L.				
34. *erebinthos*	31. chick pea	*Cicer arietinum* L.			315f	
	Roses:					
35. *batos*	32. bramble	*Rubus ulmifolius* L. + sp.		1181f	135f	103, 105
36. *archas*	33. pear	*Purus communis* L.			41	

	Common Name	Scientific Name	Tyler	Dispensatory	Lewis	Trease
37. *mēlea*	34. apple	*Pyrus malus* L. L *Malus* sp.		287, 362		
38. *kydōnia*	35. quince	*Pyrus cydonia* L.	52	1660		352
39. *ouon*	36. service tree	*Sorbus domestica* L.		1867	41f	
40. *mespilē*	37. medlar	*Pyrus germanica* Hook.				
41. *amygdalē*	38. almond	*Amygdalus communis* L.	92–3	45	40f	305f
	Dicotyledons:					
42. persea	39. Persea tree	*Mimusops schimperi* [Cordia myia L.—Dierbach]			266	
43. *kraneia*	40. dogwood	*Cornus mascula* L.		1647	135f	
44. *sēsamon*	41. sesame	*Sesamum* sp.	92	1847f		316
45. *strychnos*	42. garden nightshade	*Solanum nigrum* L.	204f	146	55f	135f
46. *thridax*	43. lettuce	*Lactuca sativa* L.		926	446	144
47. *linozostis*	44. annual mercury	*Mercurialis annua* L.			69	
48. *lapathon*	45. dock	*Rumex patientia* L.		603	135f	89
49. *andrachnē*	46. purslane	*Portulaca oleracea* L.			89	
50. *kotyledon*	47. cotyledon	*Cotyledon umbilicus* L.				
51. *ampelos*	48. grape & wine	*Vitis vinifera* L.				89
	Phlegm, Sweet, Oils, Fatty Drugs:					
52. *akantha*	1. acacia	*Acacia* sp.	45–6	1	119f	351
53. *pelekinos*	2. axweed	*Securigera coronilla*			255	
54. *kytisos*	3. tree-medick	*Medicago arborea*			81	106f

	Common Name	Scientific Name	Tyler	Dispensatory	Lewis	Trease
55. *epikeras*	4. fenugreek	*Trigonella foenumgraecum* L.	481–2	1908	219f	103f
56. *agopyros*	5. hares tailgrass	*Lagurus ovatus* L.				
57. *anchousa*	6. alkanet	*Anchusa tinctoria* L.		1536		134f
58. *phlomos*	7. mullein	*Verbascum thapsus* L.		1927	297f	136f
59. *ixon*	8. mistletoe	*Viscum album* L.	489–9	1928	48f	88
60. *strouthion*	9. soap-wort	*Saponaria officinalis* L.		1837	224f	90
61. *bechion*	10. colt's foot	*Tussilago farfara* L.	478			144
62. *malachē*	11. mallow	*Malva rotundifolia* L.			391	116
63. *linon*	12. flax	*Linum usitatissimum* L.		757	224f	107f
64. *polypodion*	13. polypodium	*Polypodium vulgare* L.		618	133f	78
65. *glykyrrhiza*	14. licorice	*Glycyrrhizaglabra* L.	484	619	182f	487f
66. *meli*	15. honey		486	653		331
	Oils; fats					
67. *elaia*	16. olive oil		89–90	921	283	314f
	Astringent drugs: light					
68. *rhodon*	1. rose	*Rosa* sp.	115	1197f	103f	70f
69. *kentaurion*	2. great centaurea	*Centaurea centaureum* L.		1620*	52*	143*
70. *helxinē*	3. helxine(?)	1. *Parietaria officinlis* L. 2. *Helxine solieiolii* Req.			1–70 2–256	
71. *kissos*	4. ivy	*Hedera helix* L.	454		49, 86	121, 123
72. *xanthion*	5. burweed	*Xanthium strumarium* L.		1318*	374	147
73. *ereikē*	6. heather	*Erica arborea* L.				124*
74. *peristereōn*	7. vervain	*Verbena officinalis* L.	473–4*	1928	122.391	134, 137

	Common Name	Scientific Name	Tyler	Dispensatory	Lewis	Trease
75. *erythrodanon*	8. madder	*Rubia tinctorum* L.			269f*	270f
76. *philision*	9. cleavers	*Galium aparine* L.			192*	
77. *adianton*	10. maidenhair	*Adiantum capillus veneris* L.			326	
78. *skolopendrion*	11. ceterach	*Asplenium ceterach* L.				
	Astringent drugs: stronger					
79. *pentaphyllon*	12. cinquefoil	*Potentilla reptans* L. + sp.		1816	235f	
80. *stoibē*	13. thorny bunet	*Poterium spinorum* L.				
81. *myrsinē*	14. myrtle	*Myrtus communis* L.		1761		120–1
82. *rhoa*	15. pomegranate	*Punica granatum* L.		1797		558
83. *lōtos*	16. nettle tree	*Celtis australis* L.			70*	
84. *rhamnos*	17. rhamnos (?)	1-*Zizyphus vulgaris* L. 2-*Lycium europaeum* L.			2–313*	1–11 5–6
85. *melia*	18. manna ash	*Fraxinus ornus* L.		1747	293f	126, 307
86. *myrikē*	19. tamarisk	*Tamarix gallica* L.	498	1895	236	306
87. *rhous*	20. tanning sumach	*Rhus coriaria* L.		1829	218f	645f
88. *itea*	21. willow (?)	*Salix alba* L.		1834	150f	86f
89. *hypokistis*	22. hypocracy tree	*Cytinus hypocistis* L.		1660	338f	558f
90. *kinnabaris*	23. dragon's blood	*Dracaena* sp.			342	467
91. *kēkis*	24. oak gall	*Quercus* sp.		1820, 1379	245f	367
	Sharp drugs					
	a. vegetable					
92. *narkissos*	1. narcissos	*Narcissus* sp.	456** **as poison		135f	

	Common Name	Scientific Name	Tyler	Dispensatory	Lewis	Trease
93. *asphodelos*	2. asphodel	*Asphodelus ramosus* L.				
94. *skorodon*	3. garlic	*Allium sativum* L.	482	1538	123f	149
95. *prason*	4. leek	*Allium porrum* L.	482*	1538*	219*	149*
96. *krommyon*	5. onion	*Allium cepa* L.	482*	1538*	219f*	149f*
97. *mōlyza*	6. moly	*Allium subhirsutum* L. (?)	482*	1538*	219f*	149*
98. *bolbos*	7. purse-tassels (?)	*Muscari comosum* L. (?)			135	
99. *skillē*	8. squill	*Scilla maritima* L. *Urginea maritima* L.	179	1305	184f	151
100. *aron*	9. cuckoo-pint	*Arum maculatum* L.				338
101. *drakontion*	10. dragon arrowroot	*Arum dracunclus* L.				338*
102. *helleboros leukos*	11. white hellebore	*Veratrum album* L.	251	1486	188f	151f
	Dicotyledons					
103. *helleboros melas*	12. black hellebore	*Helleborus niger* L.	180	1711	31f	506f
104. *batrachion*	13. crowsfoot	*Ranunculus* sp.	456		70f	684
105. *anemōnē*	14. poppy anemone	*Anemone coronaria* L. + sp.		1818	313f	684
106. *staphis agria*	15. stavesacre	*Delphinium staphisagria* L.		1869	309f	684
107. *melanthion*	16. fennel flower or black cumin	*Nigella sativa* L.				
108. *glykysidē*	17. peony	*Paeonia officinalis* L.			314*	
109. *isatis*	18. woad					100f
110. *kardamon*	19. cress	*Lepidium sativum* L.				
111. *lepidion*	20. lepidium	*Lepidium latifolium* L.				
112. *thlaspi*	21. shepherd's purse	*Thlaspi Bursa pastoris* L.				

	Common Name	Scientific Name	Tyler	Dispensatory	Lewis	Trease
113. *napy*	22. mustard	*Sinapis nigra* L. + sp.	72f	869f	94f	524
114. *euzōmon*	23. rocket salad	*Eruca sativa* Mill.				
115. *erysimon*	24. hedge mustard	1-*Sisybrium polyceratium* L.; 2-*Erysimum officinalis* L.			2–36	
116. *leukoion*	25. wall flower	*Cheiranthus cheiri* L. + sp.		1623	184f	100f
117. *telephion*	26. sedamine	*Sedum telephium* L. ?		1838		558
118. *krinanthemon*	27. houseleek	*Sempervivum tectorum* L.			344*	
	Cucurbitaceae					
119. *ampelos agria*	28. bryony ?	*Bryonia* sp. ?			281	
120. *elatērion*	29. squirting cucumber	1-*Momordica elaterium* L.; 2-*Ecballium elaterium* L.		1–1758 2–1675	2–281	2–119
121. *kolokynthis agria*	30. wild colocynth	1-*Cucumis colocynthis* L.; 2-*Citrullus colocynthis* L.		2–359	2–281	1&2–119
	Compositae					
122. *knēkos*	31. safflower?	*Carthamus tinctoris* L.				542f*
123. *chamaileōn melas*	32.?	*Cardopatium corymborum* + *Carthamus corymbosus* + *Brotera corymbosa* +				
124. *kammaron*	33. aconitum	*Doronicum pardalianches* L. + sp**	450–1	107f	374	617f
	**species uncertain but it is an aconite bearing plant					
125. *skammōnia*	34. scammony	*Convulvulus scammonia* L.		717	257*	472

	Common Name	Scientific Name	Tyler	Dispensatory	Lewis	Trease
126. *epithymon*	35. cuscuta	*Cuscuta europaea* L.				137
127. *tithymallos*	36. spurge	*Euphorbia* sp.		1688	253f	108f
128. *peplion*	37. peplis spurge	*Euphorbia peplis* L.		1688*	253*	108*
129. *peplos*	38. peplus spurge	*Euphorbia peplus* L.		1688*	253*	108*
130. *hippophaes*	39. spiney spurge	*Euphorbia spinosa* L.		1688*	253*	108*
131. *kyparissos*	40. wolksmilk	*Euphorbia cyparissias* L.		1688*	253*	108*
132. *krōton*	41. castor oil plant	*Ricinus communis* L.	87–89	1957	94f	316f
133. *knestron*	42. thymelaea	*Daphne gnidium* L.		1756	323*	177*
	Miscellaneous					
134. *daphnoides*	43. laurel daphne	*Daphne laureola* L.		1756	323*	177*
135. *aristolochia*	44. aristolochia	*Aristolochia* sp.		1840f	134f*	577f*
136. *kyklaminos*	45. cyclamen	*Cyclamen graecum* L. + sp			135*	
137. *polykarpon*	46. knotgrass ?	*Polygonum hydropepper* L.		1606	119f*	333*
138. *kapparis*	47. giant spider flower	*Capparis spinosa* L.			169f*	100*
139. *anagallis*	48. pimpernel	*Anagallis arvensis* L.		1807*	252	
140. *pēganon*	49. rue	*Ruta graveolens* L. + sp.		1831f	81f	110f
141. *aktē*	50. [identified by Dierbach as *Sambucus niger* L. but probably general word for grain]					
142. *leukonion melas*	51. gilliflower	1-*Matthiola incana*; 2-*Galanthus nivelis*	[id. so uncertain that refs. would be too speculative]			
143. *balanos aigyptios*	52. Egyptian acorn	?				

	Common Name	Scientific Name	Tyler	Dispensatory	Lewis	Trease
	Insects					
144. *kantharis*	1. blister beetle (1)	*Meloe* sp. producing cantharidin	76	238	n/a	622
145. *bouprēstis*	2. blister beetle (2)	*Meloe variegatus* Donov.	76	238	n/a	622
	Aromatics and oil drugs:					
145. *peperi*	1. pepper	*Piper* sp.		1799	250f	558–60
146. *karclamōmos*	2. cardamomum	*Elettaria cardamomum* L.	115–6	255–8	83	454–8
147. *iris*	3. iris	*Iris florentina* L.			282	515
148. *kalamos euōdēs*	4. calamus	*Acorus calamus* L.		1610	212f	155f
149. *kypeiros*	5. nut grass	*Cyperus rotundus* L.			374*	156
150. *schoinos enosmos*	6. camel grass	*Cymbopogon schoenanthus* Spreng.			94	408
	Dicotyledons:					
151. *daphnē*	7. laurel; bay	*Laurus nobilis* L.				92
152. *kinnamōmon*	8. cinnamon	*Cinnamomum* sp.	121f	328f	250f	435f
153. *kasia*	9. cassia	*Cinnamomum cassia* L.?	121f	328f	250f	435f
	Labiataceae:					
154. *elelisphakon*	10. sage	*Salvia officinalis* L.		1834	257f	135
155. *aithiopis*	11. Ethiopian sage	*Salvia aethiopis* L.	121f*	1843*	257*	135*
156. *horminon*	12. sage	*Salvia horminum* L.	121f*	1843*	257*	135*
157. *hyssōpos*	13. marjoram	*Origanum hirtum*, Hebr. L.	491*	1425*	259*	134*
158. *mindē, hedvosmon*	14. green mint	*Mentha sativa* or *Viridis* L.	120*	1014*	83f	408f

	Common Name	Scientific Name	Tyler	Dispensatory	Lewis	Trease
159. *sisymbrion*	15. bergamot mint	*Mentha citrata* Ehrh.	120*	1014*	83f*	408f
160. *glēchōn*	16. pennyroyal	*Mentha pulegium* L.	492–3	1750	83*f	134f*
161. *thymos*	17. conehead thyme	*Thymus capitatus* Hoffm. and Link.	130*	1425*	84f*	134f*
162. *thymbra*	18. savory	*Satureia thymbra* L.			331f	135
163. *kestron*	19. betony	*Stachys officinalis* (L.) Trev.			390	134
164. *prasion*	20. hoarhound	*Marrubium vulgare* L.	487	1747	307	134, 138
165. *pseudodiktamnos*	21. false dittany	*Ballota acetabulosa* L.				134
166. *diktamnos*	22. dittany	*Origanum dictamnus* L. or *Amaracus distanus* Beath.		1426	342	
167. *origanon*	23. marjoram	*Origanus heracleoticum* + sp.	491	1426*	342*	134, 138
168. *polyknēmon*	24. ?					
169. *herpyllos*	25. creeping thyme	*Thymus serpyllum* L.	130*	1426*	246*	675*
170. *kalaminthē*	26. catmint	*Nepeta cataria* L.	476	1618	250	134, 138
171. *ōkimon*	27. basil	*Ocimum basilicum* L.			370	134, 138
172. *epipetron*	28.?	*Sedum* sp. ?				
173. *polion*	29. hulwort	*Teucrium polium* L.			390*	
174. *amarakos*	30. marjoram ?	*Origanum majorana* L.	491		257	134, 138
	Compositae:					
175. *abrotanon*	31. southernwood	*Artemisia abrotanum* L.			389	514*
176. *apsinthion*	32. wormwood	*Artemisia absinthium* L.	500	1211	84f*	514*

	Common Name	Scientific Name	Tyler	Dispensatory	Lewis	Trease
177. *artemisia*	33. various wormwoods	*Artemisia* sp.		1211*	84f*	514*
178. *bakkaris*	34. wild ginger unguent	*Asarum europaeum* L.				
179. *konyza clysosmos*	35. fleabane scabwort	*Inula* sp.		1723		143, 328
180. *konyza euosmos*	36. fleabane	*Inula* sp.		1723		143, 328
181. *euanthēmon*	37. ?					
182. *polyophthalmos*	38. ox eye	*Anacyclus* spp.				
183. *parthenion*	39. feverfew	*Pyrethrum parthenium* L.		1798f	197	651–3
184. *helenion*	40. catmint or elecampane	1-*Calamintha incana* L. 2-*Inula helenium* L.		2–1723		2–143, 328
	Umbellifereae:					
184. *seseli massaleōtikon*	41. Massilian hartwort	*Seseli tortuosum* L.				
185. *annēson*	42. anise	*Pimpinella anisum* L.	135f	1550	121f	122f
186. *selinon*	43. celery	*Apium graveolens* L.				421
187. *marathron*	44. fennel	*Foeniculum vulgare* L.	134	566		414–7
188. *hipposelinon*	45. alexanders	*Smyrnium olus-atrum* L.				
189. *krithmon*	46. samphire	*Crithmum maritimum* L.				
190. *hippomarathron*	47. horse fennel	*Prangos ferulacea* L.				
191. *kachrys*	48. parched barley	[Dierbach's mistake]				
192. *koriannon*	49. coriander	*Coriandrum sativum* L.	115	365	83f	418
193. *kaukalis*	50. hartwort	*Tordylium apulum* L.				
194. *daukos*	51. wild carrot	*Daucos carota* L.		1616	81f	
195. *kyminon aithiopikon*	52. cumin	*Cuminum cyminum* L.				421
196. *anēthon*	53. dill	*Anethum graveolens* L.		1670	81f	418
197. *staphylinos*	54. candy carrot	*Athamanta cretensis* L.				

	Common Name	Scientific Name	Tyler	Dispensatory	Lewis	Trease
198. *peukedanos*	55. hog's fennel	*Peucedanum offin.* L.			81f	122–3
199. *sion*	56. parsnip	*Sium nodiflorum* L.			50*	
200. *thapsia*	57. wild carrot	*Thapsia garganica* L.		1927*	333	
201. *narthēx*	58. common fennel	*Ferula communis* L.	134	566	85f	465
202. *panakes*	59. all-heal plant	?				
203. *ammōniakon*	60. Libyan fennel	*Ferula marmarica* L.	134*	566*	85f*	465*
204. *sagapēnon*	61. Persian fennel	*Ferula persica* Willd.	134*	566*	85f*	465*
205. *chalbanē*	62. all heal fennel	*Ferula galbaniflua* Boiss and Buhse	134*	566*	85f*	465*
206. *silphion*	63. silphium	1-*Ferula tingitana* L. 2-*Ferula asa-foetida* L. 3-*Ferula cyrenaica***	134*	566	85f*	465*
		**as proposed by John Scarborough, *Pharmacy's Ancient Heritage: Theophrastus, Nicander, and Dioscorides* (Lexington, Ky., 1985), 76. *F. cynenaica* Diosc. would be classed as an extinct species of *Ferula* by Scarborough.				
207. *amōmon*	64. amomum	1-*Napaul cardamon* 2-*Amomum subulatum* 3-*Cissus vitiginea* L.	1–257 2–257		 3–338f	 2–457
208. *agnos*	65. chaste tree	*Vitex agnus-castus* L.			257f	134, 137
209. *nardos*	66. nard	various plant species, incl. 1-*Nardostachys jatamansi* and 2-*Valeriana* sp.	2–499f	2–1922	1–340 2–168	2–460f
210. *melilōtos*	67. melilot	*Melilotus officinalis* L.		1750	192f	
	Resins:					
211. *asphalton*	1. asphalt			1800f	n/a	
212. *dais*	2. pine	*Pinus* sp.	132f	1063f	214f	421f

	Common Name	Scientific Name	Tyler	Dispensatory	Lewis	Trease
213. *pitus*	3. pine	*Pinus* sp.	132f	1063f	214f	421f
214. *arkeuthos*	4. juniper	*Juniperus* sp.	115	733	300f	408f
215. *kedros*	5. juniper	*Juniperus* sp.	115	733	300f	408
216. *kyparittos*	6. funeral cypress	*Cypressus sempervirens* L.		1836		
217. *styrax*	7. storax	*Styrax officinalis* L.	159–60	1315	85f	307
218. *ebenos*	8. ebony	*Diospyrus* sp.			232f	
219. *terminthos*	9. terebinth	*Pistacia terebinthus* L.	465f	1389	83f	421f
220. *schinos*	10. mastic	*Pistacia lentiscus* L.	149	785	249f	466f
221. *balsamon*	11. balsam	*Commiphora opobalsumum* Engl. + sp.	158–161	1592	245f	463
222. *libanos*	12. frankincense	*Boswellia* sp.			161	464
223. *smyrna*	13. myrrh	*Commiphora* sp.	157–8	1592	245	463
224. *hyperikon*	14. St. John's wort	*Hypericum crispum* L + sp.		1720	81**	99, 686
				**provokes allergies		
225. *tragion*	15. stinking tutsan	*Hypericum hircinum* L.		1720*		99, 686
226. *kisthos*	16. rock rose	*Cistus* sp.			338f	118–9
227. *ladanon*	17. gum cistus	*Cistus creticus* L.			338f*	118–9
228. *aspalathos*	18. ?					
229. *triphyllon*	19. trifolium	*Psoralea bituminosa* L.		197*	313*	
230. *aigeiros krētikē*	20. Greek poplar	*Populus* sp.		1088	151f	86
231. *chamaileōn*	21. ?					

	Common Name	Scientific Name	Tyler	Dispensatory	Lewis	Trease
232. *kastorios orchis*	22. castoreum from beaver.				n/a	
	Narcotics:					
233. *aira*	1. darnel	*Lolium temulentum* L.		1744	70f**	
			**provokes allergies			
234. *krokos*	2. saffron crocus	*Crocus sativus* L.		1651	325f	515
235. *kōnion*	3. hemlock	*Conium maculatum* L.	452	1644	49–50	615f
236. *hyoskyamos*	4. henbane	*Hyoscyamus niger* L.	206f	673f	192f	542–5
237. *mandragora*	5. mandrake	*Mandragora* sp.	209	1746	330f	552f
238. *mēkōn*	6. opium poppy	*Papaver somniferum* L.	225f	923f	161f	569f
	Minerals:					
239. *theion*	1. brimstone	sulfur		1370f	n/a	465
240. *nitron, litron*	2. nitrum	soda carbonate	270–1**	1263	n/a	
		**sodium compounds				
241. *titanos gypsos*	3. gypsum	calcium sulfate		1611	n/a	
242. *miltos*	4. red earth	iron oxide ?		717	n/a	
243. *gē keramitis*	5. potter's earth					
244. *gē smēktris*	6. fuller's earth or purgative earth	sepiolite?, a hydrated magnesium silicate		772**	n/a	
				**magnesium compounds		
245. *kissēris*	7. pumice			1142	n/a	

	Common Name	Scientific Name	Tyler	Dispensatory	Lewis	Trease
246. *styptēria*	8. alum			51	n/a	
247. *hals*	9. salt	sodium chloride		1265f	n/a	
	Metals:					
248. *molibdos, chrisitis, etc.*	*1. lead*	*lead sulfate + other lead compounds*		744	n/a	
249. *chalkos* 7 other terms for copper	2. copper compounds	copper compounds		362f	n/a	
250. *sidēros* + others	3. iron	iron compounds		362f	n/a	
251. *arsenikon*	4. gold arsenic	arsenic trisulfide		109f	n/a	
252. *sandrachē*	5. red arsenicrealger			109f	n/a	
253. *tetragōnon*	6. antimony	various compounds		95f	n/a	
	Appendix:					
254. *spongos*	1. sponge	**sponge spicules		601		343**
255. *cholē*	2. gall	**from plants		1772**		367**
256. *keras*	3. horn					
257. *hysōpēra eria*	4. oily wool					

XV

METHODOLOGY OF HISTORICAL DRUG RESEARCH

Ellis Peters' medieval murder mystery takes place in an English monastic setting during the twelfth century. The novel's hero is Brother Cadfael, the dispenser of drugs for his community, who cleverly solves a crime. The plot revolves around the title of the book, *Monk's Hood*, which is a deadly herbal poison and, at the same time, a beneficial drug, if used correctly in non-toxic amounts.[1] Similarly, another historical novelist, Jean M. Auel, enthralls her readers by telling, in the series called *The Earth's Children*, about the exploits of a cave woman during the Ice Age which lasted from 35,000 to 25,000 years before the present. The heroine has uncanny influence in her tribal community in part because of her skill in knowing the medicinal usages of plants. Auel includes fewer details about specific plant drugs than Ellis Peters in her medieval novels.[2] Auel's cave herbalist keeps her secrets from vulgarization, just as medieval alchemists did. A pivotal proposition in both novels is that premoderns had a excellent knowledge of the medicinal usages of herbs and other substances, a knowledge that we have mostly forgotten and do not acknowledge as having existed for any meaningful purpose.

In contrast to the pictures presented by these novelists, a popular image is that in the distant past those engaged in medical practice were so misinformed about the nature of anatomy, physiology, pharmacy, and disease that they probably did more harm than good. Obnoxious remedies, bleeding, and drastic purges come readily to mind. Today, we classify drugs by their actions such as analgesics, laxatives, antibiotics, and the like. Classical and medieval medicine classified drugs by the symptoms they relieved in therapy. Historically the intent of the physician was to regulate humoral

---

1. New York, Ballantine Books, c. 1980.

2. Jean M. Auel's titles are: *The Clan of the Cave Bear* (New York: Crown, 1980); *The Valley of Horses* (1982); *The Mammoth Hunters; The Plains of Passage* (1990).

or bodily secretions. The goal was to restore a natural equilibrium, out of balance either through injury, disease, regimen, or nutrition.

In an earlier study of the drugs in the Hippocratic corpus, the earliest extensive medical writings in Greek, 89.5% of the 257 identifiable drugs in the corpus are found in at least one of four modern pharmaceutical or pharmacognosy guides.[3] According to this study, the drugs (as defined by modern medicine) that were available to be discovered had already been discovered by the time medical writings appear.

Much the same drugs span the ages and cultures but the medical theories on which they were administered by various medical systems were different. In other words, a laxative is a laxative regardless of whether prescribed by a Chinese physician of the Ming dynasty, a Hippocratic physician, an African shaman, or a clinician in a London hospital. The consistency of drugs would lend some credit to Jean Auel's fictional cave woman who knew the medicinal herbs. Given that most of the plants which the human digestive system is capable of metabolizing into energy, that is to say food plants, were discovered by the time we have written records, it should be no surprise to learn that drugs had a similar evolutionary and distant discovery.

The relatively stable working pharmacopoeia points to folk transmission of beneficial drug properties from various ethnic groups and even across continents. Beginning with the Hippocratic medical writers as early as the fifth century B.C., writings about drugs served as a means of transmitting data from generation to generation. To be sure, through these documents we learn what they once knew. Even with the documents, a primary means of information transfer about drugs continued to be oral tradition.

While oral and written sources were the conduits for data transfer, ethnopharmacists observe that independent discovery of drugs is a factor as well. Studies show that among native American tribes one tribe seemingly learned about the qualities of plants without direct

----

3. John M. Riddle, "Folk Tradition and Folk Medicine: Recognition of Drugs in Classical Antiquity," in: *Folklore and Folk Medicines*, John Scarborough, ed. (Madison: American Institute of the History of Pharmacy, 1987), p. 37.

transfer, even between tribes that were contiguous.[4] In many cases, however, as other essays in the volume demonstrate, the transfer of information about new drug discoveries is established on linguistic evidence. For instance, the discovery of camphor, a Malay word, in or around the sixth century, is recognized in Western Europe by the ninth century with the use of the Malay term.

ACONITE, A POISONOUS DRUG

Monkshood and its poison, aconite, provide an opportunity to examine the historical conjectures that an historian can make based on evidence. The plant is a relatively easy case study. First, in the ancient texts two plants went under the name *aconitum*. Dioscorides' *aconitum* was the plant we call leopard's bane or *Doronicum pardalianches* L., plus possibly other species of the *doronicum* genus in the Compositae family.[5] What Dioscorides called "the other aconite (ἀκόνιτον ἕτερον)" is what we called monkshood, *Aconitum napellus* L. (Ranunculacea family), and even here, other species of the same plant may have been included, such as *A. vulparia* Reichenb. or wolfsbane, and *A. anthora* L or yellow monkshood.[6] Dioscorides wrote that *aconitum* or leopard's bane was employed in eye medicines, but he said nothing more specific than that. In what proved to be an important statement about monkshood, Dioscorides described a poison that, when mixed with meat, killed animals, such as panthers and wolves.

Monkshood -- the "other *aconitum*" -- is botanically described by Dioscorides but, inexplicably, he ascribed no medicinal properties to it. This is strange because Dioscorides wrote about medicinal plants, and here in this chapter -- and in the *only* chapter in a five-book work -- he has an entry for which no medicinal usages are given. He said that aconite was mixed in raw meat in order to poison wolves. Why Dioscorides chose to include monkshood at all is conjectural but it is reasonable to assume that some people in Dioscorides' day may have

---

4. Lyda Averill Taylor, *Plants Used as Curatives by Certain Southeastern Tribes* (Cambridge, Mass.: Harvard University Press, 1940), pp. 66-71.

5. Dioscorides. *De materia medica*. 4. 76.

6. *Ibid*. 4. 77.

regarded it as a medicine. Dioscorides may have wanted to include it in his work, lest by its omission a reader take it medicinally. Dioscorides' motive may have been no more than to relate the fact that it was only a poison.

Pliny (d. 79 A.D.) gave more information about monkshood than did Dioscorides but Pliny does not extend the medicinal usages. Scholars believe that Pliny's *aconitum* is *A. napellus* or monkshood, but there could be two levels of error here: Pliny could have intended either leopard's bane or both leopard's bane and monkshood.[7] Assuming that Pliny's *aconitum* at least included monkshood, we can proceed with the information that he gave. Pliny wrote of the legend that the poison aconite sprang from the foam around the dog Cerberus' mouth when Hercules dragged him from the Underworld.[8] In Pliny's time the plant was said to grow in Heraclea in the Black Sea region where it marked the entrance to the Underworld. Pliny said that humans learned the plant's properties by observing the results of animals eating it. Ingested aconite will kill a person "unless in that being it finds something else to destroy." Our ancestors observed, Pliny said, that wild animals use the plant to cure their ills: "it is shameful that all animals except man know what is health-giving for themselves."[9] In seeming contradiction to the previous statement, however, Pliny noted that "our ancestors" regarded the poison aconite as a "very health-giving ingredient of preparation for the eyes."[10] This is the same detail as given by Dioscorides but, in his case, the plant for the eye medicines was leopard's bane, not monkshood.

A famous series of murders allegedly were committed using aconite as a poison. In the Roman republic, Calpurnius Bestia was accused of killing his wives by aco-

---

7. The index of plants in the Loeb Pliny (2nd ed., 1980, vol. 7, p. 487) which is a composite opinion by a number of scholars, last revised by A. C. Andrews, identifies *aconitum* as monkshood; whereas Jacques André (*Les noms de plantes dans la Rome antique* [Paris: Société d'Édition "Les Belles Lettres", 1985], p. 4) more correctly, in my opinion, believes that it could be either or both plants, the same as in Dioscorides' work.

8. *Natural History*. 27. 2. 4-5.

9. *N.H.* 27. 2. 5. (W. H. S. Jones, trans.).

10. *N.H.* 27. 2. 9.

nite poisoning.[11] In Ellis Peters' historical novel, Brother Cadfael rubbed a mixture of the ground root of monkshood (aconite), mustard oil and flax seed oil on the skin of a old monk because it "works wonders for creaking old joints."[12] According to modern reports, aconite liniment acts as an anodyne, febrifuge, and sedative. Its active ingredient, aconitine (an alkaloid), also depresses the central and peripheral nervous system.[13] Ellis Peters, therefore, is quite right in that if a monk in the twelfth century had rubbed aconite liniment on an older person's skin, a beneficial effect would have been noticeable.

In the novel's plot, a young apprentice, who, we learn later, came from a dispossessed family, witnessed Cadfael's therapy and overheard him say that internally the ointment was a powerful, deadly poison. Subsequently the apprentice stole a small amount from the jar (for that is all that was needed) and sneaked it into the food of his victim, the person who now possessed his family estates. This provides the murder mystery for Brother Cadfael to solve. The novelist, Peters, is correct about aconite being known as a poison in the twelfth century. Aconite was even given to execute criminals and to poison arrows.[14] One mg. is known to have killed a horse and 2 mg-4 mg is a lethal dose in humans.[15] The question, however, is whether beneficial usages for aconite were known in the twelfth century; in the case of the novel, would Brother Cadfael have had it in his pharmacy cupboard?

Already we examined what was said by Dioscorides,

---

11. *N.H.* 27. 2. 4. L. Calpurnius Bestia was either the tribune in 63 B.C. who was involved in the Catilinarian conspiracy, or the aedile mentioned by Cicero (*Phil.* 13. 26) as one of Clodius' attackers. Vid. F. Münzer, Nos. 24, 25, in: *Paulys Real-Encyclopädie der classischen Altertumswissenschaft* (Stuttgart: Mezler, 1897), 5, 1367.

12. *Monk's Hood* (1980 ed.), p. 25.

13. James A. Duke, *CRC Handbook of Medicinal Herbs* (Boca Raton: CRC Press, 1985), pp. 13-4.

14. M. Grieve, *A Modern Herbal*, 2 vols. (New York: Dover, 1971), 1, 6-11; Duke, *CRC*, p. 12.

15. Duke (1985), p. 13; Jay M. Arena, *Poisoning. Toxicology, Symptoms, Treatments*. 4th ed. (Springfield: Thomas, 1979), p. 350.

the greatest authority during antiquity and the Middle Ages. Neither monks nor lay persons were limited to Dioscorides' text during the Middle Ages, however. The great physician Galen related much the same information as had Dioscorides by distinguishing between ἀκόνιτον or leopard's bane and monkshood -- "the other *aconitum*". Galen adds an important comment: monkshood has the same properties as leopard's bane.[16] By inference, Galen was saying that monkshood was suitable for eye medicines. There is no way to know whether the eye medicines spoken of by Galen and Dioscorides were effective, inasmuch as neither informs us about the other ingredients or the purpose of the administration.

The ancients' knowledge about aconite poisoning was common, judging by the number of references to it.[17] There are frequent references to antidotes for aconite poisoning.[18] Nicander (late 2nd century B.C.) wrote a treatise on antidotes, called *Alexipharmaca*. Aconite is the first poison Nicander listed, where he said that, put into the mouth, it is "deadly".[19] He gave for monkshood a synonym, "woman-killer (θηλυφόνος)", which points to a male's nefarious usage. Symptoms of aconite poisoning are well described by Nicander. Great attention was given to antidotes, beginning with gypsum.[20] Modern toxicologists say that there is no true antidote for aconite poisoning and the treatment is entirely symptomatic.[21]

Brother Cadfael, being a person of moderate learn-

----

16. Galen. *De simplicium medicamentorum temperamentis ac facultatibus*. 7. 1. 19-20 (K. G. Kühn ed., 11, 820); Galen gave χαμαιάκτης as a synonym for monkshood whereas Dioscorides (*De materia medica* 4. 77) gave λυκοτόνον as a synonym.

17. See references by P. Wagler, "Ἀκόνιτον", in: *Real-Encyclopädie der classischen Altertumswissenschaft* (1894), 1, 1178-83.

18. Such as, Pliny. *N.H.* 20. 23. 50, 22. 8. 18, 23. 23. 43, 47.92, 60. 135; 25. 103. 163.

19. Nicander. *Alexipharmaca*. 12-42 (A. S. F. Gow- A. F. Scholfield, eds.); on Nicander, see John Scarborough, "Nicander...", *Pharmacy in History*, 19 (1977): 3-23, 21 (1979): 3-34.

20. *Alexipharmaca*. 42-115.

21. Arena, *Poisoning*, p. 350; Duke, *CRC*, p. 13.

ing, could have known about the plant called *aconitum*, but we cannot be certain which of the two possible plants he may have known. The English vernacular name, monkshood, was not used during the Middle Ages, and two other plants are indicated as passing under the term *aconitum*, namely *Digitalis purpurea* L. and *Lolium temulentum* L.[22] Because the English name monkshood came later to be associated clearly with *Aconitum* (whatever the species), it is a reasonable conjecture that a twelfth-century Benedictine monk in England would have known the plant by the same name, *aconitum*, that we now give to it in scientific nomenclature.

Again, the question: would Cadfael have been likely to know about its positive active medicinal properties as an applicant? Dioscorides' work was translated into Latin by the sixth century. On monkshood, the translation was faithful to the Greek and, therefore, adds no information on its usage.[23] However, there is a hint about the usage for *aconitum* as an eye medicine. The Latin text said that *aconitum* was a *colliriis anodinis* or "pain relieving collyrium". The translation of the Greek term ὀφθαλμικαῖς ἀνωδύνοις unequivocally means "pain-reliever for the eyes." The Latin term *collirium* normally meant a medicine for the eyes but was more general and could mean a topical applicant elsewhere on the body or even a suppository and, later in the Middle Ages, a salve.[24] Therefore, the Latin translation of Dioscorides indicates that leopard's bane, similar to monkshood, had known beneficial usages, not dissimilar to how Brother Cadfael administered it. Probably by the twelfth century the meaning of the Latin term *aconitum* meant monkshood, not leopard's bane.

Unless Brother Cadfael had this particular translation of Dioscorides' *De materia medica* in his Benedictine library, he would not have learned about monkshood from Dioscorides, or, at least, not directly. The Latin

----

22. Tony Hunt, *Plant Names of Medieval England* (Cambridge: D. S. Brewer, 1989), p. 6.

23. Dioscorides. *De materia medica*. Latin trans. in: Hermann Stadler, ed., "Dioscorides Longobardus", *Römanische Forschungen*, 11 (1899): pp. 42-3 (Bk. 4. 73-4).

24. *Oxford Latin Dictionary* (1982), s.v.; *Revised Medieval Latin Word-List from British and Irish Sources*. R. E. Latham, ed. (London: Oxford University Press, 1965), s.v.

translation was a product of Benedictine scriptoria[25]; however, given the small number of manuscript copies in existence, the textual reference is an unlikely source for Cadfael to learn about *aconitum*'s use in salves. Even with this assumption, we need to supply yet another assumption, that one could substitute leopard's bane for monkshood. According to Dioscorides, Pliny, and Galen, there were good grounds for doing so.

There were other written sources on monkshood that he could have used. None of the Roman or early medieval sources that I could find make the claim about its beneficial usages.[26] Constantine the African's *De gradibus*, Platearius' *Circa instans*, and Macer's *De virtutibus herbis*, popular medical works prior to Cadfael's life (fictional though it is), have no mention of the *aconitum* plant. The influential writer, Isidore of Seville (7th c. A.D.), wrote about the plant in passing and told only of its poisonous nature.[27] Gerard of Cremona's translation of Avicenna's *Canon of Medicine* does not list the plant by its Latin name.[28]

By the eighteenth century, however, aconite was employed as a topical medicine.[29] In our times, aconite rescued the central character in Aleksandr I. Solzhenitsyn's *Cancer Ward*, widely believed autobiographical, who was saved by taking one drop of an alcohol extract from monkshood root with a glass of water. The second day the dosage was increased to two and progressively until ten drops a day. Thereafter, the dosage was gradually reduced and the procedure was repeated several times.[30]

---

25. On the Old Latin translation, see John Riddle, "Dioscorides," in: *Catalogus Translationum et Commentariorum* (Washington: Catholic University Press, 1981), 4, 20-3.

26. For instance, see the concordance prepared by Carmélia Opsomer, *Index de la pharmacopée Ier au Xe siècle*, 2 vols. (Hildesheim: Olms-Weidmann, 1989), 1, 16. Oribasius discussed *aconitum* but he followed Galen and Dioscorides.

27. Isidore. *Origines*. 17. 9. 25 (W. M. Lindsay ed.).

28. Venice ed. 1507; fasc. reprint, Hildesheim: Olms, 1964.

29. Wolfgang Schneider, *Lexikon zur Arzneimittelgeschichte*, 5 vols. (Frankfurt a. M.: Govi, 1974), 5, pt. 1, pp. 40-3.

30. Aleksandr I. Solzhenitsyn, *The Cancer Ward*. Rebecca Frank, trans. (New York: Dial, 1968), pp. 276 ff.

As celebrated as monkshood was historically, the evidence is not strong enough for believing that a monk in the twelfth century would have had monkshood in one of his apothecary jars as a liniment. If it was present at a monastic house, likely it would have been in the barn where its use was to poison wolves and other predatory animals. Just the same, while there is no evidence, it is not unreasonable that a person could have made the discovery about its useful properties and had information orally transmitted. Pliny's and Dioscorides' texts and the more explicit wording in the Latin translation of Dioscorides convey evidence that monkshood's qualities as an anodyne in salves was known, but none of these sources gave any details about the preparation and its usages. If Pliny was not describing a practice in his day, he was ominously prophetic when he said that in every poison there can be found beneficial qualities and that monkshood will poison the body if the poison cannot find some thing else on which to apply its venom. Solzhenitsyn appreciates monkshood's property in that regard. Rather than being prophetic, Pliny was relating things he heard or, more likely, read, but he did not incorporate the details in the *Natural History*. In summary, Pliny, Dioscorides, and Galen all alluded to monkshood being used in salves but none of them gave the details.

Aloe: A Case Study

Aloe affords an example of just how difficult it is to generalize about pre-modern drugs' effectiveness. Aloe is a familiar plant, many people having a pot of it for both ornamental and medicinal usages in their homes. For our purposes, let us put aside the question of which species of aloe the Western Europeans would have been using historically, even though it is important in judging the effectiveness of a drug made from it. Let us then assume -- it is reasonable to do so based on the evidence -- that, when aloe was prescribed, it was a species of the aloe which is recognizably pharmaceutically active.[31] Modern Western pharmacopoeias recognize aloe for its cathartic action due to a stimulation of peristalsis, probably as a result of irritation of mucous

---

31. An excellent examination of aloes in antiquity is by John Scarborough, "Roman Pharmacy and the Eastern Drug Trade. Some Problems as Illustrated by the Example of Aloe," *Pharmacy in History*, 24 (1982): 135, 137-43.

membrane especially in the upper bowels. Modern popular use of aloe is for burns, wounds, dermatitis, and various ulcerated skin problems.

Let us now compare these two generic, modern uses with medieval uses. First, there were the classical authorities whom medieval physicians consulted. Dioscorides said that aloe had a power of binding, inducing sleep, drying, thickening of bodies, and loosening the bowels. When two spoons of it are taken with water or warm milk, it purges the stomach. Three oboli (approx. 1.5 grams) and one spoonful of aloe stops hemoptysis (spitting of blood). Also it cures jaundice; placed on wounds, it heals them; it brings boils to a head and prevents them; it heals ulcers in the genital area, especially being good for the irritated prepuce; with wine, it cures lumps (κονδυλώματα) and anal hemorrhoids; it stops bleeding from hemorrhoids; it promotes scars of the πτερύγιον (a triangular thickening of bulbar conjunctiva on the cornea); it makes bruises and black eyes vanish; it helps ψωροφθαλμία (an itch in the eye or eye lids attributed to excessive dryness); it helps a headache when placed on the forehead with vinegar and rosaceum; with wine it prevents hair from falling out; and it is good for the tonsils, gums, and the mouth in general.[32] Galen repeated Dioscorides' usages, but he added that aloe aids the nose as well as the mouth.[33]

The popular early medieval tract, *Properties of Simple Drugs*, that is ascribed to Galen, listed aloe under purgatives. While generally giving some of the same or nearly the same usages, Pseudo-Galen had fewer usages than did Dioscorides and Galen. Generally, however, the tract is more specific in giving directions for administration. As an example, the tract says that, as a laxative, aloe is best given after the evening meal.[34] Because its action is in the upper bowels, which causes evacuation in about eight to twelve hours, the information in the tract complies with modern expectations. Another Pseudo-Galenic tract, *On Simple Drugs*, dating from about the same period, said: "aloe has a warming power, and it comforts and dries the stomach [upper digestive tract]. It cures wounds and it is placed on

---

32. Dioscorides. *De materia medica*. 3. 22.

33. Galen.*De simplicium medicamentorum temp. ac fac*. 6. 23 (Kühn ed., 11, 821-2).

34. Cambridge, Gonville and Gaius College, Ms 379, s. xii, fol. 57r.

lumps [or, tumors] in the nose, mouth, or eyes."[35] The drying and comforting action may be a recognition of a stimulation by peristalsis. If one had constipation, surely it would be comforting. If not, perhaps it would not be. In any case, one must infer the action intended, and such judgments are subject to error.

Throughout the Middle Ages, aloe was employed for many purposes, most of which coincide with Dioscorides' usages. The patriarch of Jerusalem recommended it to King Alfred the Great (871-899) of England, when he journeyed to the Holy Land.[36] Allegedly Emperor Otto III (983-1102) of the Holy Roman Empire died of an overdose of aloe.[37] Here we have a "drug" about which we can have some assurance concerning its medicinal action, but still how does one answer the question: did they employ the drug correctly? An answer must have numerous qualifications. For most herbal drugs, we need to know the exact species, the morphology of drug preparation, the time of harvesting, the correctness of diagnosis, conveyance (such as wine or water), and the exact amount of dosage and frequency and site of administration, before we can be prepared to attempt a definitive answer. Such information is not to be found in the documents.

With all of these qualifications, the fact is that aloe is a laxative and it was used for this purpose during the Middle Ages. A similar determination can be made about many of the substances used in medieval pharmacy. There was rational drug usage.

The case study on aloe shows just how difficult it is to generalize about a drug's effectiveness. A modern textbook on medicinal chemistry names thirteen individual patient variable factors affecting drug metabolism, ten variable factors related to drug administration, and thirteen variable factors related to external environmental factors.[38] In respect to aloe, the number of varia-

---

35. St. Gallen, Stiftsbibliothek, Ms 762, s. ix, fol. 138.

36. Friedrich A.Flückiger and Daniel Hanbury, *Pharmacographia: A History of the Principal Drugs of Vegetable Origin Met with in Great Britain and British India* 2nd ed. (London: Macmillan, 1879), p. 680.

37. *Ibid.* I have been unable to verify Flückiger's statement in the sources.

38. Andrejus Korolkovas and Joseph P. Burchhater, *Essentials of Medicinal Chemistry* (New York: Wiley, 1976), pp. 7-8.

bles has already been mentioned that affect a plant drug's effectiveness. Since we do not know such things as the soil conditions and extraction method employed, we can never know with certainty.[39] However, we can know within reason.

Core Drugs and Their Effectiveness

There is a core of around 300 drugs that constantly appear in the medical documents, be they Greek, Latin, Chinese, or other ancient languages.[40] Until the nineteenth century, there was a remarkable consistency about the drugs used and a resistance to changes in natural product drugs. A typical medicine chest of an eighteenth-century physician was not very different in the drugs it contained from a thirteenth-century physician's chest except the medieval physician would not have had the drugs from the New World, such as balsam of Peru, quaiacum, sasparilla, and tobacco. Physicians of these two widely separated centuries would readily recognize and be likely to have had in their cupboards: almond oil, aloe, anise, barley water, bees' wax and honey, zinc oxide, celandine, centaury, cinnamon, cumin, fennel, ginger, hyssop, mastic, myrrh, opium, nutmeg, various spurges, white hellebore or veratrum, parsley, pennyroyal, plantain, rosemary, rue, and wormwood, to name a few. A more knowledgeable specialist would know that drugs in current use derive from natural sources, e.g. atropine from *Atropa belladonna*, morphine from the poppy, quinine from cinchonna bark, emetine from ipecacuanaha root, strychnine from *Nux vomica*, santonin from wormseed, digitalis from common foxglove, and resperine from periwinkle. The medicinal usage for each of these substances, while known only as a part of a plant, was discovered by folk medicine long before medicine and chemistry isolated the compounds.

In contrast, many drugs are "new" to modern times in another sense. By 1979, 80% of the twenty-five single-ingredient drugs most frequently prescribed in the United States were introduced after 1950. One-half of them

---

39. Edward M. Croom, Jr., "Documenting and Evaluating Herbal Remedies," *Economic Botany*, 37 (1983): 13-27.

40. For Chinese drugs, see Xu Ren-Scheng, Zhu Qiao-Zhen and Xie Yu-Yuan, "Recent Advances in Studies on Chinese Medicinal Herbs with Physiological Activity," *Journal of Ethnopharmacology*, 14 (1985): 223-53.

were introduced after 1960.[41] That is one way to look at the situation. Another: of the 300 million *new* prescriptions written in 1963, more than 47% contained a drug of natural origin either as the sole active ingredient or as one of two or more active ingredients.[42] Many of our primary drugs are chemically synthesized from natural products, usually plants, and manufactured by processes no longer directly involving their natural homes. Thus, if one knows the chemical name, he or she might not know that its actual medicinal effects were discovered by our remote ancestors.

As discussed above, the thirteenth-century physician would recognize the common drugs of his first-century counterpart, except the medieval physician would have a few more drugs available, such as senna and camphor, because they were medieval discoveries. For that matter, one can find these drugs in popular modern herbals, such as Ingrid Gabriel's *Herb Identifier and Handbook* (London, 1975).[43] Most of the items in this herbal were a regular part of the pharmacy of the Middle Ages.

The written documents show a larger drug list than what must have been available from the dispensary of the average herbalist, druggist, or physician.[44] The normal monastic drug cupboard would not have had the thousand or so items listed in the written documents. Evidence exists that inventories of druggist's shops of later periods (12th- 16th centuries) are much smaller than the number of drugs thought efficacious in the medical writings of the same period.[45] There must have been a loosely defined but generally recognizable "core" pharma-

---

41. Michael C. Gerald, *Pharmacology. An Introduction to Drugs.* 2nd ed. (Englewoods Cliffs: Prentice-Hall, 1981), p. 7.

42. Barber (1967), p. 11.

43. An excellent study that begins with a modern herbalist and traces how he acquired his knowledge is by John Crellin and Jane Philpott, *Herbal Medicine Past and Present*, 2 vols. (Durham: Duke University Press, 1990).

44. Philip M. Teigen, "This Sea of Simples--The Materia Medica in Three English Recipe Books," *Pharmacy in History*, 22(1980): 104-8.

45. S. D. Goitein, "The Medical Profession in the Light of the Cairo Geniza Documents," *Hebrew Union College Annual*, 24(1963): 189.

cy.[46] For instance, there was general recognition of usages for the following laxatives in an approximate order from mild to strong: acorus or sweet flag, aloe, colocynth, castor oil, and scammony. If one of these was not available, a physician could substitute. He knew to be careful with the amounts and to take into consideration the condition of the patient. This sensitivity derived more from experience than books, just as Galen, Ibn Sīnā, and other authorities indicated. Just to assist, however, there existed in the Middle Ages treatises called "Quid pro quo," or "This for that," which were lists of drug substitutes. A typical "Quid pro quo" assisted memory; it could not replace reliance on empirical observation.

DRUGS AND THEIR EFFICACY

Did medicine prior to the modern period have results beneficial to most of the people? Were pre-modern drugs effective? One physiologist-sociologist, L. J. Henderson, expressed what is probably a widely held hypothesis: prior to 1912 (the year he saw as the turning point to modernity) a random physician and a random patient with a random disease had chances no better than 50-50 of benefiting from the encounter, except for the doctor's fee.[47] Henry F. Dowling estimates that prior to 1700 there were fewer than two dozen "effective drugs."[48] Perhaps this is the time to define what is meant by "effective". To be effective, I mean some action more extensive than a psychological or placebo reaction because, if it acts in such a manner, then all substances would be potentially equally effective so long as they did not correspondingly

---

46. A study of 13th c. spicers and apothecaries has the names of 107 drugs in active use. See G. E. Trease, "The Spicers and Apothecaries of the Royal Household in the Reigns of Henry III, Edward I and Edward II," *Nottingham Mediaeval Studies*, 3(1959): 19-52. An Elizabethan apothecary's inventory has about 57 drug items but some few are compounds, such as *oxycroceum*, a plaster composed of saffron, tar, colophony, wax, turpentine, galbanum, ammoniacum, myrrh, frankincense and mastic. See R. Sharpe France, "An Elizabethan Apothecary's Inventory," *The Chemist and Druggist* (September 9, 1959), p. 50.

47. Bernard Barber, *Drugs and Society* (New York: Russell Sage Foundation, 1967), p. 4.

48. *Medicines for Man* (New York: Norton, 1970), p. 14.

harm.[49] To be effective, a drug must have some measurable and perceptive means by which a person would be relieved, assisted, or cured from a physical or mental difficulty.

In the 1970's medical science had to change its procedures for testing the effectiveness of drugs. Prior to the decade, the standard test was a single-blind procedure: two groups of patients having a similar medical problem would be formed; one group would receive an inert, harmless substance and the other group would receive a similar-appearing drug which was the substance to be tested. The results were inaccurate because some how the physician or drug dispenser was conveying impressions to the patients of what was expected. The mere expectation, conveyed in the most discreet, subtle and sensitive means, was sufficient to alter the test results. To avoid this psychological and very real factor, modern methodology for drug experimentation demands that neither patient nor experimenter know which is the experimental drug and which the placebo. Since the effect is of such importance, historians assume that a major factor in medicine's effectiveness in the past is through the placebo factor. I cannot quarrel with the position that some of the effectiveness of early medicine lies in the placebo effect, but I believe that we can go beyond the recognition towards a deeper analysis.

A very important factor in therapeutics is the quality of the relationship established between the patient and his or her medical attendant. This association is a situation of human interaction. Historians readily accept that most patients and medical people in the past had satisfactory relationships, otherwise people would not have continued with them. Because patients and physcians developed strong trust relationships, medicine was effective. To be sure, the argument is circular: because benefit was perceived, medicine was effective. To many medical historians, no further judgment can be made. The hypothesis is faulty, I think, that only psychological factors account for early medicine's effectiveness. Because many, if not most, people in all periods of the past regarded as satisfactory the product of their therapeutic relationships with medical people (including physicians), medicine in all periods would be equally effective. I doubt that medical historians

49. For a modern pharmacist's definition of a drug, see Robert M. Julien, *A Primer of Drug Action*. 4th ed. (New York: Freeman, 1975), esp. p. 14.

actually can argue persuasively that in all periods of time in all cultures, medicine was equally effective (and, conversely, ineffective). We certainly hold with conviction and reason that modern medicine with its drugs, electronics, and chemical diagnostic technology, is better that medicine of the nineteenth century.

In studying ancient and medieval medicine, there is no way to ascertain whether it is "most" people or just "many" people who were happy with their medical attention. Had the result of therapy been otherwise, it is a reasonable supposition that people would not have continued to enter physician-patient relationships. We know that they did because there were always during the classical and medieval periods people called physicians (using a variety of terms) who made medical practice a livelihood. This is also a circular argument. Historians know that the nature of historical documentation will not yield statistical data about attitudes between patient and physicians on anything but an anecdotal basis.

A critically important and reasonable supposition is that most medicine was self-administered or family-administered, just as it is today. Cuts, sores, indigestion, earaches, headaches, and similar minor problems were normally not a reason to go to a physician. Most therapy is conducted by drugs, just as it is today. When we judge a drug's effectiveness historically, we judge not merely the established medical personnel but the common lay person's ability to make rational decisions.

In summary, we concede two factors in judging medicine's effectiveness: the placebo effect and its attendant patient-physician relationships. I am calling both of these psychological and I acknowledge their importance. Still a person curious about early medicine wants to know: when a patient visits a doctor, were the diagnosis and the therapy based on it beneficial to the patient in ways other than psychological? This article will not examine the question about what the ancients knew about disease and consequently will not be concerned with diagnosis. Most diagnoses were based on symptoms and most therapy was by drugs and that too was based on symptoms. The question is not whether, if a physician prescribed a laxative or an analgesic, those actions were merited but, instead, whether, if given, the substances had the intended affect.

Drug Effectiveness and History

Modern physicians recognize the complexity of factors involved in medicine in their own time and are understandably reluctant to attribute qualitative judgments in other time periods, especially those that span cultures as well. How can historians make judgments about medical practices a thousand or more years ago? As we have seen first with Brother Cadfael's poison/medicine and with the history of aloe, it is possible to arrive at reasonable conclusions, not those beyond a shadow of a doubt but within the bounds of reasonable probability. The historian plies his craft following the same procedure used to determine reasonable probability in a court of law.

Medical history is one of the few fields where judgments are not made. When all variables are taken into account, judgment is modestly suspended. Historians of the exact sciences have no difficulty in judging their science counterparts in the past during the same periods where medical historians tread lightly. If a mathematical problem in a Sumerian text was incorrectly conceived or an error occurs, the historian does not hesitate to record it as a mistake because it is recognizable. In other fields of historical inquiry, historians attempt to supply rationale to their data. Similarly an economic historian will attempt an analysis of the purpose, implementation, and outcome of a government's policy towards business, currency or international trade. The historian will provide an evaluation based on his understanding of economic rules, although those rules are as fragile as are medical guidelines. Having made a detailed study of an economic policy, the reader expects some assessment about the policy's effectiveness. Indeed, were we to read an economic history with no interpretative appraisal given, we would regard the work as deficient.

Similarly if a scientist, such as Aristotle, incorrectly pronounces the rules of motion, the historian notes the error. This is not to say that a modern historian cannot understand science from the standpoint of someone in Aristotle's fourth century B.C. He can, but he also knows that the laws of nature, physics in this case, were the same then as now and so, when Aristotle made an incorrect observation from nature, he erred. Given that Aristotle's Hellenic models were different, he nonetheless made a misjudgment in observation about the relationship between the movee and mover. Indeed, historians of anatomy can easily understand how Galen, for instance, erred in his description of the heart, but, even so, they do not hesitate to point out both the error and its historical consequence. Conversely, if Galen had "correctly" described the heart, the event would be celebrated.

When writing the history of drugs, the historian is compelled to arrive at some assessments of the nature of the documents. Magic and superstition cannot be disregarded, and they cannot only be viewed in the context of our culture. When our modern knowledge falls short of being able to evaluate the documents, an historian can only make note of his inadequacy. However, when a medical prescription makes sense to us, one should say so, all the while acknowledging that there are many variables that could affect a conclusion. One consequence of non-evaluative medical history is that, when in the distant the discovery of an important new drug was made, one that affects the lives of millions of people, the event goes unmarked as well as unsung. In contrast, discoveries during our era are commemorated, such as the Salk vaccine, penicillin, and the contraceptive pill. Discoveries of opium based drugs, effective analgesics and antiseptics, laxatives, and antipyretics pass the pages of world history with hardly a word as to the event or its consequences. One example of an important drug discovery is quinine that made it possible for the European incursions into southern Africa.[50] Another example is the importance attached by classical medicine to avoid narcotics, hallucinogens, and drug dependence. A final example is the use of contraceptives and early-stage abortifacients in the Roman Empire that brought with it a decline in the population. Ultimately many, if not most of problems faced by the Empire were a direct consequence of what was a crisis in population size.[51]

A danger lurks in judging the quality of medical care in the past, namely historical positivism. That is to say, we should never evaluate the past on the basis of what modern science and cultural values regard as truth. Each culture, each time period, should be viewed entirely on its own grounds. Just the same, we cannot avoid the use of reason in understanding the past and that reasoning invokes the rules of nature the way we, the interpreters, understand the rules. Inevitably, whether intentional or unaware, the interpreter of medical history makes a judgment about the quality of medicine he or she describes. All factors cannot, however, be analyzed

---

50. Daniel R. Headrick, *The Tools of Empire. Technology, and European Imperialism in the Nineteenth Century* (New York: Oxford University Press, 1981), pp. 66-76.

51. John M. Riddle, *A History of Oral Contraceptives and Early Abortions* (Cambridge: Harvard University Press, forthcoming).

because present knowledge is not full knowledge adequate for an understanding. Where we find gaps in our knowledge of ancient and medieval medicine, we simply acknowledge that we do not know what the rationale for certain medical practices may have been. In some cases, however, the historical documentation is sufficent for hypotheses.

By refusing to evaluate pre-modern medicine and pharmacy, we cut ourselves off from our past. A common view holds that modern science and technology have made such advances that physicians are no longer connected with their Hippocratic counterparts. Such notions are unhistorical, however. The deeper one searches the clues in the records of the past, the more one sees that the modern physician is closer to his ancient counterpart than just the ethics presented in the Oath to Hippocrates. We freely acknowledge that our ancestors can instruct us about values and, possibly, esthetics, but we deny that they can also tell us how to do things. The art of medicine is long, said Hippocrates, and so it is that our present medical truths (that includes drugs) are based on principles found embedded deep in the past. The historians' task is to understand the past by evaluating it. In the process, the historian binds the present both with the past and with the future.

INDEX

(The Roman numeral refers to the Chapter and it is followed by the page number.)

I. Manuscripts:

Augsburg, Stadt- und Kreisbibliothek, Ms 121, I-112
Bamberg, Staatsbibliothek, Ms Med. 6, IV-205-9
Berleburg, Schlossbibliothek Ms F. 4, I-115
Berlin, Königliche Bibliothek, Ms lat. 88, I-120
Berlin, Staatsbibliothek, Ms 968, III-41
Ms lat. 60, I-112
Ms lat. 75, I-112
Bern, Stadtbibliothek, Ms 410, III-45
Ms 556, I-116
Ms A 91 11, III-42
Bologna, Bibl. Universitaria, Ms 1887, I-118
Breslau, Universitätsbibliothek, Ms III. Q. 4, I-118
Ms lat. 2317, I-118
Brno, Bibl. Univ. Knihovna, Ms Mk 107, VI-175
Ms Mk 46, III-45
Brussels, Bibl. Royale, Ms 8902, Ms III-45
Cambridge, Corpus Christi, Ms 243, III-40
Cambridge, Gonville and Caius, Mss 336 and 725, I-119
Cambridge, Jesus, Ms 51, III-42
Ms Q. D. 2 (44), III-41-2; IV-209
Cambridge, Pembroke, Ms 111, III-48
Cambridge, Trinity, Ms 1122, III-45
Ms O 2 48, IX-46
Ms O I 77, I-119
Ms 1351, III-41
Cambridge, University Library, Ms Kk III 25 (2040), III-42, 48
Cheltenham, Phillips Ms 386, XI-283, 285
Clermont-Ferrand, Bibl., Ms 171, III-41
Copenhagen, Kõngelige Bibl., Ms 1653 (760), VI-175
Douai, Bibl., Ms 217, III-42
El Escorial, Ms III R 3, XIII-101
Ms T II 12, III-96, 98-9
Erfurt, Stadtbibliothek, Ms Amplon. 222, I-118
Ms Amplon. 550, III-41
Ms Amplon. F 303, III-42
Ms Amplon. O 77, III-44
Ms Amplon. Q 217, III-44
Erlangen, Universitätsbibliothek, Mss 423, III-44; 434, III-45; VIII-231-2
Florence, Bibl. Medicea Laurentiana, Ms Ashburn. 1520, III-42, 44;VIII-231
Ms Plut. 73 16, IX-46, 70
Ms Plut. 73 23, XI-283
Ms Plut. 73 41, IX-46
Ms Strozz. lat. 73, IX-70
Florence, Biblioteca Nazionale, Ms XV. 150, I-116, 120
Florence, Biblioteca Riccardiana, Ms 1219, I-116
Glasgow, Hunterian Museum, Ms 468, III-42
Glasgow, Hunterian Library, Ms T. 4. 13, II-190
Gotha, Landsesbibliothek, Ms A. 501, I-120
Graz, Universitätsbibliothek, Ms 1249, III-45
Heilbronn, Stadtbibliothek Ms M. 2002 Q, I-115-8, 120
Ms M. 2002 Q, I-112
Karlsruhe, Bibliothek, Ms Augiensis 120, II-192
Krakow, Bibl. Jagellonica, Ms 816, I-121
Ms 817, III-44
Ms 6392, VIII-229
Leiden, Univ. Lib., Ms B.P.L. 1283, IX-46
Ms Voss Gr. F 58, XIII-96-7
Leipzig, Universitätsbibliothek, Ms 1179, I-112-3, 118
Liège, Bibl. de l'Univ., Ms 77, III-44; VIII-230
London, British Museum, Ms Add. 8928,

IX-47
Ms Add. 8929, IX-46
Ms Add. 16566, III-42
Ms Add. 22719, VIII-234
Ms Add. 32622, III-41
Ms Arundel 164, III-45
Ms Arundel 251, III-41
Ms Arundel 323, III-45
Ms Arundel 342, III-42
Ms Arundel 18210, III-45
Ms Cotton Vitellius C III, IX-70
Ms Egerton 1984, III-45; VIII-231-2; 234
Ms Egerton 2852, III-41
Ms Harley 585, II-192; IX-70
Ms Harley 2378, VI-175
Ms Harley 3353, III-42
Ms Hatton 76, IX-70
Ms lat. 1471, III-42
Ms lat. 5294, IX-46
Ms Royal App. 3, IX-70
Ms Sloane 84, XI-283, 286
Ms Sloane 231, III-42
Ms Sloane 284, III-44
Ms Sloane 340, III-41
Ms Sloane 1975, IX-46, 50, 70
Ms Sloane 2008, III-41
Ms Sloane 2320, I-119
Ms Sloane 2428, III-45; VIII-232, 234
Ms Sloane 3281, III-41
London, Wellcome, Ms 116, III-44
Ms 531, III-42
Milan, Ambrosiana, Ms I 65 sup, VIII-231
Modena, Biblioteca Estense, Ms lat. 606, I-117
Montpellier, École de Méd., Ms 277, III-41-42, 44; VIII-230
Ms 503, III-42
Munich, Staatsbibliothek Ms lat. 337, IV-208;IX-43-4
Ms lat. 372, I-118, 120
Ms lat. 441, I-111
Ms lat. 444, III-41
Ms lat. 963, I-120
Ms lat. 13582, III-45
Ms lat. 14851, III-48
Ms lat. 18444, III-42
Ms lat. 23479, III-42
Naples, Biblioteca Nazionale, Ms XII E 31, VIII-231
Ms suppl. 28, XIII-101
Oxford, Bodleian, Ms 130, IX-46
Ms 177. III-41
Ms Ashmole 1471, III-41-2, 44-5; VIII-231
Ms Ashmole 1475, III-46; IX-71
Ms Auct. D 4 15, III-48
Ms Canonicus lat. 178, III-48
Ms Digby 13, III-41-2, 48
Ms Digby 37, III-41
Ms Digby 79, III-45
Ms Digby 147, III-41
Ms Digby 153, III-41
Ms Digby 193, III-45
Ms Douce 291, III-39
Ms Harley 76, III-42
Ms Harley 4986, XI-283
Ms Harley 5792, XI-283
Ms Hatton, 76, III-41
Ms Rawlinson 545, VIII-232
Ms Rawlinson A. 273, III-41
Oxford, Corpus Christi, Ms 221, III-45
Oxford, Exeter, Ms 35, III-42
Padua, Biblioteca del Seminario, Ms 194, XIII-96
Paris, Arsenal, Ms 1080, VIII-231
Ms 3174, III-42
Paris, Bibliothèque Nationale, Ms fr. 2009, III-4
Ms fr. 14969, III-41
Ms gr. 2182, XIII-96, 98
Ms gr. 2183, XIII-96, 98-9
Ms gr. 2185, XIII-98
Ms lat. 523a, III-45; VIII-231
Ms lat. 6755, III-45
Ms lat. 6819, IV-209
Ms lat. 6820, IV-207
Ms lat. 6862, IX-46
Ms lat. 7027, XI-283
Ms lat. 7475, III-44
Ms lat. 8454, III-41-2
Ms lat. 9332, IV-208; IX-43
Ms lat. 11210, III-42
Ms lat. 11218, XI-283
Ms lat. 12233, I-120
Ms lat. 12955, IV-208; IX-43
Ms lat. 14470, III-48
Ms lat. 16702, III-42
Ms lat. nouv. acq. 873, III-46, 48
Ms lat. nouv. acq. 13955, IX-46
Paris, Mazarine, Ms 3599, I-119, 121
Paris, St. Geneviève, Ms 2261, III-42
Prague, Universitätsbibliothek, Ms I F II, I-116
Ms III C 2 (629), III-45

Ms V B 22 (839), III-42
Ms VII G 25, III-42
Ms IX A 4, I-117
Ms XI C 2 (2027), III-44
Ms XII F 11, VI-175
Salamanca, Biblioteca Universitaria, Ms 2659, XIII-96, 98-9
Savignamo, Biblioteca dell' Accademia, Ms 26, III-42
St. Gallen, Stiftsbibliothek Ms 44, II-186, 194-5
Ms 751, IX-46
Ms 762, XI-283, 285
Tours, Bibliothèque, Ms 892, III-42
Turin, Nazionale Bibl., Ms D. III. 5, III-39
Valladolid, Universidad de Valladolid, Ms 10046, III-42
Vatican, Bibliotheca, Ms Barberini 343, III-42, 46, 48
Ms lat. 707, III-44
Ms lat. 724, III-45; VIII-231-2
Ms lat. 822, III-45
Ms lat. 2403, III-42
Ms lat. 4251, III-41
Ms lat. 4482, III-44
Ms lat. 5373, VI-175
Ms lat. 10046, III-41-42
Ms Pal. graec. 77, XIII-96-7, 99, 101
Ms Pal. lat. 1088, XI-283
Ms Pal. lat. 1144, III-45; VIII-231
Ms Regina lat. 21, III-48
Ms Regina lat. 45, III-48
Venice, Bibl. Marciana, Ms G Z 97, XIII-96
Ms L VI LIX, III-41-2
Ms Z 271, XIII-96, 98-9
Ms Z 272, XIII-96, 101
Ms Z 273, XIII-101
Ms Z 597, XIII-96
Ms 2317, III-45
Ms 2442, III-45
Vienna, Hofbibliothek, Mss 2378, III-48; 5312, I-118
Vienna, Nationalbibliothek, Ms gr. 1, IX-44-5, 50; XIII-97, 99-100
Ms gr. 16, XIII-99, 101
Ms lat. 93, IX-46, 48-50, 59, 70, 74
Ms lat. 1365, VIII-231
Ms lat. 2301, III-42
Ms lat. 2317, I-118; VIII-231
Ms lat. 2442, III-45
Ms lat. 2898, III-42
Ms lat. 3408, III-45
Ms lat. 5311, III-45
Ms lat. 5371, VI-175
Ms lat. 5512, III-42
Ms lat. 11235, III-42, 45
Ms lat. 12901, III-42
Ms Pal. lat. 2317, I-113
Wiesbaden, Landesbibliothek, Ms 61, I-112, 115
Wolfenbüttel, Herzogliche Bibliothek, Ms 217, I-119
Ms Helmstadt 429, I-118
Ms Helmstadt 783, I-119
Ms Helmstadt 784, I-116, 119
Ms 5312, I-118
Zürich, Zentral-bibl., Ms C101, III-41

II. Index of terms:

Plant and animal names are variously listed by their scientific and English names. When a translation are left in the original.

Aaron's rod, IX-75
Aaron, III-40; VIII-233-4
abortifacient, X-425
abortion, VIII-209; IX-62-3; XI-294
abrotanum, IX-81
abscesses, XI-292
Abu Mansur, XII-322
Abyssinia, see Ethiopia
Acacia sp., XIV-49
acantha, IX-61
acanthus Arabian, XIII-101
Acantus mollis, IX-73
Acarna gummifera, IX-73
acetum, I-113
Achillea millefolium, IX-78
Achillea sp., IX-78
achor, X-424
Ackerknecht, Edwin, XIV-34, 39
aconite, XIV-39; XV-2-9
Aconitum napellus, *A. napellus*, XV-3
aconitum, XIV-53, XV-1-9
acorn, XI-310; Egyptian, XIV-50; Sardian, X-425
Acorus calamus, XIV-55
acorus, XV-14
Adamantius, V-10
Adiantum capillus veneris, IX-74; XIV-51
Aelian, V-5
Aesculapius, IX-51
Aetius of Amida, II-186, 191; III-47; V-10-2; XI-293
Afodisius, II-186
Africa, Thomas, X-417
agates, VIII-210
Agricola, VIII-216, 221
aigeros, V-7
Ajuga chamaepitys, IX-73
akantha, XII-323
Al-Hahiz, VI-184
Albertus (Magister), I-118
Albertus Magnus, III-40, 44-5, 48, 50; VIII-2033-34
Albertus Magnus (Pseudo-), III-48
Albrecht van Borgunnien, I-117
alchemy, VIII-203-6, 223
Alcuin, II-189, 195
Alexander of Tralles, II-186, 197; V-10
Alexander of Macedonia, II-186
Alexander, I-121
Alexander Severus, X-411
alexanders, XI-302; XIV-37, 57
Alexandrian library, VIII-214
Alexandrian romances, III-40
Alexandrian science, X-420
Alexiasm, XIV-39
Alfonso X (el Sabio), III-43-45
Alfred the Great, XV-11
Alisma gummifera, IX-79
Alisma plantago, XII-323
alkaloids, X-417
alkanet, XIV-50
all-heal plant, XIV-58
Allium cepa, XI-304; XIII-101; XIV-52
Allium porrum, XI-306; XIV-52
Allium sativum, XIV-52
Allium sp., XI-304; XIII-100
Allium subhirsutum, XIV-52
Allium ursinum, XI-306
Allium vineale, XI-306
almond oil, XV-12
almond, X-427; XI-294-5; XIV-37, 49; sweet, XI-310
aloe, II- 187, 190-4; VI-167; XV-8-12, 14
alopecia, X-413-4
Alphabetical Latin Dioscorides, IV; IX-71
alphos, XII-325
Alsace, VIII-217
alum, XIV-61
Amaranthus blitum, XI-302; XIV-47
amber, I-111-22; V-3-17; VI-174; VIII-210
ambergris, I-111-22; V-11-17; VI-167
amethysus, VIII-234
ammonicum, II-187
ammonite, VIII-210
ammonium chloride, II-187
amomum, II-187; XIV-58
Amomum subulatum, XIV-58
amulets, I-115;III-41, 49-50; V-3, 5; VII-211; IX-63; XIII-96, 98
amygdalin, XII-328
Amygdalus communis, *A. sativa*, XI-310; XIV-49
Anacyclus sp., XIV-57
Anagallis arvensis, IX-81
anagallis, IX-66
Anchusa tinctoria, *A. officinalis*, IX-81; XIV-50
anchuse, IX-81
Anicia Juliana, XIII-99
Andelhausen, VIII-221
Anemone coroniaria, XIV-52
Anethum graveolens, XI-

302; XIV-57
Ani papyrus, V-4
Anicia Juliana Ms, XIII-97
anise, X-427; XIV-37, 57; XV-12
Annagallis arvensis, XIV-54
anodyne, X-427; XV-7
anthelmintic use, X-422
Anthemis arvensis, IX-75
Anthemis cotula, IX-75
Anthemis tinctoria, IX-75-6
Anthemis valentian, IX-76
Anthimus, X-408
anthrax, XII-326
anthropology, XIV-34
antidotaria, II-185; VI-167
antidotes, X-419; XIII-100
antifertility, XIII-96-7
antimony, XIV-61
Antipater, V-7
Antirrhinum majus, IX-75
antispasmodic, II-193
Antonius Musa, Pseudo, IX-51
Apium graveolens, XI-300; XIV-57
apostêma, XII-325
apotheca, II-196; VI-168
apparment, II-194
appetite, loss, X-417
apple, Assyrian, X-422
apple, bitter, (see also bitter) IX-54; X-421-2; XI-306; XIV-49
apple, Median, X-422
apple, X-421-2
apricot, XI-308; XII-328
Apuleius, Pseudo, V-10; VI-163; IX-46-7, 51, 56, 66-7; X-408; XI-293; XII-328; XIII-99
aqua rosarum, I-113-4
arancii, I-113
Archigenes, V-10
Aretaeus of Cappadocia, V-8; V-11
Arisarum vulgare, IX-78
Aristolochia baetica, XIII-100
Aristolochia clematitis, IX-74; XII-328; XIII-99-100
Aristolochia pallaida, XIII-99
Aristolochia sempervirens, XIII-99
Aristolochia sp., XIV-54
aristolochia, see also birthwort, XIV-54
aristolochic acid, XII-328
Aristotle, III-45; VI-161; VIII-204-7, 215, 217; X-418, 420
Aristotle, Pseudo, VIII-233; III-44
Arnald of Villanova, VI-174
Arnold of Saxony, III-44, 48; VIII-231-3
aromatics, II-190
arsenic trisulfide, XIV-61
arsenicrealger, red, XIV-61
Artemisia abrotanum, XIV-56
Artemisia absinthium, X-427; XIV-56
Artemisia arborescens, IX-81; IX-81
Artemisia sp., XIV-57
artes mechanicae, VI-160
artichoke, XI-304
arts, culinary, VI-162
arum arrowroot, IX-79
Arum dracunculus, IX-79; XIV-52, 57
Arum maculatum, XIV-52
Asarum europaeum, XIV-57
ashwood, IX-60
asipu, XIV-35
Asparagus acutifolius, XIII-96
Asparagus officinalis, XIV-47
asparagus, IX-62; XIII-95-6; XIV-47
asphalt, XIV-58
asphodel, XIV-52
Asphodelos ramosus, *A. albus*, XIII-98; XIV-52
Asplenium ceterach, XIV-51
Assyrian texts, V-4
asthma, VIII-210
astringents, VIII-213
astrological medicine, VI-173
asu, XIV-35
Athamanta cretensis, XIV-57
Atractylis gummifera, IX-73
Atriplex hortensis, XIV-47
Atriplex sp., XI-302
Attalus II, X-419
Atropa belladonna, XV-12
atropine, XV-13
Auel, Jean, XV-1-2
autopsy, X-413, 416-9
autumn crocus, XII-319-20
Auzia, X-410-11
Avena sativa, XIV-47
Avicenna, I-113, 118, 121; III-46; VI-172, 176, 178, 180, 184; VIII-203, 205-6; XII-321, 326; XV-8, 14
axweed, XIV-49
Ayurvedic medicine, XII-327

Baader, Gerhard, IX-51; XI-283
Babylon, V-3
Babylonian medicine, XIV-38
balagius, VIII-211
balsam, II-192; XIV-59
barley water, XV-12
barley, XI-286, 291, 298; XIV-47
barrenness, XIII-96
Bartholomaeus de Ripa Romea, III-48
Bartholomaeus Anglicus, III-48; VIII-233
basil, XI-302
bay, XIV-55
bean, Egyptian, XIV-47
bean, white, XIV-48
Beccaria, Augusto, XI-283
Bede, III-42; VIII-209
bees' wax, XV-12
beet, XI-300; XIV-47
beetle, see blister
belching, X-413
Bellis perennis, IX-80
Benedictus Crispus, V-10; VI-166
Berber, IX-53; X-410
Berchtoldus (Magister), I-112-3, 118, 120
Bernard Gordon, III-41
bernstein, I-117; VI-174; see

also amber
bestiaries, III-50; V-3
Beta vulgaris, XI-300; XIV-47
Bible (Exodus), V-5
bile, red, X-417
Biringuccio, VIII-216
birthwort (aristolochia), IX-62, 74; XII-328; XIII-99
bites of animals, IX-61
bitter apple (see also apple), IX-79
black bile, XII-326
black bryony, IX-76
Black Death, VI-179
bladder stones, VIII-209
bladder, disease of, IX-66
bladder, flux of, VIII-212
bladder, useful for, XIII-97
bladder, XIII-96
Blasius of Barcelona, I-116
bleeding, stops (see also hemotopysis), IX-62
blister beetle, XII-329; XIV-55
blite, XI-290-1, 294-5; XI-302; XIV-47
blood, increases, XI-291
blood, spitting of, XI-292-3
Bohemia, VIII-221
boils, X-415; XI-291-2; XII-328
boli armenici, I-113
Bonser, Wilfrid, II-194-5; VI-165
Borago officinalis, IX-73
Boswellia sp., XIV-59
bowels, flux of, VIII-212
bowels, looseness of, VIII-210
bowels, loosens, XI-291
bowels, suffering of, V-7
brain, purify, III-49
bramble, XIV-48
Brassica oleracea, XIV-48
Brassica rapa, XI-302; XIV-48
Brassica sp., XI-300; XII-329
breast cancer, XII-329
breasts, IX-62
breathing, VIII-209
brimstone, XIV-60
Brotera corymbosa, XIV-53
Bryonia sp., XIV-53
bryony, XIV-53
buglossa, I-113; IX-67
bupthalmos, IX-58
burns, XI-291
burrage, IX-61
burweed, XIV-50
business, improves, VIII-213
bustalmon, IX-58
Byzantine medicine, XIII-95-102

cabbage, XI-294-5, XI-300; XII-329-30; XIV-48
Cadfael, XV-1-9
Caelius Aurelianus, V-9, 11; X-408, 417-20
Caesar, III-49
calamine, VIII-225
calaminth, I-113; II-194
Calamintha incana, XIV-57
calamus aromaticus, I-113
calamus, XIV-55
calcium carbonate, VIII-213
calcium sulfate, XIV-60
Calendula arvensis, IX-77
Callistratus, V-8, 11
Calpurnius Bestia, XV-4
caltrop, land/ small, IX-76
calx, VIII-222
Camaeleon albus, IX-73
camalention masculis, IX-81
camalention, IX-81
camel grass, XIV-55
camphor, I-113, 119; II-190; VI-167; XV-13
Cancer Chemotherapy National Service Center, XII-320
cancer, XII-319-330; XIII-100; XV-8
cannabis, XIV-37
cantaloupe, XI-304, 290-1; XIV-48
cantharidin, XII-329
caper, IX-80
Capparis spinosa, IX-80; XIV-54
Capsella bursa pastora, IX-75
Caranthus, XIV-38
carcinoma, nasal, XIII-98
carcinoma, XIII-100
cardamomum, II-192; XIV-55
cardiac arrest, X-418
cardoon, IX-78
Cardopatium corymborum, XIV-53
Carminis de viribus herbarum, XIII-100
carnelian, VIII-212
Carpathian mountains, VIII-217
carrot, wild (Queen Anne's lace), XI-302; XIV-39, 57
carrot, candy, XIV-57
carrot, wild/death, XIV-58
Carthamus tinctoris, XIV-53
Cartharantus, XII-327
cassia, II-187; IX-65; XIV-55
Cassiodorus, IX-56-9; X-409, 413, 428
Cassius Felix, V-10; X-408; XII-325
Castanea sativa, XI-310
Castiglioni, Arturo, VI-157
castor bean, XII-325-6
castor oil plant, XIV-54; XV-14
castoreum, XIV-60
cathartic, XV-9
catmint, IX-60; XIII-98; XIV-37, 57
catnip, Italian, V-9
Cato the Elder, IV-207; X-427; XII-329
cattail, XIII-101
caucalis, XIV-37
celandine, greater or common, IX-75; XV-12
celery, V-424, 427; XI-294, 300; XIV-57
Celsus, V-10; X-413, 416, 420; XIV-41-2
Celtic medicine, II-186; VI-164
Celtis australis, XIV-51
Centaurea centaureum, XIV-50
centaurea, great (see also

centaury), XIV-50
Centaurium umbellatum, IX-80
centaury, XV-12
centimorbia, IX-66, 80
Cerberus, XV-4
cestros, IX-65
Ceterach officinarum, IX-78
ceterach, XIV-37, 51
chamomile, yellow, IX-76
charlatans, XIV-33
chaste tree, XIV-35, 58
chastity, III-49
Cheiranthus cheiri, IX-80; XIV-53
Chelidonum majus, IX-75
chemical mixtures, VIII-208
cherry, XI-293, 308
chestnut, XI-310
chick pea, XI-286, 298; XIII-96; XIV-48
Chicorum endiva, XI-287
Chicorum intybus, XI-287
chicory, IX-77; XI-287, 302
childbirth, helps with, VIII-209
chill, intermittent, VI-173
Chinese medicine, VI-184; XII-327, 329; XIII-101
cholera, XI-291
Christian Church's influence on medicine, VI-166-7
Chrozophora tinctoria, IX-77
chryselectrum (-on), V-10, 12; VIII-210
Chrysanthemum coronarium, IX-76
Chrysippus, X-426
Church Fathers, VI-167
Cicer arietinum, XI-298; XIV-48
Cichorium endiva, XI-302
Cichorium intybus, IX-77; XI-302
Cilicia, XIII-97
cinchonna, XV-12
cinnamon, II-186-190, 192, 194; XIV-55; XV-12
Cinnamomum cassia, XIV-55
Cinnamomum sp., XIV-55
cinquefoil, XIV-51
Cissus vitiginea, XIV-58
Cistus creticus, XIV-59
Cistus sp., XIV-59
cistus, gum, XIV-59
citron, X-422; XI-308
Citrullus colocynthis, IX-79; XI-300; XIV-53
Citrus medica, XI-308
citrus, I-113
Claudius, V-5
cleavers goosegrass, IX-81
cleavers, XIV-51
climate and herbs, IX-54-5
clove, II-194
Clune, Francis J., XIV-39
Cockayne, Thomas, VI-165
cocliaria, IX-65
colchicine, XII-319-20, 322; XIII-98
Colchicum autumnale, XII-319-20
colds (catarrh), II-193
colicotis, X-415
collyrium, XV-7
colocynth, wild, IX-54; XIV-53
colocynth, XIV-35, 37; XV-14
colofonia, II-187, 189
Cologne, VIII-225, 228-30
colt's foot, XIV-50
Coluccio Salutati, VI-182
Columella, X-427
Commiphora opobalsumum, XIV-59
Commiphora sp., XIV-59
complexion, skin, IX-66
compound medicines, VI-173
condiment, IX-61
Condorelli, Sebastian, X-409-10, 412
condylomata, XII-325
conehead thyme, XIV-56
consilia, VI-159, 179-180
Constantine the African, III-47; IV-205-9; VI-169-170, 183; VIII-207, 212; XI-295; XII-322, 325-6; XIII-102; XV-8
contraceptive, VIII-209; IX-62; XIII-96; XV-18-9
Convulvulus scammonia, XIV-53
copper, VIII-218-9, 224, 227; XIV-61
coral, VIII-213
corallorum rubeorum, I-113
core drugs, XV-12-4
coriander, I-113; XI-295, 302; XIV-37, 57
Coriandrum sativum, XI-302; XIV-57
Cornus mascula, XIV-49
Cornwall-Devon, VIII-220, 222
Cortusius, Jacob, IX-44
Corylus avellana, XI-310
Cosmas and Damian, VI-166
cost of medicines, I-111
Costa ben Luca, III-48; VIII-211-2, 233-4
Costofforus of Oxford, I-116
costus, II-192, 194
Cotyledon umbilicus, XIV-49
cotyledon, XIV-37, 49
cough, V-7, XI-293
Courcelle, Pierre, XI-283
cow basil, XIII-102
Crataegus azarolus, XI-308
Crataegus oxyacantha, IX-73
Crateuas, XIII- 98-100
creeping jenny, IX-66, 80
cress, garden, XI-306
cress, XIV-37, 52
criminals, medical uses of, X-419
Crithmum maritimum, XIV-57
crocus (see also saffron), I-113; II-188
Crocus sativus, XIV-60
crowsfoot, XIV-52
cuckoo-pint, XIV-52
cucumber, XI-294-5; XIV-37, 48
Cucumis colocynthis, XIV-53
Cucumis melo, XI-304; XIV-

48
Cucumis sativus, XIV-48
Cucurbita maxima, XIV-48
cucurbita, see gourd
Cucurbita agrestis, IX-79
Cucurbita caprariam, IX-79
Cucurbita silvestrem, IX-79
cumin, black, XIV-37
cumin, IX-73; XIV-52, 57; XV-12
Cuminum cyminum, IX-73; 57
Curae boum, X-413
Cuscuta europaea, XIV-54
cuscuta, XIV-54
cyanogenic glycoside, XII-328
cyanosis, VI-173
Cyclamen graecum, XIV-54
cyclamen, XIV-54
Cydonia oblonga, XI-306
Cymbopogon schoenanthus, XIV-55
Cynara cardunculus, IX-78; XI-304
cyperos, V-9
Cyperus rotundus, XIII-99; XIV-55
cypress, funerial, XIV-59
Cypressus sempervirens, XIV-59
cysts, IX-62
Cytinus hypocistis, XIV-51

damasonion, XII-323
Damigeron, III-39, 41-2; IV-206; VIII-233
Daphne gnidium, IX-77-8; XIV-54
Daphne laureola, XIV-54
Daremberg, Charles, VI-158
darnel, XIV-60
date palm, XIV-47
daucos (see also Queen Anne's lace), XIV-37
Daucus carota, XI-302; XIII-97; XIV-57
Daucus gingidium, XIII-97-8
De holera arboresque pomiferas, X-411-3
De horti, X-411
De locis in homine, XIV-36
De morbis, XIV-36
De mulierum affectionibus, XIV-36, 39
De natura mulierbri, XIV-36
De observantia ciborum, XI-284, 289, 296-311
De taxone liber, IX-51
De victus ratione, XI-283
De virtutes herbarum, XI-283
decurion, X-410
degrees, VI-173
Delphinium staphisagria, IX-78; X-417; XIV-52
Delphinium consolida + sp., IX-80
Democritus, XIV-42
Demostratus, V-11
DeNavarro, J. M., V-5
Desiderius, Abbot, VI-177
Devon, VIII-217
diarrhoea, VIII-209
Didymus, XIII-96
Dierbach, Heinrich, XIV-36
Dietetics, XI-284
digestive tract, X-424
Digitalis purpurea, IX-76; XV-7
digitalis, XV-13
dill, XI-302; XIV-57
Diodorus of Sicily, V-4
Diokles of Carystos, V-6; X-421, 426
Dioscorides, Alphabetical Latin, IV-204-9; X-409
Dioscorides, II-188; III-39, 42, 47; V-5-7, 10-11; VI-162; VIII-232-3; X-413-6; 421-6, 428; IX-51, 57, 63, 67; X-413-6, 421-6, 428; XI-287, 293-5, 296-311; XII-320, 324-9; XIII-95-102; XIV-37-38, 40-1, 43, 59; XV-3-9, 10
Dioscorides, Old Lat. Translation, XI-288-9, 296-311; XIII-99, 102
Dioscorides, Pseudo, IX-43-81
Diospyrus, XIV-59
Dipsacus fullonum, IX-79
Dipsacus laciniathus, IX-79
Dipsacus silvestris, IX-79
discutient property, XII-326
Diseases V, XIV-36
dispersing property, XII-326
dispositions, improve, IX-66
dittander, XIII-98
diuretic, X-415; XI-292; XIII-97
dock, XI-286, 296, 302; XIV-49
dog rose, IX-66, 81
dogs mercury, IX-75
dogwood, XIV-49
Dolichos Lablab, XI-298
Doronicum pardalianches, XV-3
doronicum, I-113
doum palm, XI-310
Drabkin, I. E., X-409
Dracaena sp., XIV-51
dragon arrowroot, XIV-52
dragon's blood, XIV-51
dragonstone, VIII-210
dropsy, X-415
drug costs, I-119
drug effectiveness, XIV-34, 36-8; XV-2, 17-20
drug testing, XV-15
drug theory, X-414-5, XI-289
drug trade, VI-168, 174-5
drug, experimentation, XIV-40-1
drug, property, XIV-35
drug, theory, XI-289
drug, trade, VI-175
drug-food conceptionalization, XI-284
drugs, self-administered, XV-16
drugs, use of animals, XV-4
Dustin, A. P., XII-319
Dynamidia, XI-283-311
dynamis, X-414
dysentery, V-7; VIII-210, 213; X-414; XIII-96

eaglestone, VIII-210
earache, X-413, 424
earth, fuller's, XIV-60
earth, potter's, XIV-60
earth, purgative, XIV-60
earth, red, XIV-60

Ebers papyrus, V-4
ebony, XIV-59
Ecballium elaterium, XII-324; XIV-53
Echium vulgare, IX-78
eczema, X-417
education, medical, VI-159-160
Edwin Smith papyrus, V-4
eggs, XIV-47
Egyptian science, XIV-33
Ehrlich, Paul, XII-319
Elbe, VIII-217
elecampane, XIV-57
electron, V-3
electrum, I-117; VI-174
Elettaria cardamomum, XIV-55
elf-enchantment, II-194
emerald (see also smaragdus) III-210; VIII-210
emetic, X-415-6, 424
emetine, XV-12
Empedocles, VIII-204
enchantments, II-194
endive, XI-302
England, VIII-220
ephêles, XII-328
epilepsy, III-41, 49; VIII-213, 226; IX-47, 66; X-415
epsêlis, XII-325
Equisetum telmateia, IX-77
ergot, XIV-378
Erica arborea, XIV-50
eruptions, subcutaneous, X-424-5
Eruca sativa, XIV-53
Eruca sp., XI-306
Ervum lens, XIV-48
Eryngium, campestre, IX-80
Erysimum officinalis, XIV-53
erysipelata, XII-325
erysipilis, X-424
Erzgebirge, VIII-220-1
esophagus, weakness in, X-417
Ethiopia, II-188
ethnopharmacy, XIV-38
Eudemus the Chian, XIV-39
Euphorbia characia, IX-77
Euphorbia cyparissias, XIV-54
Euphorbia peplis, XIV-54
Euphorbia peplus, XIV-54
Euphorbia sp., (see also spruge) XII-326; XIV-54
Euphorbia spinosa, XIV-54
Eusebius, IX-57
Evans, Joan, III-40
Evax, III-42, 46; IV-206; VIII-214, 233
Ex herbis femininis, Old English transl., IX-56, 71
Ex herbis femininis, VI-163; IX-43-81
exacolitus, VIII-211
exact sciences, XV-17
exanthema, X-424
eye disorders, II-194; III-40; X-423
eye glasses, III-49
eye trouble, X-423
eye, itch of, XV-10
eye, relieves pain of, XV-7
eye, tumor, IX-60
eyeglasses, III-46
eyes, darkness of, XI-292-3
eyes, troubles with, III-40

Führer, Herman, III-39
faith healers, XIV-33
Faraxen, X-410
Farrar, George, XIV-36
female herbs, IX-43-81
fennel, all-heal, XIV-58
fennel, common, XIV-58
fennel, hog's, XIV-58
fennel, horse, XIV-37
fennel, Libyan, XIV-58
fennel, Persian, XIV-58
fennel, XI-304; XIV-52, 57; XV-12
fenugrecum, II-187
fenugreek, XIV-50
ferrous oxide, VIII-212-3
fertility of fields, increases, III-49
Ferula asa-foetida, XIV-58
Ferula communis, XIV-58
Ferula cyrenaica, XIV-58
Ferula galbaniflua, XIV-58
Ferula marmarica, XIV-58
Ferula persica, XIV-58
Ferula tingitana, XIV-58
fetus, expels, IX-62; XI-294
fever (incl. tertian, quotidian, etc.), VIII-209; XI-288; XIII-98-99
feverfew, XIV-57
Ficus sp., XI-308; XIV-48
fig, XI-308; XIII-96, 101; XIV-48
figwort, XII-324
filacterium, VIII-210
Fistulas, XIV-36
flatulency, V-7
flax, see linum
flax, XIV-50
fleabane scabwort, XIV-57
fleabane, XIV-57
fleas, IX-64
fleas, prevents, IX-62
fleawort, V-7
flint, VIII-206
flowers, IX-64; X-423
Foeniculum vulgare, XI-304; XIII-96; XIV-57
folk transmission, XV-1
font rod, IX-75
food, XI-284, 296
Forbes, Thomas, III-50
foxglove, XV-12
foxmange, X-413, 415
Francis of Assisi, VI-184
frankincense, I-113, 119; II-188, 192; VI-167; XII-324; XIV-59
Fraticelli, Vanda, XI-286
Fraxinus ornus, XIV-51
freckles, XII-328
Frederick II, II-196
frees one from enemies, XIII-100
freestone, VIII-206
Freiberg, VIII-220, 228-30
friar's cowl, IX-63, 78
fruits, X-411
Fuchs, Leonard, IX-44
Fulbert of Chartres, II-189
furuncles, XI-291

Gabriel, Ingrid, XV-13
gaggrainai, X-415-6
Galanthus nivelis, XIV-54
galbanum, II-192
Galen, II-186-7, 192; III-39,

46-7; IV-206-7; V-6-7, 9, 10, 12; VI-164-5, 170, 174, 180, 182; VIII-206-7; IX-67; X-413-4, 416-7, 419-21, 423, 426; XI-283, 288-9, 294-5; 321-6; XIII-99-100; XV-6, 8 10, 14
galena, VIII-219
Galium aparine, IX-81; XIV-51
gall, XIV-61
gallenga (galingale), II-192, 194
Gallus (Magister), I-117
gangrainode, XII-326
gangrene, XII-328
Gargilius Martialis, V-10; IX-57; X-408-29; XI-285-8; XI-293-311
gariofilum, I-113, 119; II-192, 194
garioguinem, II-194
garlic, XI-288; 304; XIV-35, 52
Geber, VIII-224
gecolitus, VIII-211
Geniza documents, VI-175
gentian, X-427
Gentilis, II-186
geological formations, VIII-216
geology, VIII-227
Geoponica, XIII-95-6
Gerard of Cremona, III-44; VI-172, 176-177; VIII-233; XV-8
germander speedwell, IX-76
Germanic medicine, VI-164
Germany, VIII-220
giant spider flower, XIV-54
giggidion, XIII-97-8
Gilbert, W. S., X-420
gilliflower, XIV-54
ginger, II-189-90, 192, 194; V-9; XV-12
ginger, wild, XIV-57
Giordano of Pisa, III-46
Giovanni Santa Sofia, I-119
Gladitsia farnesiana, IX-81
Glossae medicinalis, V-10
Glycyrrhiza glabra, IX-78; XIV-50
goitre, V-9
gold arsenic, XIV-61
gold, VIII-216, 218-9, 228
Goltz, Dietlinde, XIV-38
goosefoot, XI-296
Gordon, Benjamin Lee, VI-166
Goslar, VIII-219
gossan, VIII-222
gotyumber, II-194
gourd, IX-53; XI-294-5, 300; XIV-48
gout, III-40; XI-287-8; XIII-98-9
grape, XI-286, 308; XIV-49
Grattan, J. H., VI-165
Graupen, VIII-220
Gregory of Tours, II-197
ground olive, IX-78
growths, X-415, 425
Guilliretus, Stephanus, XI-285
gums, good for, XV-10
Guy de Chauliac, VI-182
gypsum, XIV-60

hair, loss, X-417; XV-10
hair, stimulates growth, X-426
Haly Abbas, VI-172, VI-176-7
happiness, confers, VIII-209
hare tailgrass, XIV-37, 50
harioli, II-196
hartwort, XIV-37, 57
hawthorn, IX-60, 64, IX-73
hazel nut, XI-310
head, purges, XI-293
headache, IX-65; X-424; XV-10
heart attacks, VIII-209
heart, ailments of, V-10
heather, XIV-50
Hedera helix, XIV-50
hedge mustard, XI-286; XIV-53
heliotrope, IX-65
Heliotropium europaeum, IX-77
helkos, XII-325-326
hellebore, black, XIV-37, 52
hellebore, white, X-417; XIV-37, 52; XV-12
Helleborus niger, XIV-52
Helxine solieiolii, XIV-50
helxinet, XIV-50
hemlock, XIV-37, 39, 60
hemoptysis, V-7; IX-61; XV-10
wounds, heals, XV-10-1
hemorrhoids, VIII-209-10; XV-10
henbane, X-427; XIV-37, 60
Henderson, L. J., XV-14-5
Henri de Mondeville, VI-182 XII-327
Henricus de Bremis (Ribbenicz), I-116
Heracules panaces, IX-75
herbs, gender, IX-43-8
Hercules, XV-4
Hermes, VIII-208, 214, 223
hernias, X-423
herpes, X-424
hexecontalithos, III-50
Hibiscus sylvestris, X-424
hiena, VIII-210
Hildegard of Bingen, II-191; III-48; VI-171; XII-322-3
Hippocrates and Hippocratic Corpus, II-186; VI-207; V-6-7; VI-160, 164-5, 182; IX-51; X-412; XIV--33-40, 43, 46-61; XV-1
Hippocrates, Pseudo, XI-283-311
Hippocratic ethics, XV-19
Hispanic medicine, VI-164
Historia Augusta, X-411
Hodgkin's disease, XII-327
holly, sea, IX-60
Homer, V-4
honey, Attic, XI-292
honey, XIII-98; XIV-50
honeysuckle, IX-80
Hordeum vulgare, XIV-47
horn, XIV-61
horoscope, VI-173
horse bean, XI-286; XII-327-8
horse fennel (see also fennel), XIV-57
horseradish, X-427
horsetails, IX-62, 77

household remedies, X-428
houseleek, IX-65, 74, 77; XIV-37, 53
Howard, Ernest, IX-67
Howell, E., X-409
Hrabanus Maurus, III-42
humoral balance, III-49; VI-172
humors, spitting up of, V-7
Hunain ibn Ishaq, VI-176
hyacinth, tassel, IX-78
hyacinth, XI-286, XIII-100
Hyacinth comosus, IX-78
Hydrastis canadensis, XIV-38
Hyoscyamus niger, XIV-60
Hypericum hircinum, XIV-59
Hypericum perforatum + sp., IX-79
Hypochoeris glaba, IX-77
hypocracy tree, XIV-51
hypomelidus, X-425
hyssop, XV-12

iatroi, XIV-39
Ibn Ahmad ibn al-Awwaan, X-409
Ibn al-Nadim, VI-181
Ibn Sarabi, see Serapion
Ibn-Hedijadi, X-409
Ibn-Sina, see Avicenna
ileocolitus, X-415
illustrations, manuscript, IX-44-5
Indian medicine, VIII-211; XII-327
Indians, Native American, XIV-39
indium, II-194
infections from scratching, X-417
inflammatio, XII-321
Inquiry into Plants, XIV-39
intelligence, increases, III-49
Internal Affections, XIV-36
intibus, XI-287
Inula conyza, IX-76
Inula helenium, XIV-57
Inula sp., XIV-57
Inula vis cosa, IX-76
ipecacuanaha, XV-12
Iris florentina, XIV-55
iris, Illyrian, V-7
iris, XIV-55
iron oxide, III-40; XIV-60
iron, VIII-216, 226; IX-60; XIV-61
Isaac Judaeus, IV-207
Isatis tinctoria, XIII-102
isatis, wild, XIII-101
Isidore of Seville, II-192; III,42; IV-206; V-5; IX-56, 58-9; X-409; XI-284; XV-8
isiferitis, IX-62, 77
ivy, XIV-50

jaundice, VIII-209; XI-288, 292; XIII-96
Jerome, V-5
jet, see also kacabre, VIII-210
Jewish medicine, VI-166
Joannes de Penna, I-112, 115
Johannes de Noctho, I-115-6
Johannes Jacobi, I-113
John of Gaddesden, I-121; III-41
John of Procida, I-121
John of Saxony, I-120
Joly, Robert, XI-283
Jones, W. H. S., XIV-34, 41
Juba, V-8
Juglans regia, XIV-48
Julian the Apostate, V-9
Juliana Anicia Codex, IX-44-5
juniper, XIV-35, 37, 59
Juniperus sp., XIV-59
Justinian, IX-57
Juvenal, I-111

Kästner, Heinrich, IX-44; IX-67
kacabre (jet ?), VIII-210
karabre (see also amber), VI-174, VIII-232
karkinoma, XII-328
karkinos genomenos, XII-326
karkinos, XII-321, 324-5
kidney trouble, III-40
knotgrass, IX-64, 74; XIV-54
Kollesch, Jutta, X-409
kondylomata, XV-10
Kyrannides, III-42

Lacnunga, II-191
lactation, X-413; XI-291
Lactuca sativa, XIV-49
Lagurus ovatus, XIV-50
lapidaries, VIII-203-34
larkspur, field, IX-80
laudanum, I-113, 119
laurel daphne, XIV-54
laurel, XIV-55
Laurus nobilis, XIV-55
Lavandula stoechnas, IX-74
lavender, French, IX-74
laxative, X-425; XV-10
lead sulfate, XIV-61
lead, poisoning, VIII-226-7
lead, VIII-216; XIV-61
Leechbook of Bald, VI-169
leechbooks, II-185
leeches, II-196
leek, XIV-52
leichene, XII-329
lemons, X-421-2
lentil, XIV-37, 48
leopard's bane, XV-6-7
Lepidium latifolium, L. sativum, XIII-98; XIV-52
Lepidium sativum, XIV-52
lepidium (-on), XIII-98; XIV-37, 52
lepra, XII-329
lethary, X-415
lettuce, XI-290-1, XI-294-5; XIV-37, 49
leuke, XII-323
leukemia, XII-327
Lewis, Walter, and M. Elvin-Lewis, XIV-37
libanus (see also frankincense), II-187
liberal arts, VI-160
Liberale, Giorgio, IX-44
lice, X-413, 416-20
licentiousness, moderates, VIII-209
lichen, XII-325-6
licorice, IX-78; XIV-37, 39,

50
liggourion, see lyngourion
lightning, prevents, VIII-213
lignum aloes, I-113, 119
Ligurians, V-5
linseed, XI-286
linum (flax), II-187, 189
Linum isitatissimum, XIV-50
liparea, VIII-214
liquid amber, XIV-37-8
liver, X-427
Lloyd, Geoffrey, XIV-40-1
logos, XIV-41
Lolium temulentum, XIV-60; XV-7
Lombardy, XI-288
Lonicera periclymenum, IX-80
loosestrife, yellow, IX-80
Lopez, Robert, II-195
lousewort, IX-78
lower digestive tract, XIII-97
Lübeck, VIII-228-30
lumps, cures, XV-10-1
lupin, XI-286
Lupinus albus, XIV-48
Lycium europaeum, XIV-51
Lynchnis coronaria, IX-81
lyncurium, V-8
lyngourion, V-5
lyngurion, I-117
lynx, V-4-5; VIII-210
Lysimachia vulgaris, IX-80
Lythrum salicaria, IX-76

Macer Floridus, VI-171; IX-71; X-409; XV-8
Machinery for Reducing Dislocations, XIV-36
MacKinney, Loren C., VI-165
mad dog bites, IX-60
Madagascar, XII-327
madder, XIV-51
magi, XIV-41-2
magicians, XIV-33
magnesium silicate, XIV-60
Mai, Angelo, XI-285
maiden spleenwort, IX-74
maidenhair fern, IX-74; XIV-51
Mainz, II-195
malignant humors, IX-61
mallow, XI-294-5; XIV-50
Malva rotundifolia, XIV-50
malva, X-424
Mandragora officinarum, IX-74
mandrake, IX-74; XIV-60
manna ash, XIV-51
marbles, VIII-206
Marbode of Rennes, III-42, 44, 46, 48; VI-171; VIII-209, 212, 233; X-409
Marcellinus, IX-57
Marcellus Empiricus, II-192, 197; V-9-12; X-408; XIV-42
Marcus Aurelius, V-7
marjoram, IX-60, 74; XIV--55-6
Marrubium vulgare, XIV-56
Martial, I-111
Martianus Capella, VI-159
Martin of Aragon, I-116
Masawaih, Abu Zakariya ibn Masawaih, II-190-1
Masawaih, see Mesue
Massilian hartwort, XIV-57
mastic, I-113; II-187-8, 192, 194; VI-167; XI-292; XIV-59; XV-12
Matthaeus Platearius, VI-174; IX-71; XII-322, 327; XV-8
Matthaeus Silvaticus, VI-174
Matthew Paris, VIII-220
Matthiola incana, XIV-54
Matthiolus, Petrus Andreas, IX-44
mayweed, IX-75-6
Mazzini, Innocenzo, X-409-10, 412, 426; XI-286
meadow saffron, XIV-39
Medicago arborea, XIV-49
medical practice, VI-180
medicine, religious and secular, XIV-35
medlar, XIV-37, 49
melanchoia, X-415
melancholy, VIII-209
Melilotus officinalis, XIV-58
meliot, XIV-58
Meloe sp., XIV-55
Meloe variegatus, XIV-55
menstruation, reduces bleeding, VIII-210
menstruation, flux of, VIII-212
menstruation, VIII-213; XIV-37
mental attitude, IX-66
Mentha citrata, XIV-56
Mentha pulegium, XIV-56
Mentha sativa, XIV-55
Mercurialis annua, IX-75; XIV-49
Mercurialis perennis, IX-75
mercury plant, IX-50, 64
mercury, annual, IX-75; XIV-49
mercury, poisoning, VIII-227
Mesopotamian science, XIV-33, 35
Mesue (the Younger), see Masawaih, I-121; III-46; VI-174; XII-325
metal alloys, VIII-216
metal, disease of, VIII-225-6
metals, formation of, VIII-217-8
metals, VIII-212
mezereon, Mediterranean, IX-50, 77-8
micturation, difficulty of, XIII-96
midwivery, XIV-41
midwives, II-196
milk, XIV-47
millet, Italian, XIV-47
millet, XI-286
Mimusops schimperi, XIV-49
minerals, VIII-203-34
miners and mining, VIII-216-8
mint, bergamot, XIV-56
mint, green, XIV-55
mint, XI-292, XI-294
miracle drugs, II-187
misces, IX-65
mistletoe, XIV-37, 50
Mithridates VI, X-419
moles, XII-328
moly, XIII-100; XIV-52

Momordica elaterium, XIV-53
money making, III-49
moneywort, IX-80
monkshood, XV-1-9
Montpellier, School of, VI-181
morphine, XV-12
Morus nigra, XIV-48
Moschion, X-414
mouthwash, X-423
mulberry, XI-294-5; XIV-48
Mulholland, James, VIII--203-34
mullein, great, IX-75
mullein, XIV-50
Muretania, X-410
Muscari comosum, IX-78; XIII-100; XIV-52
muscular contractions, XIII-96
musk, I-113, 115, 119; II-190
mustard, XIV-53
Mycenae, V-3
Mylabris phalerata, XII-329
myrrh (murra), II-187-8, 192, 194; VI-167; XIV-37, 39, 59; XV-12
myrtle, XIV-51
mystic powers, VIII-215

Nabateans, II-193
Napaul cardamon, XIV-58
Narcissus sp., XII-325; XIV-51
narcissus, XII-325; XIV-51
nard, XIV-58
Nardostachy jatamansi, XIV-58
Nature of Women, XIV-36-7
nature, XIV-35
Neapolitan lozenge, V-7
Nef, John, VIII-216
Nelumbrium speciosum, XIV-47
nenufaris, I-113
Nepeta cataria, XIV-56
Nero, III-46, 49
nervous disorders, II-193
nettle tree, XIV-51
nettle, XII-324; XIV-48
Neuclerius, II-186
Newby, Gordon, IX-51-2, 72
Nicander, X-413; XV-6
Nicholas of Montpellier, VI-181
Nicholaus Myrepsos, VI-174
Nicholus de Burgo, I-118
Nickel, Dietthard, X-409
Nicolas, VI-171
Nicolaus of Alexandria, VI-174
Nicolaus von Udine, I-112-3
Niedermann, Max, X-408-9
Nigella sativa, XIV-52
nightshade, black, IX-76
nightshade, garden, XIV-49
nightshade, XII-324
Nikostratos, V-7
nitrogen mustards, XII-319
nitrum, XI-288; XIV-60
nomai, XII-328
nomas, X-415-6
nucis muscatae, I-113
numeri, VI-173
nut grass, XIII-99; XIV-55
nut, XIV-48
nutmeg, XV-12
Nutton, Vivian, X-408; XI-284; XIV-42
Nux vomica, XV-12
Nymphaea nelumbo, XIV-47

oak gall, XIV-51
oak, XIV-48
oats, XIV-47
occult powers, VIII-214
Ocimum basilicum, XIV-56
odor therapy, I-116
odors, removes, IX-62
odors, X-417
oidêmata, XII-320-1, 323-5; XIII-100
olive oil, III-49-50; XIV-50
olive, IX-62
Olympia Thebena, X-421
On Visions, XIV-36
onion, XIII-101; XIV-35, 52
onkos, XII-321
Onopordon acanthium, XIII-101
onyx, VIII-210
Ophrys apifera, XII-323
ophthalmus, VIII-210
opium poppy, XIV-60
opium, II-187, 189, 192; V-7; XV-12
Opopanax chironium, IX-81
orache, XI-290-1, 294-6, 296, 302; XIV-47
oranges, X-421
orchis, XII-323
Oribasius (-os), V-9; XI-283; XI-285; XII-322
Oribasius, Pseudo, IV-206
Origanum hirtum, XIV-55
Origanum majorana, IX-74
Origanum vulgare, IX-74
Osol, Arthur, XIV-36
Osyriua reniformis, IX-79
Otto III, XV-11
Ovid, V-5
ox eye, XIV-57

Padus (river), V-6
Paeonia officinalis, XIV-52
Palladiius, X-409
Panicum italicum, XIV-47
Panicum miliaceum, XIV-47
pansy, IX-64
pansy, mountain, IX-80
pantheros (-us), III-50; VIII-210
Papaver somniferum, IX-79; XIV-60
parasites, intestinal, XI-295
Parietaria officinalis, XIV-50
Paris, University of, I-119
Paris, VIII-206, 225, 228-9
parotis, XII-325
parsley, II-187, 189; X-427; XV-12
parsnip, XIV-58
passions, checks, VIII-209
patient-doctor relationships, XV-16
Paul of Aegina, II-186, 191-2; V-10; XII-322, 325
Pausanias, V-4
Pazzini, A., VI-158
pea, XI-286
pea, yellow, XIV-48
peaches, XI-293-4
pear, X-426; XI-286; XIV-48
pearl, VIII-210

pediculosus, X-416
Pediculus humanus, X-418
pelletierine, X-422
penicillin, XV-18
pennyroyal, XIV-56; XV-12
peony, XIV-52
peplis spurge, XIV-54
peplus spurge, XIV-54
pepper, II-187-8, 190, 192, 194; V-9; VI-167; IX-65; XIV-55
pepperwort, XIII-98
peranites, VIII-211
percrum, II-194
perdicius, XI-292
peri diaites, X-412
Periplus of the Erythraean Sea, V-11
periwinkle, XV-12
Persea tree, XIV-49
pessary, XIII-96
Pestschriften, I-111-22; VI-159, 179
Peter of Abano, IV-207-9; VI-174, 184
Peter of Spain, VIII-207
Peter the Deacon, VI-169
Peters, Ellis, XV-1,
petroselinum (rock parsley), II-187, 189
Peucedanum officinalis, XIV-58
Phaethon, V-6
phagedaina, XII-326
phantasies, prevents, III-49
phantoms, prevents, VIII-209
pharmakopoloi, XIV-39
Phaseolus vulgaris, XIV-48
Philemon, V-11
phlegm, IX-66
phlegmone, XII-321
Phoenician language, IX-53
Phoenix dactylifera, XIV-47
phrenitis, XIII-96
phthiriasis, X-413-20
phumata, XII-320-1; XIII-100-1
physician, military, X-411
physicis, VIII-208
picea (pitch), II-187, 189
pimpernel, XIV-54
Pimpinella anisum, XIV-57
pine thistle, IX-79
pine, XIV-58-9
Pinus sp., XIV-58-9
Pirenne thesis, II-185
Pirenne, Henri, II-195
piretrum, I-113
pistachio, XI-286
Pistacia lentiscus, XIV-59
Pistacia terebinthus, XIV-59
Pisum ochres, XIV-48
Pisum sativus, XIV-48
placebo effect, XV-16
Placitus, V-10
Plantago lagopus, IX-79
Plantago major, IX-79
Plantago psyllum, IX-76
Plantago sp., XIII-98
plantain, common, IX-79
plantain, XIII-98; XV-12
Plato, V-4
Plinii Medicina, XI-285
Pliny the Elder, I-115, 117; II-187, 192; III-42, 46; V-3-5, 8, 11-2; VI-161; VIII-216, 228; IX-47, 58, 67; X-413-4, 416, 423; XI-283, 287, 289, 293-5; XII-324, 327; XIV-41-43; XV-4, 8
Pliny (Pseudo-), Medicina (-ii), IX-58; X-408; XI-285
ploughman's spikenard, IX-62, 76
plums, XI-286; X-425
Plutarch, V-4
poison, XV-1-9
poisons, combats, (see also antidotes) X-424
polenta, XI-286
Polygonum aviculare, IX-74
Polygonum hydropepper, XIV-54
polyp, XIII-98
polypharmacy, I-113
Polypodium vulgare, XIV-50
polypodium, XIV-50
polyps, nasal, XII-328
pomegranate, X-421-4; XI-290; XIV-51
pomicar, II-194
poplar, Greek, XIV-59
poplar, V-6
poppy anemone, XIV-52
poppy, IX-79; XIV-37
poppy, XV-12
Populus sp., XIV-59
Porphyra laciniata, IX-81
Portulaca oleracea, XIV-49
portulaca, I-113
Potentilla reptans, XIV-51
Poterium spinorum, XIV-51
potter's earth (see also earth), XIV-37, 60
praecordia, X-415
Prangos ferulacea, XIV-57
Praxagoras, X-426
Primus de Gorlicio, I-113
protective medicine, I-112
prunes, X-425-6; XI-290, 294-5
psôra, XII-325-6
Pseudo-Galen, XV-10-1
Psoralea bituminosa, XIV-59
psorophthalmia, XV-10
psychotherapy, VIII-213
psyllium plantain, IX-76
psyllium, IX-61-2
pterygion, XV-10
Ptolemaic kings, X-413, 418-9
Ptolemy, III-45
pumice, XIV-60
Punica granatum, XIV-51
purgative, X-425; XV-10
Purgatives, XIV-36
purse-tassels, XIV-52
purslane, XIV-49
Purus communis, XIV-48
Pyrethrum parthenium, XIV-57
pyrite, VIII-219
Pyrus cydonia, XIV-49
Pyrus germanica, XIV-49
Pyrus malus, XIV-49
pysllium, IX-63-4

quacks, XIV-33
qualities of actions, X-414
Quercus sp., XIV-48, 51
quicksilver, VIII-219
Quid pro quo, VI-175; XV-14
quince, X-421; XIV-49

quinine, XV-12, 18
Quintus Serenus Sammonicus, X-408
Qusta ibn Luqa, see Costa

radish juice, X-416-7
radish, X-413-23; XI-288, 290; XIV-48
ramai, VIII-210, 213
rams' horns, XIII-95
Ranunculus sp., XIV-52
Raphanus sativus, XIV-48
Ravenna, IX-52; XI-283
Raymond Lull, III-41, 46, 48
receptaria, II-185
red bulbs, IX-54, 78
Reeds, Karen, IX-72
Regensburg, VIII-229
Regimen, XI-284
reopontico, II-194
resperine, XV-12
rhamnos, XIV-51
Rhazes, V-7; VI-178, 181
Rhine, VIII-217
rhizotomoi, XIV-39
Rhus coriaria, XIV-51
Ricardus Anglicus, VI-176
Riché, Pierre, IX-52; XI-283
Richer of Rheims, VI-170
Ricinus communis, XII-325-6; XIV-54
Rickettsia prowazeki, X-418
Ritter, Edith K., XIV-35
Rivers, W. H. R., XIV-34
robbery, prevention of, VIII-208-9
rock crystal, VIII-210
rock-parsley, V-9
rocket, XIV-37, XIV-53
Roger Bacon, VI-174, 176, 178; VIII-207
Rosa canina, IX-81
Rosa sempervirem, IX-81
Rosa sp., XIV-50
rose champion, IX-81
rose oil, IX-66
Rose, Valentin, IV-206; IX-58; X-408-9, 412; XI-285-6
rose, rock, XIV-59
rose, XIV-50
rosemary, XV-12
rough spots on skin, XII-328
rubeus sandalus, I-119
Rubia tinctorum, XIV-51
Rubus ulmifolius, XIV-48
rue, X-424; XIV-54; XV-12
Rufinus, XII-326
Rufus of Ephesus, V-7
Rumex patientia, IX-79; XIV-49
rustics, II-196
Ruta graeveolens, XIV-54
rutin, X-424

Sacred Disease, XIV-33
safflower, XIV-53
saffron (see also crocus), II-192; XIV-60
sage, Ethiopian, XIV-55
sage, II-194, IX-45-9, 73; XIV-55
Sahl ben Bist ben Habib, III-45
Salerno, School of, IV-207; VI-170, 179-181
saliva, blood in, VIII-212
Salix alba, XIV-51
Salk vaccine, XV-18
salt, XIV-61
Salvia horminum, XIV-55
Salvia officinalis, IX-73; XIV-55
Sambucus niger, XIV-54
Sambucus, Johannes, IX-44
samphire, XIV-37; XIV-57
sandalum, I-113
sanguines draconis, II-194
santonin, XV-12
sapphires, VIII-208, 210
Saponaria officinalis, IX-80; XIV-50
sarcoma, XIII-100
Sarton, George, III-40; V-9; VI-158; XIV-34
savory, XI-294; XIV-56
saxifrage, V-9
Saxony, VIII-221
scabies, IX-66
scammony, XIV-53; XV-14
scamonia, II-187-9
Scarborough, John, IX-72; X-408, 428; XI-284
scarlet pimpernel, XIV-54
Schipperges, Heinrich, VI-175
scholastic medicine, VI-175-184
Schottus, J., XI-285
sciatica, XIII-96
science and magic, VIII--214-5
scientia, VI-160
Scilla maritima, IX-79; XIV-52
*Scolymus carduncul*us, IX-78
Scolymus hispanicus, IX-78
scorpion, X-415
Scribonius Largus, V-10; X-413; XII-325
Scrophularis peregrina, XII-324
sea holly, IX-80
sea squill, IX-79
secrets, betray, VIII-209
Securigera coronilla, XIV-49
sedamine, XIV-53
sedition, restrains, VIII-209
Sedum telephium, XIV-53
Sempervivum ochroleucum, IX-77
Sempervivum tectorum, IX-74, 77; XIV-53
Seneca, VI-160
senna, XV-13
sepiolite, XIV-60
Serapion (d. 1074), III-46; XII-325
service tree, XIV-49
Servus, X-409
sesame, XI-286; XIV-49
Sesamum sp., XIV-49
Seseli tortuosum, XIV-57
seselis, V-9
Sextius Niger, IX-67; X-421, 424
Sextus Papyriensis, V-10
Sextus Placitus, IX-51
sexual activity, stimulates, XIII-98
sexual desire, stimulates, X-413
sexuality of stones, VIII-211
Shapiro, Arthur K., XIV-34

shepherd's purse, IX-75; XIV-37, 52
Sideritis hirsuta, IX-75
Sigerist, Henry, II-185-6; IV-206; VI-158; IX-67; X-409
silphium, XIV-58
silver, VIII-216-8
Simon of Genoa, VI-174; IX-71
Sinapis nigra, XIV-53
Singer, Charles, II-185, 192; V-7; VI-157-8, 165; IX-54, 67
Sisymbrium polyceratium, XIV-53
Sisymbriumm sp., XI-293-4
Sium latifolium, IX-81
Sium nodiflorum, IX-81, XIV-58
sleep, causes, X-427
sluggishness, XI-291
smaragdus, III-46
Smyrnium olusatrum, XIV-57
snake bites, IX-60
snakeweed, IX-790
snapdragon, IX-64, 75
soap-wort, IX-80; XIV-50
soda carbonate, XIV-60
sodium chloride, XIV-61
Solanum nigrum, IX-76; XIV-49
solanum, XII-324
Solinus, III-42
Solzhenitsyn, A. I., XV-8
Somilia, II-188
Soranus, V-9-10; XIV-40-3
Sorbus domestica, XIV-49
sores, XI-295
sorrel, IX-62, 79; XI-294-5
southernwood, IX-81; XIV-56
spelt, XIV-47
sphalerite, VIII-219
spica (-um), II-194
spice nard, IX-65
spider bites, XIII-95
spiney spurge, XIV-54
spleen, englargement of, IX-65
spleen, IX-65; X-427
spleenwort, IX-62-3, 78
spodius, I-113
sponge, XIV-61
spots on skin, XII-328
sprains, XIII-96
spurge, large Mediterranean, IX-77
spurge, XII-326; XIV-39, 54; XV-12
sputum, rusty, VI-173
squill, IX-63
squirting cucumber, XII-324; XIV-53
St. John's wort, IX-79; XIV-59
St. Michael at Litomerice, VIII-221
Stachys officinalis, XIV-56
Stadler, Hermann, IX-51, 58
Stannard, Jerry, VI-165
stavesacre, IX-78; X-417; XIII-101; XIV-37, 52
sterility, XIII-96
Steudel, Johannes, II-185
stomach ache, VIII-209; IX-47
stomach disorders, II-193; V-10, 12
stomach, good for, X-424
stomach, kills worms in, X-413
stomach, upset, XI-291
stomach, XIII-97
Stone, William S., XII-319, 330
stones, bladder, VIII-209
stones, formation of, VIII-217
stones, kidney, expel, X-415
stones, kidney, VIII-209
stones, sculptured, III-50
storax (-ce), I-113; II-187, 189, 192, 194; XIV-37, 59
storms, prevention of, III-49; VIII-208, 213
Strabo, V-5
strangury, V-10; XIII-96
strychinine, XV-13
strychnos, XII-324
stuttering of tin, VIII-223-5
styptic power, VIII-212; XI-290
Styrax offficinalis, XIV-59
succinus, VIII-210
sucinum, I-117; V-5, 9
Sudhoff, Karl, I-111; IV-205; VI-158
sulfur, VIII-218; XIV-60
Sumerian texts, V-4
suppurations of diaphragm, X-415
sweet flag, XV-14
synthetic drugs, II-193
Syria, XIII-97

Talbot, Charles H., VI-165, 169, 178
talisman (see also amulet), XIII-98
Tamarix gallica, XIV-51
tamerisk, XIV-51
Tamus communis, IX-76
Tamus viridis, IX-76
tanning sumach, XIV-51
tapeworm, X-422
Tapper, Ruth M., X-409
Taraxcum officinale, IX-77
tarragon, IX-50
teasle, common, IX-79
teeth, X-423
terbenthum, I-113
terebinth, II-187, 189; XI-294-5; XIV-59
terra sigillata, I-113
Teucrium chamaedrys, IX-74
thêriodai, XII-328
Thapsia garganica, IX-75; XIV-58
thapsia (*also*, *thlapsia*), XIV-39
Theodore Priscianus, II-192; V-10
Theodorus, XI-283
Theophilus, VIII-224
Theophrastus (-os), III-39, 42, 46; V-5, 7; X-413-4; IX-47; XIII-96; XIV-39, 43
Thetel (Zael), III-45
thistle, golden, IX-78
thistle, IX-62
thistle, Scotch, XIII-101
Thlaspi Bursa pastoris, XIV-52
Thomas of Cantimpré, III-

40, 44-5, 48; VIII-231-4
Thomas, II-186
Thorndike, Lynn, VI-170; VIII-231
thorny burnet, XIV-37, 51
Thrasyas of Mantineia, XIV-39
thura, see frankincense
thus, see frankincense
thyme honey, IX-65
thyme, II-194; IX-73; XIV-35
thymelaea, XIV-54
Thymus capitatus, XIV-56
Thymus serpyllum, IX-73
Tiberius, VIII-214
tin, see also "stuttering of"
tin, VIII-216, 220
tonsils, good for, XV-10
toothache, IX-66; XIII-95
topaz, VIII-210
Tordylium apulum, XIV-57
toxcity, X-424
toxicity of drugs, VIII-212; XII-322, 326
Traba natans, IX-76
translators, Latin, VI-177
traumata, XII-326
tree-medick, XIV-49
Tribolos terrestris, XIV-47
tribulus, XIV-47
trifolium, XIV-59
Trigonella foenumgraecum, XIV-50
Triticum spelta, XIV-47
Triticum vulgare, XIV-47
trocisus, V-10
Troy, V-3
tryptophan, XIV-38
Tschirch, Alexander, II-191
tufa, VIII-206
tumors, IX-60-1; XI-292, 294; XII-320-330; XIII-101
tumors, ear, XI-293
tumors, eye, XI-293
turnip, XI-290; XIV-37, 48
Tussilago farfara, XIV-50
tutsan, stinking, XIV-59
tutty, VIII-224-4
Tyler, Varro, XIV-36-7
Typha latifolia, T. angustifolia, XIII-101
typus, X-418-20

ulcers, intestinal, X-415
ulcers, malignant, XII-328
ulcers, X-415; XI-295; XII-328; XIV-36
Ulva latissma, IX-81
United States Dispensatory, XIV-36
upper digestive tract, XIII-97
ureter, XIII-96
Urginea maritima, IX-80; XIV-52
urination, promotes, X-413
urine, bloody, VI-173
urine, smell of, IX-62
Urtica pilulifera, U. urens, XII-324
Urtica sp., XIV-48

Vaccaria pyramidata, XIII-102
vade mecum, VI-178
Valeriana sp., XIV-58
Varro, VI-159-160; X-427
vegetables, X-411
Venice, VIII-215
Veratrum album, X-417; XIV-52
Verbascum sinuatum, IX-75
Verbascum thapsus, IX-75; XIV-50
Verbena officinalis, IX-80; XIV-50
Veronica chamaedrys, IX-76
vervain, IX-80; XIV-50
Vespasian, II-186
vetch, bitter, XII-327-8; XIV-48
vetch, XI-286
veterinary medicine, X-412-3
Vicia ervilla/ Vicia fava, XII-327-8; XIV-48
vicianin, XII-328
victory, bestoes, VIII-212
Vinca major, XII-327
vinca, XIV-38
Vincent of Beauvais, III-44
vinegar, XI-288
Viola odorata, IX-81
viper's bugloss, IX-78
vipers, horned, X-415
virites (stone), VIII-210
Viscum album, XIV-50
Vitex agnus-castus, XIV-58
Vitis vinifera, XIV-49
Vitruvius, VIII-226-7
vocima, XI-292
Voigts, Linda, IX-51

Walafrid Strabo, II-194; VI-166
wall flower, IX-64; XIV-53
wall germander, IX-74
warts, IX-66
water (as drug), XIV-47
water parsnip, IX-81
watermelon, XI-290
Wattenberg, Lee, XII-328
weak, makes one, XI-291
weber dandelion, IX-77
Wellmann, Max, IV-206; XIII-97
Welsh medicine, VI-166
wheat, XI-286
White, K. D., X-428
willow, XIV-37, 51
wine, XIV-49
Winter, Pierre, VI-158
witch-doctors, XIV-33
Withania somnifera, XIV-38
woad, XIII-102; XIV-52
wolf's bane, XIV-39
wolfsmilk, XIV-54
woman-killer, XV-6
Women's Disorders, XIV-36
wool, oily, XIV-61
worms, X-417
wormseed, XV-12
wormwood, shrubby, IX-81
wormwood, X-427; XIV-37, 56-7; XV-12
wounds, head, XI-292
wounds, IX-47
wounds, joins, IX-61
wounds, stops bleeding, IX-61
Wyckoff, Dorothy, VIII-204, 217, 221, 232-3

Xanthium strumarium, XIV-50

yellow loosestrife, IX-66
Ysaac, Benjamin, III-46

Zael (Thetel), III-45; VIII-231
zamalention masculis, IX-81
zamalention, IX-81
zedoary, II-191, 194; VI-167
Zeus, V-6
zinc oxide, XV-12
zinc, VIII-224-5
zinzibar (ginger), II-187
Zizyphus vulgaris, XIV-51
zodiac, III-45; VI-173
Zubrod, C. Gordon, XII-319